Intermittent fasting success stories from followers of Gin Stephens and her *New York Times* bestseller *Fast. Feast. Repeat.!*

"I have gone on to lose 46 pounds in four months and I feel healthier than I ever have in my entire life. My energy is through the roof, my sleep has improved immensely, and I am no longer getting 3–4 headaches per week. Actually, I haven't had a headache since I started all this back in January. So many coworkers have been curious about what I did to make such a dramatic change in such a short time that I have let them borrow my copies of Gin's books. There is actually a waiting list that I have in my office for who gets the books next. I LOVE IF and after trying so many different crazy weight loss diets over the years, I finally feel like I have found a lifestyle instead of a diet that finally works. I have reached my goal weight, I am effortlessly maintaining, I feel FREE, and I am truly LIVING MY BEST LIFE NOW! Thank you, Gin!"

—Jen T.

"I love this way of life! It is going on a year and I can't wait to share your book and celebrate what I have done over this past year. At this point I have lost 32 pounds and many inches, I feel gorgeous in my own body, and I do not plan to ever give this up. I thank heaven for finding you and your books and all the others you have shared with me through your podcasts. I listen every week to the new ones and many times relisten just to catch something I may have missed. I'm now sharing this journey with others, and my mom and my sister do their own version and my closest friend has lost over 10 pounds in the last two months during her journey. This very week I have had two people at work look me up to tell me that after I shared they too read your book and are starting their own journey. I give you all the credit for your words reaching me, touching my head and my heart! Thank you so much!"

"Like Gin, I have tried many diets during my adult years after putting on weight after the birth of my two daughters. I am 5'3", 64 years old, and was at my highest: 242 pounds. I began OMAD (one meal a day) on October 19, 2018, and have since lost 50 pounds. I have been amazed at how easy this has been, and I believe that is because I have been able to deny myself nothing. I love my carbs and eat dessert every day! I have hit a plateau the last couple of months, so this week have begun ADF (alternate daily fasting), which has been a bit challenging but is working to move the number on my scale. I love my new WOL (way of life) with OMAD, which will be my sweet spot for life. Thanks, Gin, for such an easy-to-understand book. I am proud to share my success with anyone who asks how I've lost the weight. We are changing the world!"

—Sarah S.

"To date I have gone down five pants sizes and from an XL shirt to a medium. All because of clean fasting! I still eat carbs. I still have dessert (though I try to not do it as often). There is no forbidden food. The only limitation of this lifestyle is the time limit of the number of hours in which I consume food. Can it really be that simple?! I'm here to tell you it is!"

—Michelle

"Gin Stephens is one of my heroes. This lifestyle might be the short-est span of my journey to date, but I'm reasonably certain it will be with me for the rest of my life."

—Leah

"As I hit my one-year Fastiversary, I now dare to declare myself in maintenance. My body continues to change and recompose as my fat-to-weight percentage shifts downward. I am no longer shack-led by exercise. I will always work out regularly because it makes me strong, energetic, and flexible, but not as a weight loss tool and nowhere as frantically as before. I feel like with IF, I can finally relax into myself. The best part? I have returned to my home cuisine, which I enjoy eating with my family every night. My food—whole-meal grains and millet, lots of dal, nuts, and seeds, fermented food, all kinds of fruit and vegetables, full fat yogurt and cheese—has no restrictions. Thank you, Guru Gin and wonderful fasting family. You are all so far away from me but you finally led me back home."

—Rajee

"I am such an avid supporter of IF as a solution to the worldwide health issues related to obesity that I now have a support group I set up in New Zealand, and I teach all my patients about this way of life. I bought a hard copy of Gin's book to share with people and promote it as life changing because it really is!!! Thanks, Gin!!!!!"

—Sarah K.

"Within the first week of fasting, all of my medical issues disappeared. No lie. It really happened that fast. I had unbelievable sleep, I stopped falling all over the place, and most important, I stopped crying. I couldn't believe it. Oh, right. I almost forgot . . . seven months in and I've lost 40 pounds. I truly love Gin's book because the information saved my life. Gin and this group became my world. To them I will be forever thankful."

—Jeethah

"Biggest lesson learned: If Gin tells you something, like don't buy too many new clothes in size large because soon you will be in mediums or smalls, or maybe try delaying your desserts for a couple of weeks, you can fight against it if you want to, but in the end she will be right and you will wish you'd listened sooner!"

—Lyn H.

Also by Gin Stephens

Delay, Don't Deny

Delay, Don't Deny: Digging Deeper

Delay, Don't Deny: Life Journal

Feast Without Fear

Fast. Feast. Repeat.

CLEAN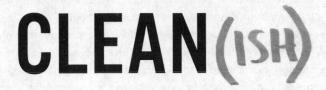(ISH)

EAT (MOSTLY) CLEAN, LIVE (MAINLY) CLEAN,
AND UNLOCK YOUR BODY'S NATURAL
ABILITY TO SELF-CLEAN

GIN STEPHENS

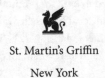

St. Martin's Griffin

New York

The information in this book is not intended to replace the advice of the reader's own physician or other medical professional. You should consult a medical professional in matters relating to health, especially if you have existing medical conditions, and before starting, stopping, or changing the dose of any medication you are taking. Individual readers are solely responsible for their own health care decisions. The author and the publisher do not accept responsibility for any adverse effects individuals may claim to experience, whether directly or indirectly, from the information contained in this book.

Library of Congress Cataloging-in-Publication Data

Names: Stephens, Gin, author.
Title: Clean(ish) : eat (mostly) clean, live (mainly) clean, and unlock your body's natural ability to self-clean / Gin Stephens.
Description: First. | New York : St. Martin's Griffin, 2022. | Includes bibliographical references and index.
Identifiers: LCCN 2021042269 | ISBN 9781250824158 (trade paperback) | ISBN 9781250824165 (ebook)
Subjects: LCSH: Nutrition—Popular works. | Diet—Popular works. | Self-care, Health.
Classification: LCC RA784 .S736 2022 | DDC 613.2—dc23
LC record available at https://lccn.loc.gov/2021042269

CONTENTS

PART 1 ▶ WHAT GOES *IN*: YOU ARE WHAT YOU EAT (AND WHAT YOU ABSORB)   27

AUTHOR'S NOTE

We all want to improve our health so we can age well, prevent disease, and feel good in our bodies . . . and maybe even lose a few pounds. To do so, most of us have tried to "clean up" our diets and our lives, but it's hard to know where to start or how far we really need to go. In my *New York Times* bestseller *Fast. Feast. Repeat.*, I taught you how to fast (*completely*) clean as part of an intermittent fasting lifestyle.

Now, whether you're an intermittent faster or not, I want to show you how to become clean(ish) where it counts: eat (*mostly*) clean and live (*mainly*) clean as you unlock your body's natural ability to self-clean. Instead of aiming for perfection (which is impossible) or changing everything at once (which is hard and never leads to lasting change), you'll cut through the confusion, lose the fear, and embrace the freedom that comes from becoming clean(ish). As you learn how to lower your toxic load through small changes, smart swaps, and simple solutions, you'll breathe a (clean) sigh of relief and embrace your own personal evolution toward becoming clean(ish).

Why get clean(ish)? As a part of my personal health and wellness journey, I have gradually "cleaned up" what I eat based on how foods make me feel, and I have discovered that the *better* my nutritional choices, the *better I feel*. Feeling good is a powerful motivator, indeed! Soon, the changes I was making to how I was eating began to carry over into other aspects of my life. The more I learned, the more changes I made along the way. I'm confident that each change is having a lasting impact on my overall health and wellness.

Clean(ish) means that we develop a focus on real foods and a healthier home environment that is free of obvious toxins, yet without becoming overly dogmatic or fixated on an unattainable level of perfection. By living clean(ish), we can focus our efforts where it matters while still living an enjoyable lifestyle. The *ish* makes it doable.

I want to warn you ahead of time: after reading the first few chapters, you may be a little bit (or maybe even a *lot*) angry. How did we get into this mess? What can we *do* about it?

Let's come together as citizens of the world to insist that we have cleaner and safer foods, personal care products, and household cleaners, as well as a cleaner and safer environment in general. Becoming clean(ish) doesn't just help us individually, but it can help us all.

Clean(ish) living is not about partisan politics, but you may feel like getting a little vocal after reading this book. No matter who you vote for or whichever side of the political aisle you embrace, I know we can agree that every human on earth deserves to live a healthy life. It should not be dependent upon socioeconomic status, disposable income, or zip code, either. I believe that health is our birthright, not just a political talking point. We have the power to vote with our wallets, and as we make changes to what we buy and which companies we support, the current trends toward a larger selection of cleaner and safer options will continue, and these options will become more affordable over time. That's already happening.

One by one, we can join together to demand that we head toward a safer and cleaner future that we envision together. Our planet, our kids, and our grandkids depend on us.

But for now: let's figure out how to become clean(ish) together, using the tools we have before us *today* . . . because every small change we make adds up.

FOREWORD
BY DR. TIM SPECTOR

A tuna and sweetcorn sandwich, orange juice, and a bag of crisps were my healthy lunch of choice for ten years whilst working at a busy teaching hospital in London. My workload left little time for thinking about food choices. If asked whether I thought my lifestyle and diet were good, I would have said "yes." It was only after a six-hour climb to an Italian peak in 2011 that my health bubble burst. I developed double vision and high blood pressure due to a mini-stroke in the eye and for the first time in my life, my body started to work against me. Although I recovered, my blood pressure remained consistently high and I decided to take a closer look at my lifestyle and, in particular, my nutritional choices to improve my health. This journey into the science of food changed my views on what good nutrition was.

One of the most important, but still often ignored, health findings of the last decade is the realization that the trillions of microbes in our gut have a vital function for our health. They are mainly good guys, are essential for digesting food, control our metabolism and the calories we burn, provide vital vitamins and enzymes, and keep our immune system happy. These microbes are also unique and highly individual to each and every one of us, providing our own personal chemical factories. The higher the microbial diversity, the more the ratio of beneficial microbes and the higher the correlation with good health.

I helped fund the nutritional science company ZOE, which is based in Boston and London, in 2017. ZOE was built on the power of gut microbes and personalized nutrition. But before we could offer advice, we needed to collect data. We set up a study called PREDICT, which is deemed the largest and most innovative nutrition study to date. Our research showed that each of us, even identical twins, have very different biological responses to the same food. We also found that the microbes in our gut play a unique role. As these microbes are essential for our health, making and having access to good nutritional choices are vital so we can keep both ourselves and our microbes healthy. After doing the ZOE PREDICT study I learned that my usual sandwich lunch was terrible for my metabolism and gave me large sugar spikes in my blood, and that I could avoid this stress on my body by switching to healthier alternatives and building up my gut microbes.

This is where it gets tricky. What is healthy food when so many products on our supermarket shelves fight to convince us with their low-cal, low-fat, high fiber, extra vitamin, high protein stickers and labels? What they don't tell you is that these extra ingredients make you eat more, make you tired, and increase your appetite. They also don't tell you that the chemicals in these foods are bad for your gut microbes and reduce their diversity.

This is why books like *Clean(ish)* are so important. In the following pages, Gin Stephens thoughtfully provides insight into how most of our calories come from ultra-processed foods and how so many of the multiple ingredients used by the food industry are not even recognizable at all. So many of these foods and ingredients are full of chemicals that, at best, do nothing to nourish our bodies and, instead, are likely to fuel diabetes, obesity, heart disease, and, even according to our latest research with the ZOE Covid Study, increase our risk of developing Covid-19. A key tenet of my philosophy about food is diversity and embracing all healthy ingredients or whole food groups. This is something that *Clean(ish)* also supports, as it shines a light on what foods will have a positive impact on you and which ones will do nothing beneficial for you. You'll also gain some insight into just how many of the products we use to clean our homes and to beautify ourselves can be wreaking havoc on our health, often via our microbes.

Clean(ish) is not just about being cleaner. It's also about being better informed, so you, the reader, can make the right lifestyle decisions to improve your overall health—not only for the next week, month, or year . . . but for good.

—Tim Spector, MD OBE
Professor of Epidemiology
Author of *Spoon-Fed: Why Almost Everything We Have Been Told About Food Is Wrong*

IS THIS THE RIGHT BOOK FOR *YOU*?

Is your health poor, and getting worse over time, but you aren't sure why? Do you have a feeling that you aren't living your most vibrant life, but you don't really know what to change? Do you know that you *want* to make some changes and become more "clean" (and maybe even more "green"), but you aren't sure where to start? Are you stuck at a weight that is higher than you want? Have you tried everything (yes, even intermittent fasting) and yet still can't get your body to drop the last ten (or twenty . . . or one hundred) pounds? Or do you feel puffy and inflamed, and know that you need to do *something,* but you aren't quite sure what? Getting clean(ish) can help.

Right off the bat, I want to let you know that this *may not* be the book for you, though it may be just what you need.

Let's get the first part out of the way. How will you know that this book is *not* for you?

- **This book is *not* for you if you think that the rise of chemicals in our foods and environment is A-OK and that anyone who has a different opinion is an alarmist.**

  If you feel this way, I understand that it may be challenging to convince you otherwise. I have learned that it is very difficult for most of us to change our paradigms completely, and so perhaps you are convinced that everything is fine and that we really do not need to worry about pesticides, GMOs, and the increase of chemicals in our foods, personal care items, and cleaning products.

  But! Are you willing to have an open mind and learn about things you may not be familiar with like obesogens, endocrine disruptors, PBTs, and POPs, as well as how we can make a few simple changes that can make a difference in our long-term health and, therefore, a difference in the quality of our lives? If so, this book *is* for you!

- **This book is *not* for you if you think that unless everything is pure and 100 percent "clean" you should never ingest it or put it on your body or even look directly at it in the store.**

    I totally get it. Once you learn that many things around us contain ingredients that might be toxic to the body or not the ideal choice for health, worry can take over your thoughts. Health and wellness can become all-consuming, and there is a dark side to thinking "clean" that we want to avoid, because the quest for a healthy lifestyle can ultimately become an unhealthy obsession. Our goal is to be clean(ish), not strive for a level of unobtainable perfection that leads to a stressful and unhappy life.

    But! Are you ready to filter through all the noise in your head and let go of any need for perfection that you may be holding on to? Are you willing to dig in and examine your current thoughts and behaviors and consider whether you are being more restrictive than is necessary for health? If so, this book *is* for you!

- **This book is *not* for you if you have deeply held beliefs that no one on earth should ever eat _____.**

    In this book, I am going to encourage you to release yourself from what I like to call *diet brain,* which happens when you have strict rules about the types of food you "should" be eating. We are living in a state of food confusion and dietary dogma that is so extreme that you could fill in the blank in the statement above with almost any word you could imagine, and then find a plan, book, or program that espouses the belief that no one should be eating said item.

    While I'm pretty sure we can all agree with a general statement that some foods have more nutritional value than others, the emphasis of this book is to live life in a way that is clean(ish) rather than stuck in a restrictive paradigm.

    But! Even if you do have a deeply held belief of this sort, are you ready to consider that perhaps you could broaden your ideas around what foods are "healthy"? If so, this book *is* for you!

- **This book is *not* for you if you are looking for a one-size-fits-all plan or prescriptive diet to follow.**

  You are in charge at all times here. With that in mind, *you* are going to learn how to become clean(ish) on *your own terms*. I believe (and the latest science agrees) that we are all different when it comes to what foods work best for our individual bodies. That being said, there is an overall *pattern of eating* that is linked to positive health outcomes, and the majority of nutrition research scientists, nutritionists, and physicians agree on certain foundational ideas (despite what you see in the news headlines, on Instagram, through Twitter, or in your Facebook news feed).

  But! After reading this book, you may feel empowered to take the reins of your own diet and lifestyle approach and understand that you never need to search for a prescriptive diet plan again. Are you ready to design your own clean(ish) plan? If so, this book *is* for you!

- **This book is *not* for you if you are hoping for complex descriptions of biochemical pathways, definitive scientific conclusions, or scare tactics. There are other books you'll enjoy more.**

  I am going to discuss the general consensus of what some of the best minds of today *believe is likely to be true* and give you specific steps that you can follow to become clean(ish). But keep in mind that I am not a doctor or scientist, so I am going to leave the complicated scientific explanations to them. I'll cover the basics, and I will also point you toward some excellent resources if you want to dig deeper, but I am not going to be overly science-y or claim that we know everything about these topics. Some of the science is murky, and many of the conclusions are not as cut-and-dried as we may hope. Okay, and it's true that some of what I am going to tell you may be scary. It's normal to be alarmed when you learn the truth about what's truly in your food (and lurking in your environment). Keep in mind these aren't scare tactics, however. Knowledge is power. Once you understand what chemicals may be harming your health (and how you can lower your overall toxic load), you are ready to take action.

But! Are you ready to accept that even without science that is completely settled, there is enough evidence to indicate that cleaning up our foods and lifestyle can have positive health benefits, both now and as we age? If so, this book *is* for you!

Now that we have that out of the way, I hope that you have decided: **YES! This book *is* for me!**

If so, keep reading! I hope that you'll find a lot of value here within these pages.

HOW TO USE THIS BOOK

- **As you read, you'll want to take it slowly.** This is not a read-at-one-sitting type of book. It's designed with pauses between chapters for you to take some time to think about what you've read and consider how to implement changes into your life as you feel ready.

- **Make time to reflect and/or take action.** At the end of each chapter, you'll find end-of-chapter prompts and activities. To make the most of this process, set aside time to complete the reflections/actions that are provided.

    Change doesn't happen from the *reading,* it happens from the *doing.* The reflections and actions are the keys that ensure you'll actually apply what you have learned.

    You have a couple of options for completing the end-of-chapter activities:

    ⊚ Get a notebook and dedicate it as your personal Clean(ish) Journal and do all your writing there using the prompts I have included in the book. I recommend that you choose a blank notebook that will be reserved for all your clean(ish) reflections. If you're like me, picking out a pretty notebook for a new project always makes me more enthusiastic about the project itself.

    Or

    ⊚ If you prefer a more structured approach, I have created a resource that has everything you need all in one place. Visit **ginstephens.com /cleanish** to download and print the pdf version of all the pages that you'll need for the end-of-chapter reflections/actions, as well as the work you'll do in part 3 of the book. These pages will give you all the space you need to complete the various activities.

- **Be empowered!** You are the navigator of your own journey. Identify changes that feel doable and start with those. Rather than all or nothing, remember that every little step gets you to your destination in the end.

INTRODUCTION

Welcome! I'm glad you're here and that you're ready to explore the process of becoming clean(ish).

Do any of these descriptions sound like you?

- Are you worried about the chemicals that are ubiquitous in our modern environment and feeling inspired to make changes in both what you eat and how you live?

- Are you confused about what foods are "clean," and if some foods are not "clean," then does that mean they are "dirty"?

- Do you want to be able to eat foods that you love (and that taste good) without doing a math problem first? Are you tired of restricting whole food groups and have the feeling that there has to be a better way? Are you completely *over* counting and tracking?

- Are you stuck in diet-brain mentality, particularly after scrolling your social media feeds? Does it all leave you so confused that you aren't sure what to eat anymore? Should you be carnivore? Or raw vegan? Or maybe something in between? *(Spoiler alert: YES . . . the magic is in the "in between.")*

- Are you tired of living in fear, worrying that every decision you make might be a mistake?

- Are you wondering about all the health claims being made about foods and products these days (Non-GMO? Organic? Grass-fed? All-natural?) and unsure which really *matter*?

- Are you interested in taking things up a notch when it comes to the foods you choose, with a goal of increasing the amount of nutrients you eat?

- Do you want to learn about your body's amazing abilities to "clean up" a lot of this mess and how to promote more self-cleaning, just as nature intended?

- Are you looking for simple swaps that can make a big difference?

- Are you longing for a sense of balance in your life?

- Are you ready to develop a personalized action plan that you can begin to implement today, add to over time, and maintain for the long term?

- And finally: Do you want to know the basic concepts, but without some of the overly scientific deep diving found in many other books about nutrition and health?

I have written this book to address all those issues and more. The book is founded on several principles that I would like for us to agree on up front:

- We are bombarded with a larger variety of chemicals (through our environment, as well as through our foods, our personal care items, and our cleaning products) today than ever before.

- In general, what we are eating now is different from what people ate prior to the modern era.

- A combination of poor nutrition and toxic overload is creating all sorts of problems within our bodies.

- Our bodies are designed to protect us against toxins so we can exist in a state of wellness, and we can help our bodies self-clean by making changes in what we eat and how we live.

- Even if you're not well today, there are steps you can take now that will help your body heal, leading to better health outcomes in the long run (and fat loss, if you want it).

I'm going to talk about each of these concepts in more detail, but not exhaustively. That's because each topic is so robust that it could be a separate book. In fact, there *are* fantastic books about each of these topics, and after reading this one, you'll probably want to do some more reading about the topics that interest you most.

This is a book about overall health and wellness, and is not a "diet book" in the traditional sense of the word. That being said, the current obesity epidemic is related to the concepts you'll learn about in this book, and I will explain as we go.

Think of the rise of obesity as the tip of the health-and-wellness iceberg. What lies beneath the surface of the water is the massive state of our overall poor health: it's huge, it's dark, and it's murky.

The obesity crisis is one of the most visible parts of what's going on with our health in general. So, let's first have a conversation about obesity.

Are you ready for some shocking news? According to the CDC:[1]

Obesity is a common, serious, and costly disease.

- *The prevalence of obesity was 42.4 percent in 2017/2018.*

- *From 1999/2000 through 2017/2018, the prevalence of obesity increased from 30.5 percent to 42.4 percent, and the prevalence of severe obesity increased from 4.7 percent to 9.2 percent.*

- *Obesity-related conditions include heart disease, stroke, type 2 diabetes, and certain types of cancer that are some of the leading causes of preventable, premature death.*

- *The estimated annual medical cost of obesity in the United States was $147 billion in 2008 US dollars; the medical cost for people who have obesity was $1,429 higher than those of normal weight.*

Yikes . . . We are inching up on the halfway mark, when 50 percent of adults will be considered obese. How many more years before that shocking statistic becomes a reality? And keep in mind that we are talking about the number that are *obese,* and not just the percent of people who are overweight. The same CDC report from 2018 shared that more than 73 percent of Americans over the age of twenty were considered to be overweight. That means that only about *one in four* members of the adult population was within a normal weight range at the time this report was released.

After smoking, obesity is considered to be the leading cause of preventable death, and the rise of obesity rates is not just happening in the United States. In fact, it's so prevalent that many are considering it to be a pandemic.[2]

Did the whole world suddenly decide to stop trying to maintain a healthy weight? Did we all just give up? Or has something changed?

No, we haven't given up . . . but we are *confused* about how to solve the problem. In many ways, we are trying harder than we ever have before in human history and yet still failing. I read one estimate that said Americans spend over $60 *billion* each year on weight-loss products. If money could solve the problem, we would be solving it left and right. I certainly spent enough money over the years on weight-loss solutions (that didn't work long term and mostly didn't even work in the short term).

What if I told you that the answer isn't in spending money on weight-loss products? After all, if it were, we would all be slim. Instead of buying products, supplements, and programs, what if you could make some changes in what and how you eat (as well as *when* you eat) and not only would you finally be able to lose weight but your body would be healthier in the long run? Also, what if you learned that it doesn't need to cost you more money than you are currently spending on food and you might even be able to spend *less* overall?

Does it sound too good to be true? Keep reading.

We live in a blame-the-victim society. If we would just stop eating so much, we would be able to lose weight. *Are* we eating more food now?

Well, yes. We actually are. According to the Food and Agriculture Organization of the United Nations, the average American used to eat around 2,880 calories a day in 1961, but by 2017, that was up to an average of 3,600 calories per day.[3]

So . . . it seems like the answer is what we have always been told. We are eating too much. Eat less. Problem solved.

Except that we have tried that.

We have all tried the *eat less, move more* approach, and as long as we white-knuckled it, counted calories, and avoided carbs, fat, meat, grains, sugar, alcohol, and more, we have been able to lose some weight. A few really dedicated dieters are able to lose weight and keep it off long term (about 5 percent, according to some esti- mates . . . though there is some dispute as to the exact numbers), but most of us haven't been successful long term using those tired and old diet strategies. We lose some weight, regain it, try again . . . Yo-yo dieting at its finest.

Did something happen to humans back in the middle of the twentieth century that changed us? Something that turned us into gluttons who no longer have the willpower to stop eating?

Actually, yes.

- We are bombarded with chemicals in a way that humans never have been before. Chemicals like endocrine disruptors and obe- sogens play a role in not only the rising rates of obesity but in the decline of our overall health. I'll explain in the "Better Living Through Chemistry" chapter.

- Our personal care items and cleaning products are full of toxic chemicals, and we are putting hundreds of individual chemicals on our bodies every single day, just through our skin care and personal hygiene routines. These products are contributing to our overall toxic load and having negative effects on both our weight and our overall health.

- What we eat and drink has changed, and not for the better. Many people eat very little actual *food* these days, but instead are subsisting on food-like substances that don't nourish our bodies and actually leave us *hungrier* than before we ate them. I'll explain it to you in the "Food, Glorious Food" and "Take a Break from Fake" chapters.

I will discuss each of these topics and more within this book, and you'll leave equipped with tools that help you target each one of them, on your own terms.

Before we begin, I want to introduce myself. You may be someone who has been a part of my intermittent fasting community for years (I opened my first online support group in 2015, and we grew to be a thriving community with hundreds of thousands of members from around the world), you may be a listener of one of my three top-ranked podcasts (*Intermittent Fasting Stories, The Intermittent Fasting Podcast* with cohost Melanie Avalon, and *Life Lessons* with cohost Sheri Bullock), or you may have read one of my other books (*Delay, Don't Deny: Living an Intermittent Fasting Lifestyle, Feast Without Fear: Food and the Delay, Don't Deny Lifestyle,* or the *New York Times* bestseller *Fast. Feast. Repeat.: The Comprehensive Guide to Delay, Don't Deny Intermittent Fasting*). If so, you likely already know a lot about my diet history and my journey down the intermittent fasting path.

But maybe you have never heard of me before, and you picked this book up out of curiosity. For those of you who are new to my work, I want to tell you who I am and how I got here. I bet some of my story will sound like your life, as well.

And even if you have followed my work for years, I bet you're going to learn some new things about me that you didn't already know as I tell you just a little bit more about my story here.

I was born in 1969 and raised on frozen TV dinners and chicken pot pies, both of which were packaged in aluminum pans that took forty-five to sixty minutes to bake in the oven. When I didn't want to wait that long, I could open a can of SpaghettiOs and heat it up on the stove (or eat it out of the can at room temperature if I was really in a hurry). I could also make a bologna sandwich on white bread with mustard and mayo, and yes, my bologna *DID* have a first name, and it *WAS* O-s-c-a-r. If my mom felt like I was missing out on essential nutrients (lordy, that was the truth), I could chew up a Flintstones vitamin, and everything would be just fine. Even though there was nary a vegetable on my plate (I picked out the peas and carrots from the pot pies), I got all the vitamins and minerals needed to build a healthy body. At least, that is what both the vitamin and enriched-bread manufacturers told us.

When I had kids in 1998 and 1999, is it any surprise that I raised them the same way I was raised? I didn't make them eat any vegetables they didn't want to eat. I bought vitamin-enriched chocolate-flavored beverage and put it in their sippy cups. Since we had microwaves by then, I could prepare a modern microwavable TV dinner in just minutes! I bought the ones that were specifically targeted to kids, with dino-shaped chicken nuggets and a fun dessert. If they wanted to pick out the peas and carrots, I didn't even think twice about it, because I could hand them a fruity-flavored, chewable, fun-shaped vitamin shaped like their favorite cartoon characters. I was doing such a good job making sure they got all their required nutrients. (Cringe . . .)

So, with that kind of background, how did I begin my own personal journey to clean(ish)? What changed things for me?

I want to travel back in time to the year 2002 on one particular fall day. I was a third-grade teacher in Carrollton, Georgia. My older son, Cal, was four, and my younger son, Will, was just about to turn three. (Side note: I wish I could *literally* time travel back to 1997 and hand myself a copy of this book before I even became pregnant for the first time, but I can't. I would do things so much differently if I could.)

Actually, let's go back a few more years to start this story, because that's where it really begins. My second child, Will, was born in 1999, and he was a colicky baby. This is not surprising to me, knowing what I know now. While I was pregnant with him, I had one toddler already and was working full-time as an elementary school teacher, so I did a lot of driving through the Golden Arches for a quick dinner. I popped my prenatal vitamins each day, secure with the knowledge that I was providing my growing baby with the right building blocks. Yes, I was *so confused*, but I am choosing to look back on the younger-and-uninformed me with grace, because I really did not know any better.

As Will became a toddler, that colicky baby turned into a boy who was loving and kind one minute and then could turn into someone else entirely at what seemed like the drop of a hat. He had tantrums and was destructive around the house. I was an elementary teacher, and I always prided myself on my classroom management skills, but I couldn't manage my own son at home. It was humbling. (It also taught me that when children are misbehaving at school, it doesn't mean the parents aren't trying as hard as they can. That insight served me well as a teacher.)

That pivotal fall day of 2002, I remember what happened so very well. It was early in the school year, and I got an urgent call mid-morning from Will's day care. He was having a tantrum, and they wanted me to come pick him up immediately.

I had to scramble to find someone to cover my classroom so I could leave. Chad, my husband, worked over an hour away in Atlanta, so it was all up to me to take care of anything that happened during the workday. I walked into the day care, and Will was indeed pitching a fit right there on the floor of the office. I took him home, embarrassed, and hoped it would never happen again.

Guess what? It happened again the very next day. And it happened again the day after that. Except for one thing that was different on day three. That third day, the director of the day care told us not to ever come back. Ouch. We had been a part of that day care for two years, and my older son had been very successful there. Suddenly, we were no longer welcome.

At that point, it was time to scramble for another alternative. We tried a second day care. Will lasted about a month there before we were asked to leave. Since Carrollton was a small town, there weren't a lot of options available to us. Will turned three, and as luck would have it, I found a small private school that had a three-year-old classroom. We all crossed our fingers and hoped for the best.

Well, you can probably guess what happened next. Tantrums. Check. Not welcome there. Check. Even though we had already paid tuition for the whole year, that school asked us to leave. I had to hire someone to come to our home to care for Will for the rest of the school year.

In fall of 2003, we tried again at the private school. They gave us a credit for the prior-year's remaining tuition payment. (I may have begged just a little bit for them to give us another chance . . .) Will's teacher was amazing, and I remember that her name was Ms. Karen.

Ms. Karen loved Will, and Will loved Ms. Karen. She saw his loving spirit, and she also recognized how smart he was. Unfortunately for us, though, she also got to see him have tantrums and lose complete control of his behavior.

One day while I was picking him up, she mentioned that he had had a particularly bad day. She asked what seemed like a simple question at the time that ended up changing our lives for the better: "What did Will have for breakfast today?"

I remember the answer that I gave her: I had served him some Cat in the Hat cereal that morning. Fun fact: that particular cereal was only available for a short time, and this is a description of it from Kellogg's: "The limited edition The Cat in the Hat cereal contains a tasty blend of corn and oats shaped like the infamous stovepipe hat worn by Dr. Seuss' title character. An innovation in food science, the cereal represents a breakthrough in culinary technology as festive red stripes distinctly appear on the individual cereal 'hats.'"

After I explained to Ms. Karen about Will's festive breakthrough-in-technology striped-hat-cereal breakfast, she said, "Did you know that some kids don't do well with red dye, and it affects their behavior?"

Well, no, actually. I had never heard that before. Frankly, it sounded wacky. There was nothing at all wrong with his cereal. It was *Kellogg's*, which we all know is the backbone of America, am I right? It was full of vitamins and minerals, he had milk with it, and it was part of a healthy breakfast. So there.

Because I was desperate, though, I went home and googled. Actually, I probably Yahooed. It was 2003 after all, and Yahoo! was the number one search engine. If you don't believe me, you can Google it.

Sure enough, there was a great deal of chatter out there about red dye and behavior. How had I missed this? I had been a teacher for over a decade by this point, and I had never read a thing about the connection between what kids *ate* and how they *behaved*. However, the more I read, the more it made sense.

We ended up joining a group called the Feingold Organization,[4] and they still exist today at feingold.org. Dr. Ben Feingold, for whom the organization is named, was a pediatric allergist from California. Based on trends he witnessed within his practice, he developed a theory in the 1970s that a leading cause of hyperactivity in children (what we now call ADD or ADHD) was their *diet* and a few things in particular: artificial flavors, artificial colors, preservatives, and other food additives, plus a class of foods known as *salicylates*. (Many plant foods produce salicylates as a form of natural pest control. Ever known someone with an aspirin allergy? Aspirin is a member of the salicylate family.)

In addition to what these kids consumed, many were also negatively affected by things they inhaled and chemicals that touched their skin. I read everything I could get my hands on and was amazed that I had never learned any of this before. As a teacher, I had witnessed the puzzling behavior of certain kids in my classroom over the years, where some days they would be fine and other times they would melt down completely, reminiscent of my own son. Now that unusual behavior made a lot more sense. I realized that we weren't the only family dealing with this but that most parents didn't know anything about the effects of foods and chemical exposures on our kids.

Here's what is eye opening for me, and a little scary when I look back at this time of our lives. I'm pretty sure that if I had taken Will to his doctor and explained his inability to remain enrolled in any day care or private school we tried (yep, the private school kicked him out a second time after a few months), we could have easily gotten a variety of prescription medications to try. Chad and I were desperate, and it was only fortunate happenstance that Will's caring teacher sent us down a different path. I would never judge parents in the same situation as we were who *do* make the choice to include medications as a part of helping their child, because we were probably headed there as a next step. But I am so grateful to that teacher who opened my eyes. Thank you, Ms. Karen. You changed our lives.

By the way, my husband, who has a Ph.D. in medicinal chemistry, thought I had completely lost my mind when I came home with this nutty-to-him (and to me, frankly) theory. Looking back, he is just as grateful as I am that we made the changes we made, and he realizes that there is a lot of merit to the scientific theories behind it.

Based on recommendations from the Feingold Organization and other excellent resources I discovered along the way, we changed what we were feeding both Will and Cal, and we also changed the personal care products that they used (shampoo, toothpaste, soap, etc.). We also swapped out the household cleaners that we used. We didn't think *Cal* needed to make any changes in what he was eating because he was doing well in school and was very typical for his age when it came to behavior, but it would be too difficult to fix different meals, so it was easier to change things for both of them.

The difference in Will was absolutely amazing as long as we

carefully monitored what he ate and what chemicals he was exposed to. My parents and other family members became believers when they witnessed an accidental exposure at a family gathering. My sister baked two different cakes for the event. One of them contained only natural ingredients that were on plan for Will, and the other was my dad's favorite kind of cake, full of artificial flavors and other "no" ingredients. Will knew he was going to get cake later, but he didn't know that one of the cakes was not for him. Unbeknownst to us, he snuck a finger full of frosting before dinner . . . from the wrong cake. Within minutes, he was having a gigantic tantrum that seemed unexplainable . . . until we realized what had happened. My (very quiet and somewhat stoic) dad, said, "Oh, I get it now." Yep. Anyone who saw that switch being flipped from "normal Will" to "chemical-reaction-powered Will" instantly became a believer.

What was very surprising is that we also saw a positive difference in Cal's behavior and moods. This was reinforced by an incident that occurred when Cal was in kindergarten and he was prescribed a course of cough syrup that contained red dye. We gave it to him, since *he* didn't have a "problem"; Will did. Keep in mind that the only reason we made changes to what Cal ate had to do with convenience. I remember that day well. His kindergarten teacher brought him straight to my classroom midmorning, saying Cal had refused to do his work, threw it on the floor, and had a tantrum in the classroom when he wasn't allowed to go to recess. (Part of the benefits of being a teacher at your kids' school . . . they bring them straight to you if they don't behave well. It is both a blessing and a curse.)

This behavior was completely uncharacteristic for Cal, and so we were all very surprised by it. He was normally eager to do his schoolwork (he went on to skip first grade) and was an excellent student and usually well mannered with his teachers. Could it be the cough syrup? We stopped giving him the cough syrup with dye immediately, and he went right back to normal. From that point on, I realized that even kids who are "normal" like Cal could be affected negatively by these sneaky chemicals.

This changed me as a teacher, as well. I never again gave candy to my students as a reward or a treat, since most of the candy on the shelf is full of additives that I saw have a negative impact on my own sons, and I was also more conscious about what chemicals I used within my classroom (no more toxic chemical-laden sprays or plug-in air fresheners, for example). I also shared resources with parents who were open to hearing there could be an alternative to the traditional medical route for behavior issues. I'm not sure how many listened, but I hope that I was able to make a difference here and there. And as I said before, I stopped blaming the parents when kids were having a hard time. I witnessed Will struggling and out of control many times, and I was helpless to make a difference in those early years, so I understood that many of these kids were struggling with something they may not be able to control, as well.

The Feingold Organization really did change our lives. I want to point one thing out here that is worth mentioning, however: according to a 2015 review article, "The lack of well-designed placebo-controlled studies investigating the role of many of these substances makes it impossible to provide evidence-based advice for the efficacy of the removal of food additives . . . and salicylates from the diet."[5] This means that there is not enough scientific evidence to prove what Dr. Feingold and others claim to be true. It doesn't mean it isn't *true*; it simply means it isn't *proven*. While I want you to understand that difference, I know that for us, we found that changing the exposure (to food additives and environmental chemicals) for both of our kids had a profoundly positive effect on all our lives during that period of time. We were able to avoid behavior- or mood-related medication completely, and Will was able to successfully stay in school. He went from the kid who was kicked out of two day cares and one private school (the one that kicked him out twice) to a kid who qualified for the gifted program in kindergarten and then skipped second grade. Was he a perfect child? No. But he succeeded. I hate to think what might have happened if we hadn't made the changes we made.

We continued to follow the Feingold recommendations for years until we realized that Will had grown out of many of the sensitivities that he experienced when he was younger, no longer reacting the way he once had to the foods and environmental chemicals that had served as triggers when he was younger. Did he actually grow out of them, or did his body heal in other ways? We will never know for sure, but I suspect that it was actual *healing* rather than "growing out of" them. Knowing what I know now, I suspect that his gut microbiome was unhealthy from his earliest days, likely based on the chemical nonsense I ate while I was pregnant with him. He had thrush (a fungal overgrowth) as a newborn, and we were prescribed an antifungal to use orally until it cleared up. He also had lots of issues with diarrhea as a toddler and throughout early elementary school years, and I noticed that it often coincided with his negative moods.

Scientifically, we now understand that the gut is the "second brain." In fact, researchers have evidence that mood changes can be triggered by irritation in your gastrointestinal system.[6] In a 2019 review article, the authors state: "In recent years, an accumulating number of studies reported detrimental effects of some commonly used food additives on gut homeostasis, suggesting a link between their consumption and the development/worsening of human intestinal and metabolic diseases."[7] This means that evidence is strong that many of the commonly used food additives negatively affect the health of our gut microbiomes over time.

So, even though it isn't "proven" that these chemicals are related to behavior changes in children, as I already noted, we can follow this logical path: chemicals *have* been shown to affect the health of our gut microbiomes, and the health of our gut microbiomes *can* influence our behaviors and our moods. From that, the theory that these chemicals may cause behavior changes in kids (and adults!) has a solid scientific foundation, "proven" or not.

I certainly didn't have any of this understanding during the time period in question. So, guess what we did? Once we realized that Will was able to tolerate more foods, we added them all back in. We took a big sigh of relief and rejoiced that this difficult time was "over."

In hindsight and knowing what I know now, I would make different choices, of course.

You see, I still didn't understand the long-term impact of these chemicals on our health. We had a problem (Will's behavior), and we solved it (through dietary and lifestyle changes). The problem went away over time (as he either grew out of it or healed), and so we didn't "need it" anymore. Back to the SAD—Standard American Diet—we went.

Everything was fine.

Except for me. I had a big problem.

By this point of my life, I was stuck in diet yo-yo hell.

As the girl who was raised on frozen and canned convenience foods, my palate was trained from an early age to crave these ultra-processed foods. Even as I changed what I fed my kids for those important years, I continued to eat according to my early preferences. And looking back, even the "healthy" foods I fed my boys were ultra-processed: we bought organic boxed mac and cheese and organic frozen chicken nuggets. While I did buy organic applesauce for Cal and organic pear sauce for Will (since pears are low in salicylates), actual fruits and vegetables were still a rare occurrence on all our plates. In upcoming chapters, I'm going to get into details about why this is a step in the right direction but still not the overall goal.

Since I lived on ultra-processed and convenience foods, it is no surprise that I found it difficult to control my weight. I tried many fad diets along the way, including doctor-prescribed diet pills. As long as I took diet pills, I could maintain a "healthy" weight, though I now realize there was absolutely nothing *healthy* about taking diet pills to manage my weight.

Fortunately, I realized the diet pills were wreaking havoc on my body, because I just felt awful all the time. I stopped taking them, and my weight skyrocketed. For the first time, I reached the obese weight range rather than simply being overweight.

The decade spanning 2005–2014 includes my real struggle years. During that time, I continued to try everything that I could think of.

I jumped from one diet plan to another: Shakes. Low carb. The popular (yet horrific) five-hundred-calories-a-day hCG diet. Physician-assisted weight loss. Counting calories. Counting carbs. Counting bites. Not one single thing I tried during that entire decade worked long term for me. The yo-yo highs kept getting higher and higher.

During that time period, the concept of "clean eating" first hit the weight-loss industry, and several bestselling diet books came out. Since I was willing to try anything, I jumped on board the clean-eating movement more than a few times during that era in my desperate attempt to lose weight. My taste buds weren't happy because I was still hooked on the captivating flavors of the ultra-processed foods I loved. It isn't our fault—those foods were literally designed in a lab to do just that—hook us on their unnatural yet overstimulating flavors.

Since I *only* considered "clean eating" to be a way to lose weight, I eventually decided that forcing myself to eat foods I didn't like wasn't worth it and that I would find another way to lose weight that allowed me to eat whatever foods I wanted.

Enter intermittent fasting.

As I have explained in my earlier books, intermittent fasting allowed me to jump off the diet roller coaster for good. Thanks to intermittent fasting, I went on to lose over 80 pounds and reach my ultimate goal weight range, from a high of 210 pounds. (I may have actually weighed more than that at one time, because there was a period when I didn't weigh myself at all. I didn't want to face the reality of how large I had gotten, and as long as I didn't *see it* on the scale, it wasn't "real." Maybe you can relate.) Actually, I surpassed my initial goals, much to my delight and surprise. I am sitting here today, over six years later, wearing my size 0 jeans, and even as I went through the menopausal transition (I am now on the other side, hallelujah), I have maintained my size within my goal range, and I have never needed to up-size my wardrobe again.

As I lost weight, I ate "whatever I wanted" the whole time, other than a brief period of time in the spring of 2015. I was down 55 pounds and only 20 pounds away from my initial goal weight of 135, but spring was in the air. The pressing problem was that I had no season-appropriate clothes that fit my newly smaller body, and I desperately needed to go shopping. I still wanted to lose 20 pounds, however, and now I wanted to do it in a hurry. Fortunately, I read a book called *The Science of Skinny* that was very compelling, and it inspired me to clean up what I was eating. The author explained why our bodies needed to eat real food in order to reach our healthiest weight and how processed foods are detrimental in the long run, and so I stopped eating ultra-processed foods (and also delayed alcohol) for about ten weeks.

Amazingly, my rate of weight loss went *up*. After removing ultra-processed foods and alcohol from my diet, I was consistently losing about *2 pounds per week,* which is almost unheard of after already losing 55 pounds. Keep in mind that I wasn't counting calories, restricting carbs, or limiting fat . . . All I was doing was eating *real foods* until I was satisfied, and the weight seemed to melt off with no feelings of deprivation.

I rejoiced the day my scale read 135 pounds, and I was finally ready to go shopping. I was delighted to find I was a size 4 in most stores that day, which was thrilling, since I was wearing a 16W at my heaviest. (And honestly, I should have been wearing an 18W. I forced myself to wear clothes that really didn't fit, because there was something in my mind that wouldn't allow me to buy larger clothes, even though I needed them. This was just another example of how I was lying to myself when it came to my weight. Maybe you can also relate to that.)

On that day when I reached my initial goal, I also rejoiced because I could go back to eating "whatever I wanted." Sigh.

You see, "clean" always had an ulterior motive behind it. With Will, it was to control his behavior. With me, it was to lose weight. "Clean" was simply a means to an end.

As great as it felt to reach my initial goal weight, I was diet-weary by that point. Still, I felt free, and as long as I continued to live an intermittent fasting lifestyle, I was able to maintain my weight without stress. Life was good.

By the way, you don't have to become an intermittent faster to become clean(ish), but it can certainly help. Intermittent fasting activates one of your body's most powerful self-cleaning mechanisms: autophagy. More about that in the "Intermittent Fasting: A Powerful Self-Cleaning Tool" chapter. Even if you don't think you have any interest in IF, you may change your mind after you read that chapter.

In 2015, I started my first intermittent fasting support group, and it was a safe place where like-minded IFers could come together to share successes and troubleshoot when things weren't going well. The following year, I wrote my first book, *Delay, Don't Deny,* and self-published it. Much to my astonishment, people seemed to like what I had to say. The concept of *delaying* eating (through intermittent fasting) rather than *denying* ourselves of the foods we want to eat resonated with people back then, and it still does to this day. *Delay, don't deny* is a powerful mantra in more ways than one, and most of us can apply it to more aspects of our lives beyond simply food and eating.

Then, in 2017, I became a podcast cohost when Melanie Avalon and I began producing weekly episodes of *The Intermittent Fasting Podcast.* Week after week, I was digging deeper into a variety of health and wellness topics. My eyes opened to many new things along the way. The role of what we are eating began to crop up more and more in questions from listeners.

Another thing was happening during that same time period within my intermittent fasting support groups, and I like to refer to it as the "diet wars."

You see, people have *very strong opinions* about what foods are "best" to eat, and in any health and wellness communities, these opinions come out. Huge arguments ensue, in fact. Surely one side is right, and one is wrong? During my summer break from teaching, I vowed to figure out the answer to the question: What should we be eating? With so much scientific research surrounding food and nutrition, surely the answer was within the literature somewhere. It had to be. I started researching and working on my second book, *Feast Without Fear*.

This research led me back to "clean" but for an entirely different reason. Rather than choosing foods that affected behavior (for my kids) or eating in a way that would promote weight loss (for me), I was suddenly passionately interested in choosing foods that lead to positive health outcomes and longevity.

Even though I go into a lot more detail within *Feast Without Fear*, everything I learned as I wrote it can be summed up in two sentences:

- We are all different when it comes to what foods work best for our unique bodies.

- Real foods win over ultra-processed foods, every single time.

Once I realized those two things, I slowly but surely began making changes related to the foods I was eating.

It's been a process, but I am no longer someone who lives on a diet of mostly ultra-processed foods. I still *delay* rather than *deny*, even as I have become clean(ish). Every day, I still eat *whatever I want*, but what I want has dramatically changed over time. I no longer crave ultra-processed foods as the basis of my diet.

These days, I make very different choices when it comes to what I buy and what I prefer to eat. The best news of all? It doesn't feel at all like "*deny*" to avoid fake foods full of harmful or weird chemicals. I've also realized that everything I have ever enjoyed eating is available in a form that is safer for my body, so I don't feel like I am giving up a single thing—because I'm not.

After focusing on *when* I eat, and naturally shifting *what* I eat, I also started taking a closer look at the personal care items that I use on my body and the cleaning products that I use in my home, just as I did when my boys were young. I learned some shocking things about how these products affect our health (and our waistlines).

The more I learned, the more important it became to me to make changes in how I live.

You see, I don't just want to be thin—I want to be healthy. I want to be the most vibrant *me* that I can be. Living clean(ish) is my not-so-secret lifestyle weapon.

Now that you understand why clean(ish) eating and living have become so important to me, I want to take a few minutes to tell you about my educational background and why I am bringing you this book. I have already mentioned that I was an elementary school teacher, and I taught in an elementary classroom for twenty-eight years, taking early retirement in 2018. I am definitely not your typical author in the health and wellness community.

I graduated from Wake Forest University in 1990 with a degree in elementary education. Over time, I found that teaching science and math were my natural gifts, so I completed a master's degree in natural sciences from the University of South Carolina. I also realized that I absolutely loved working with gifted learners, so I earned a doctorate in gifted education. After becoming interested in health and wellness, I was inspired to attend the Institute for Integrative Nutrition, and I completed their twelve-month program to become a certified health coach. Everything I learned within that program reinforced what I had learned when I wrote *Feast Without Fear*: one of their main tenets is the concept of bio-individuality, which explains that our bodies are all unique.

At my core, I'm a teacher, not a scientist. I'm trained to deliver content to others, which has been helpful as I transitioned to my new career as both a writer and as a podcaster. Even though I'll be talking a lot about chemicals and their effects on our bodies within the pages of this book, I am definitely not a chemist (though I am married to one).

Always keep in mind that I am not a research scientist, medical doctor, or nutritionist (though I do consider myself to be *science-focused,* thanks to both my master's degree in natural science and training as a health coach, and also *research-focused,* because of my work obtaining my doctoral degree). I want to emphasize that my role here within this book is that of *teacher* and also *facilitator* as I help you design your own personal transition to clean(ish).

My goal in this book is to summarize the most relevant information I've found and to present a general picture of our modern chemical landscape in regard to both our foods and our personal care and cleaning products, and then take you through the process of developing your own personal action plan for becoming clean(ish). As I will explain in upcoming chapters, there are thousands of chemical additives in our foods and thousands more in our cosmetics and household cleaners. I am not going to list them all and conduct a safety survey of each one or explain exactly what each one does—or might do—within your body. The good news is that I don't have to do that, because there are already comprehensive databases of both chemicals and products that you can use as a reference, and I am going to share them with you here in one convenient place.

There are dozens—if not hundreds (or thousands?)—of other books about the topics I will cover here, and many of them were written by scientists or doctors, though others were written by people like me who simply want to get the word out. You may have even read many of these books. But you're here because you need *more*.

It may even be the case that you've already read many of the books about these topics, and you're convinced. You know what you *need* to do. But understanding what you need to do and actually doing it are two different things. What I am going to do is cover the basics and then give you a plan you can use. Actually, scratch that. I'm going to help *you* develop your *own* plan to become clean(ish) in a way that works for you long term.

My goal with this book is to teach (or remind) you of the *why* and then help you develop your *how*.

Some of what I will share in this book is still controversial, believe it or not. One example is the topic of GMOs, or genetically modified organisms. GMOs are living things that have had their genetic code changed in some way, and while many scientists claim they are perfectly safe for us and the environment, there are many other scientists who insist that we are damaging both the environment and our bodies in ways we don't even yet understand. In fact, a scientific journal published an article in 2015 with the title "No scientific consensus on GMO safety." That's a pretty bold statement right there in the title. How can there *not* be consensus on such an important topic?[8]

There is somewhat of an unfortunate truth when it comes to science: it seems that no matter what someone writes, someone else will dispute it. That is true in most nonfiction genres. Google the phrase "earth is really flat" and you'll see what I mean.

While most of us do agree that the earth isn't flat, not every scientist or expert agrees on what to eat, or what chemicals are safe, or what substances are dangerous, or what foods are best for weight loss, or really almost anything within the health and wellness realm.

If scientists don't all agree, then how do the rest of us know what is true or what to do?

My goal for writing this book is to cut through some of this clutter and create a clean(ish) living guide that most of us can apply to our lives.

Based on the extensive research I've done and reading all sides of the argument, I've determined that the process of becoming clean(ish) represents a realistic and achievable way of life, based on 2021 understandings. Is it possible that our understandings will change? Actually, it's certain they will. That's the nature of scientific inquiry. "*Oops—we were wrong before*" should be the motto of scientists everywhere, in fact. Just ask Copernicus, whom everyone thought was crazy when he first proposed the wacky-for-the-time concept of an earth that orbits the sun. Or Ignaz Semmelweis, whom you might never have heard of, but was ridiculed by his doctor colleagues for suggesting that they should wash their hands and medical instruments to decrease levels of infection in their patients. It wasn't until more than two decades after his death that everyone realized he was right. He didn't have any understanding of germs at the time, and people would have scoffed at the idea of living organisms so tiny that they couldn't see them, but he was clearly onto something.

So, all of that to say: it's possible that some of what I teach you here may be an overgeneralization, or I might even make an innocent mistake as I interpret the very complex and not-fully-agreed-upon science, and if so, I apologize up front. Don't let that deter you from the big picture: why we all need to embrace a move toward becoming clean(ish) and how to apply this concept to your life. Erring on the side of caution when it comes to your health is never a bad idea. Scientists call this the *precautionary principle,* and I'll talk about it more in part 3.

As I have been gathering information and writing this book, I have realized something that is ironic: the steps I've outlined here won't be stringent enough for some readers, and yet they will seem overly restrictive to others. I'm okay with that.

In this book, my plan is to share the basics within each chapter, and then to give you actionable steps. I will also give you a list of resources so you can learn more about any topics that resonate with you. Consider it to be your extra credit assignment. (I can't help it. I'll always be a teacher at heart. No, it won't count toward your final grade, because there are no grades here, but it just might help extend your life, which is worth more than any grade.)

I'm sure you have heard the saying:

If you don't make time for your wellness, you will be forced to make time for your illness.

The origin of that quote is unclear, but it's profound.

While I refuse to live in fear, I also understand that I only have one body . . . and *we* only have one earth. I don't want this book to make you afraid to live your life (although it might make you a little mad when you realize how deep these problems go). Instead of being afraid, I want you to feel empowered and optimistic. We have amazing bodies that are designed to self-clean. When we clean up what goes *in* and support our bodies' natural processes as they manage what comes *out*, we can be assured that these changes will lead to positive effects on our long-term health (and maybe even lead to the fat loss we desire, which may have been elusive up to now).

> An ounce of prevention is worth a pound of cure.
>
> —Benjamin Franklin

REFLECT: IDENTIFY YOUR *WHY*

Use your Clean(ish) Journal (or the worksheets available at ginstephens.com/cleanish) to complete these end-of-chapter prompts and activities.

It's time to identify your *why*. What do you want to accomplish as you read this book and work through the process of becoming clean(ish)?

As you read through this list, check all statements that apply to you. For each one you checked, respond to the accompanying prompt(s) in your Clean(ish) Journal.

☐ I'm worried about the chemicals that are ubiquitous in my modern environment, and I'm feeling inspired to make changes in both what I eat and how I live.

What am I especially worried about, now that I have read the introduction?

☐ I'm confused about what foods are "clean," and if some foods are not "clean," then does that mean they are "dirty"? I want to understand what foods nourish my body so I can focus on those, but without worrying about every choice I make.

Today, *before* reading this book, what does "clean eating" mean to me?

☐ I want to be able to eat foods that I love (and that taste good) without doing a math problem first. I'm tired of restricting whole food groups, and I have the feeling that there has to be a better way. I'm completely *over* counting and tracking.

What restrictive diets have I tried, and how did they make me feel while following them?

When it comes to what I eat, how do I want to live my life going forward?

What relationship with food do I want to nurture?

☐ I'm stuck in diet-brain mentality, and I'm so confused that I'm not sure what to eat anymore. Should I choose a restrictive diet, or maybe something in between? (*Spoiler alert: YES . . . the magic is in the "in between."*)

Why am I so confused about what to eat?

Where did this confusion come from?

☐ I'm tired of living in fear, worrying that every decision I make might be a mistake.

What am I afraid of?

Which decisions am I having trouble making, and why?

☐ I'm wondering about all the health claims being made about foods and products these days (Non-GMO? Organic? Grass-fed? All-natural?) and unsure which really *matter.*

When I'm shopping, how do I currently make decisions about which foods or products to choose?

What do I look for on the label?

☐ I'm interested in taking things up a notch when it comes to the foods I choose, with a goal of increasing the amount of nutrients I eat.

What foods do I already know I want to include more of in my day-to-day diet?

What foods do I already suspect I want to minimize?

☐ I want to learn about my body's amazing abilities to "clean up" a lot of this mess and how to promote more self-cleaning, just as nature intended.

What does "self-cleaning" mean to me?

What do I already know about how my body self-cleans and how to promote these processes?

☐ I'm looking for simple swaps that can make a big difference.

What are some things I already know I can easily swap out *today* to move me along the path toward becoming more clean(ish)?

☐ I'm longing for a sense of balance in my life.

What about my life is currently unbalanced?

What could I do today to help me create more balance?

☐ I'm ready to develop a personalized action plan that I can begin to implement today, add to over time, and maintain for the long term.

What's my preferred MO: Am I someone who wants to take my time and make changes gradually, do I want to jump right in and change lots of things at once, or do I prefer to be somewhere in the middle?

WHAT GOES *IN*: YOU ARE WHAT YOU EAT (AND WHAT YOU ABSORB)

In 2018, the Breast Cancer Prevention Partners (BCPP) organization and the Campaign for Safe Cosmetics released a report summarizing the shocking state of affairs in the beauty, personal care, and cleaning products industry. Their report is available for you to read in its entirety on their website, but I want to share some key summaries here with you:[1]

- There is a shocking lack of information available to consumers about what chemicals are in the products we buy.

- One of the main problems has to do with federal labeling loopholes.

- Rather than being safe, the products we buy are full of unknown and unlabeled toxins.

- Many of the personal care products they tested had more unsafe chemicals than cleaning products.

As a part of their report, they first purchased common products from the beauty, personal care, and cleaning categories: one hundred beauty / personal care products and forty cleaning products.

Then they hired two independent third-party testing laboratories, one to assess volatile organic compounds (VOCs) and the other to determine the identity/presence of a variety of chemicals within the products.

Results showed that there were between 46 and 229 unique chemicals *per product.* They found an average of 136 chemicals in each cleaning product and an average of 147 chemicals in personal care products. This means that you are exposing yourself to hundreds of different chemicals at a time, over and over again each day, every time you use personal care or cleaning products. Not all these individual chemicals are dangerous or toxic, of course, but many of them are.

Within these common products, they found carcinogens, hormone disruptors, respiratory toxins, and developmental toxins.

- *Carcinogens:* Chemicals that may cause cancer

- *Hormone disruptors:* Chemicals that interfere with normal hormone functions

- *Respiratory toxins:* Chemicals that affect the function of our respiratory system

- *Developmental toxins:* Chemicals that affect reproduction or human development in some way

Of the products they tested, body sprays had the most alarming results, with almost ninety different chemicals linked to these four categories of health hazards. The next-worst-ranked product class was shampoos, followed by cleaning products, lotion, hair-styling products, deodorant, and conditioners.

Are you as surprised as I am by these findings? I would never take one of the products I use to clean my kitchen counters and spray myself down with it. Would you? Yet the body spray you use likely has more dangerous chemicals than your kitchen counter spray. *Wow.*

The most hazardous product of all the 140 that they tested? A children's shampoo marketed to kids of color.

These were the top ten hazardous products, ranked based on the highest number of chemicals linked to cancer, hormone disruption, developmental or reproductive toxicity, and respiratory effects:

1. A children's shampoo from a hair-relaxing kit

2. A fragrance endorsed by a music, television, and film star

3. A shower, tub, and tile cleaner that is marketed as "a great cleaner that is safe and friendly to use"

4. A body lotion marketed as antiaging

5. A body spray marketed to young men

6. A perfume endorsed by a fashion designer

7. A fragrance endorsed by a pop/country star

8. A shampoo marketed as "green/sustainable"

9. An industrial cleaner / disinfectant used by custodians and firefighters

10. A perfume that's been around since 1978

In this first section of the book, I'm going to give more detail about the dangers associated with the chemicals we find in our cleaning and personal care / beauty products. Then I'll discuss the rise of chemicals in our foods. Before I get into specifics about cleaning and personal care products and foods, however, I want to give some background information about the overall proliferation of chemicals in our environment in general and explain why this all matters so much.

BETTER LIVING
THROUGH CHEMISTRY

Before we can make our own personal transitions to clean(ish) eating and living, we have to understand why it matters. That's what you'll learn in part 1 of this book.

Before I began writing this book, I was half-heartedly making what I thought were "clean" choices out of a sense of duty or obligation. I felt like it was the right thing to do, but I still didn't have a full picture of why it matters so much. The more I read and the deeper I went, however, the more concerned I became.

Most of us know in the back of our minds that there is a problem. But perhaps you (like I did, before doing my research) don't realize exactly what the problem is, how deep it really goes, or what to do about it. The good news is that the more I learned, the more empowered I felt. As I understood the scope of the problems, I knew what steps I could take right now to make a difference. Every small change adds up.

As you read this book, you'll find a section at the end of each chapter designed for you to take some time to reflect or take a few simple actions. This gives you the opportunity to take stock of your current state of affairs as you go through each chapter. In part 3 of the book, you'll put it all together and develop your personal action plan for getting clean(ish).

So, let's get started understanding some of the challenges we are facing so that we can start solving them. Knowledge is power.

If you've ever wondered, my research has convinced me that it's true: our world is in trouble.

How did we get into this mess? Let's start with the cheery phrase that marked an era: *better living through chemistry.*

It all sounded so promising. In the early days of the twentieth century, an optimistic world embraced the idea that scientific innovations were going to save us from many of the problems facing society, such as world hunger and disease. A 1935 slogan from chemical giant DuPont represents this thinking well: "*Better Things for Better Living . . . Through Chemistry.*"

DuPont wasn't working alone, of course. Many other industrial giants also personify the promises of better living through chemistry, and I'm sure you'll recognize a few of their names: Dow, Monsanto, and Bayer. These companies brought us innovations we use on a daily basis, such as aspirin, Corian, Teflon, Kevlar, Lycra, Freon, and Styrofoam. They also brought us genetically modified seeds, Roundup, chlorofluorocarbons, bisphenol A (BPA), DDT, and Agent Orange.

In many respects, they were right. We *did* see better living through chemistry thanks to these scientific and chemical advances. Crop yields went up as new plant varieties and agricultural techniques were developed. Pesticides, synthetic nitrogen fertilizers, and new breeds of high-yield corn, wheat, and rice led to a *doubling* of production.

That period of time from the 1950s to the 1960s was called the "Green Revolution," and according to the Food and Agricultural Organization of the United Nations,[1]

> *Green Revolution technology saved an estimated one billion people from famine and produced more than enough food for a world population that doubled from three to six billion between 1960 and 2000.*

When we think about it that way, it's difficult to look back and judge that period of time too harshly, even though we are looking at it through our modern lens, because they were living in a different world with different challenges. More than seventy million people died from famines during the twentieth century, and having enough food to feed the growing world population was a pressing problem that needed solving.[2] Since 1990, however, famines have been related to war and conflict rather than a shortage of available food in the world.[3] The Sustainable Food Trust tells us: "All contemporary famines are fundamentally political,"[4] meaning we may have solved the supply problem thanks to the Green Revolution, but access to our new abundance of food is still a problem in war-torn countries, even in 2021. This is the subject of a different (albeit important) book.

Now, in hindsight, it's easy to look back on some of these twentieth-century innovations and think, *The pesticides! The fertilizers! The toxic chemicals released into our ecosystem! How could they have done this?* So much of what we know now, however, we didn't understand then. Did the chemical giants understand what they were unleashing on the world? Some would argue yes, while others would say no. That's also the subject of a different book.

No matter which perspective you take—it's all been a diabolical plan brought about by big business, or it's been an innocent mistake with unexpected consequences—I think we can all agree that we are facing a mess when it comes to the chemical consequences of the twentieth-century technological advancements.

In today's modern world, along with the chemical fallout that is pervasive in the environment, we have been fed the empty promises of vitamin pills and enriched foods. We are very much "overfed and undernourished," which I will explain in more detail in a later chapter. And while it's true that we've solved many of the problems from the pre-chemistry / pre–Green Revolution age, the solutions themselves have caused new problems.

I would imagine that almost everyone reading this book lives in a part of the world where we no longer get cholera or dysentery from drinking unsafe water, but we may find toxic chemicals in our water instead. Before I get into that, I want to point out: access to safe water is still a problem in developing countries, about 2.2 billion people worldwide don't have access to safe water, and about 80 percent of illnesses in those areas are linked to poor water and sanitation conditions.[5] I'm going to say it for the third time now: that's also the subject of a different book. I think we all would agree that clean water for every human on earth is something for us to strive for, and you can find ways to take action by visiting websites such as thewaterproject.org or unicef.org/wash.

For those of us with reliable access to safe and clean tap water, we take for granted that when we turn on the water tap (or open a fresh bottle of water), out flows water that is, well, both safe and clean. But is it *really* safe, or have we traded short-term safety for long-term safety? Meaning, does our water now harm us *slowly* (through chemical exposure we may not even be aware is occurring) rather than *quickly* (through waterborne illnesses)?

That's a great question. In 2020, the consumer watchdog organization Consumer Reports performed an analysis of forty-seven bottled waters, including thirty-five that were noncarbonated and twelve that were carbonated. They tested for four heavy metals (arsenic, cadmium, lead, and mercury), plus thirty PFAS chemicals.

WHAT ARE PFAS?

Per- and polyfluoroalkyl substances are a group of man-made chemicals that are commonly found in everyday items, such as cookware, food packaging, household products, and stain repellants, just to name a few. And, according to the EPA, they are linked to low infant birth rates, negative effects on the immune system, cancer, and thyroid hormone disruption.[6]

What did Consumer Reports find? Most of the products they tested had detectible levels of PFAS, and several exceeded 1 part per trillion (ppt)—they found these levels in two of the noncarbonated and seven of the carbonated waters they tested. One of the plain waters exceeded 10 parts per billion for arsenic.[7]

All the companies who had water with detectible levels of PFAS or arsenic acted like this was no big deal, because, as they correctly pointed out, all the levels were within legally allowed limits. But since so many of the brands did have amounts lower than 1 ppt, it's certainly possible to expect all brands to do better. (And many of them scrambled to lower those numbers, due to backlash from consumers.)

Why do we want to avoid exposure to chemicals such as PFAS, when the amount is so tiny? One part per *trillion* doesn't sound like much. As I am going to explain in a moment, the issue is that many chemicals accumulate in our bodies over time, and while a tiny amount may not seem like a problem, the overall accumulation can *become* a big deal over time.[8]

Better living through chemistry, indeed. Over the twentieth century, the chemical industry created *tens of thousands* of new chemicals. The thought is absolutely staggering. Because of this, we are putting more toxins *in* and *on* our bodies than ever in human history—not to mention the ones that sneak in as we simply breathe the air in our homes. These chemicals have varying effects on our health, some of which are still unknown.

When you think about it, we're involved in a long-term chemistry experiment of sorts.

At no time in human history have we been exposed to such a chemical soup. And results are worrisome. According to the Natural Resources Defense Council, "Of the more than 80,000 chemicals currently used in the United States, most haven't been adequately tested for their effects on human health."[9]

It's alarming to realize that we are still learning about the effects all these chemicals have on our bodies. Evidence is strong that our bodies are having a hard time keeping up with the increased toxic load. Toxins clog up our livers, one of our first lines of defense. Then they get stashed into our fat cells. They even end up in your brain, which is almost 60 percent fat.

TOXINS

As you do any reading about this subject, this word keeps coming up.

Even the word is scary, but with good reason. A synonym for *toxin* is *poison*.

Before I go on, I want to have a quick vocabulary lesson.

Most of us are misusing the term *toxin* in our everyday-speak.

We say **toxin** when what we really are talking about is a **toxicant**. According to dictionary.com:

tox·in

/ˈtäksən/

noun

noun: toxin; plural noun: toxins

1. an antigenic poison or venom of plant or animal origin, especially one produced by or derived from microorganisms and causing disease when present at low concentration in the body.

tox·i·cant

/ˈtäksəkənt/

noun

1. a toxic substance introduced into the environment (e.g., a pesticide).

When you look closely at the difference between the two, you see that the word *toxin* technically only describes toxic substances that are of plant or animal origin. *A Textbook of Modern Toxicology* states, "A toxin is a toxicant that is produced by a living organism and is not used as a synonym for toxicant—all toxins are toxicants, but not all toxicants are toxins."

Let's apply that concept: anthrax or snake venom would each be an example of a toxic toxin that is also a toxicant. Confused yet?

Don't be. Here's the takeaway: when I use the word *toxin,* most of the time, I am really talking about *toxicants.* Even though referring to toxicants as *toxins* is technically incorrect in the true definition of the word, it's how the term is used in common conversation. So, if you are someone who cringes whenever someone uses the word *toxin* incorrectly when they should be saying *toxicant,* make the swap in your own head as you are reading.

Now, back to your regularly scheduled programming.

Most of us understand that toxins can make us sick. If we swallowed a known poison, we might show symptoms immediately, and we would know to seek medical help.

Unfortunately, there's another problem, which I already mentioned, and it's the buildup that comes from the accumulation of these tiny exposures of toxins over time. How is this happening? As I already explained, we are exposed through water, but we also have exposure through our foods, our beverages, our skin, and the very air we breathe—both inside our homes and workplaces and when we are outdoors.

How widespread is this problem, and is it something we need to worry about, or is this just alarmist thinking?

Well, I have bad news. It's very widespread, and the more I dug in, the more alarmed I became.

TAKING A CLOSER LOOK AT ENVIRONMENTAL EXPOSURE

In 2009, the Centers for Disease Control and Prevention (CDC) released their *Fourth National Report on Human Exposure to Environmental Chemicals.* This report was the fourth in a series of ongoing assessments to investigate the U.S. population's overall exposure to a wide variety of environmental chemicals. They update the report periodically, and the most recent update (as of the writing of this book) was in 2019.

In each new survey period, they measure blood and urine from a random sample of about 2,500 participants, looking for concentrations of the environmental chemicals themselves or their metabolites (*metabolites* are the substances produced within the body after the body processes the original chemical in some way). *Environmental chemicals* refer to any chemical compounds or elements found in air, water, food, soil, dust, or consumer products.

In the 2019 update, the CDC provided data for 352 chemicals. Of those, 6 were newly reported.

It's important to keep in mind that whether a chemical is toxic to our bodies depends on many factors. For example, the dose or concentration of each chemical is important. Small amounts may not be a problem, whereas increased exposure may lead to adverse effects. Also, chemicals in isolation may affect our bodies differently from the way they affect us in combination: it becomes a toxic soup, if you will.

As discussed in the report, the CDC found that there is widespread exposure to many chemicals of concern, such as:

Chemicals of Concern	Information and Concerns
Polybrominated diphenyl ethers	These are fire retardants that accumulate in both the environment and also in animal fat tissues . . . including the fat tissues of humans. They are linked to hormone disruption, reduced IQ in children, reduced fertility in adults, and cancer. Almost all participants had a measurable amount of this chemical in their bodies. We become exposed through everyday items, such as furniture, clothing, plastic components of electronic equipment, or even items that should be safe, such as children's car seats. While use of these chemicals is declining overall (which is good news), they remain within our environment due to widespread past use and can be found in both the dust and the air.
Bisphenol A (BPA)	You've probably heard of BPA before, and may already be actively avoiding it. It's been commonly used in food packaging and various containers, and the problem is that it leaches into the foods/beverages themselves . . . and then finds its way into our bodies. Over 90 percent of the study population had BPA in their urine. BPA exposure is linked to a variety of health conditions, such as fertility problems, heart disease, insulin resistance, diabetes, asthma, and cancer.

Perfluorinated chemicals	This class of chemicals is one we are exposed to from a variety of sources, such as nonstick cookware and stain-resistant fabric treatments. Most participants sampled had measurable levels of these chemicals.
Mercury	Mercury occurs naturally in coal and other fossil fuels, and when these fuels are burned for energy, the mercury becomes airborne and goes into the atmosphere. Then it collects through rainwater and ends up in our waterways. From there, it ends up in the fish, which passes on to us when we eat fish. Within the study population, they found that blood mercury levels tended to increase with age, declining after the age of fifty. According to the EPA, mercury is a neurotoxin. Exposure in the womb can have long-term impacts: it can affect cognitive ability, memory, attention, language, fine motor skills, and visuospatial skills.[10]
Arsenic	Arsenic contaminates water supplies either from natural deposits in the earth or from industrial and agricultural pollution. Most people become exposed through drinking water or foods, such as rice or seafood. It is linked to bladder, lung, and skin cancer and may cause kidney and liver cancer. It may also cause birth defects, reproductive problems, and harm to the nervous system and the circulatory system. In the study, researchers were able to measure both total arsenic and seven other forms of arsenic in the participants' urine. Certain populations (timber workers, for example) had higher concentrations than the general population.[11,12]
Perchlorate	This chemical is used in the manufacturing of fireworks, explosives, and rocket propellant. Ready to hear something shocking? It was found in the urine of all the participants in the study. *All.* Let that sink in for a minute. Why do we care? In large doses, it's a known endocrine disruptor, which I will explain more fully later in this chapter.
Volatile organic compounds (VOCs)	This is a large group of chemicals that are found in many products we use to build and maintain our homes, such as paint, carpet, cleaning products, and personal care products. A high percentage of the participants in this study showed detectible levels of VOCs.

These are just a few key highlights from the report, but it is available for free and in full on the CDC website.[13]

Now, thanks to this type of data that is being collected over time, we are beginning to understand just how widespread this type of toxic exposure may be. Many of these chemicals are classified as *PBTs* or *POPs,* and it's important to understand what this means for our health (and for the health of the environment in general). So, let's dive in and understand what all these letters mean.

WHAT ARE PBTS AND POPS?

Some of the chemicals within our environments are classified as *PBTs,* which means Persistent, Bioaccumulative, and Toxic. Let's look at each of these words individually to understand why we should be concerned about PBTs.[14]

- **Persistent:** These are any chemicals that resist environmental degradation. This means that they stick around. Chemicals that stick around in nature also tend to resist metabolic breakdown in animals and humans.

- **Bioaccumulative:** These are chemicals that accumulate in living organisms. This means that concentrations in tissues increase over time. Many of these chemicals are fat soluble, meaning they end up in fat deposits (of animals or humans).

- **Toxic:** As I already mentioned, the most basic synonym for *toxin* is *poison.* When a chemical is *toxic,* it may affect our bodies in numerous ways: damage to our DNA, cancer, immune system damage, or toxicity to a specific body system (having neurological, reproductive, or developmental effects, for example).

What are some examples of PBTs? Mercury is one that you're likely familiar with, and lead is another. You may have heard of dioxins. Most PBTs have complicated names that won't mean anything to you, such as hexabromocyclododecane (HBCD) or polychlorinated biphenyl (PCB). The EPA has a list of some of the worst and most recognized offenders on their website.[15]

PBTs move through or are stored in air, water, and soil, and many accumulate in the food chain. This means that they are in the air we breathe, our groundwater, and within the foods we eat.

So, where do they come from? Some of them originate from

the disposal of toxic wastes. Others come from pesticides, or air emissions. Air emissions are actually one of the most important sources today (through industry, burning, mining, landfills, and our vehicles).

Other toxic chemicals are considered to be *POPs*, which means Persistent Organic Pollutants. The World Health Organization (WHO) defines POPs as:[16]

Persistent organic pollutants (POPs) are chemicals of global concern due to their potential for long-range transport, persistence in the environment, ability to bio-magnify and bio-accumulate in ecosystems, as well as their significant negative effects on human health and the environment.

The most commonly encountered POPs are organochlorine pesticides, such as DDT, industrial chemicals, polychlorinated biphenyls (PCB) as well as unintentional by-products of many industrial processes, especially polychlorinated dibenzo-p-dioxins (PCDD) and dibenzofurans (PCDF), commonly known as dioxins.

Humans are exposed to these chemicals in a variety of ways: mainly through the food we eat, but also through the air we breathe, in the outdoors, indoors and at the workplace. Many products used in our daily lives may contain POPs, which have been added to improve product characteristics, such as flame retardants or surfactants. As a result, POPs can be found virtually everywhere on our planet in measurable concentrations.

POPs bio-magnify throughout the food chain and bio-accumulate in organisms. The highest concentrations of POPs are thus found in organisms at the top of the food chain. Consequently, background levels of POPs can be found in the human body.

> *Human exposure—for some compounds and scenarios, even to low levels of POPs—can lead to many health effects including increased cancer risk, reproductive disorders, alteration of the immune system, neurobehavioural impairment, endocrine disruption, genotoxicity and increased birth defects.*

It's important for us to understand what I just told you: that both PBTs and POPs tend to stick around and accumulate in our bodies over time.

According to the Environmental Protection Agency (EPA):[17]

> *Although scientists have more to learn about POPs chemicals, decades of scientific research have greatly increased our knowledge of POPs' impacts on people and wildlife. For example, laboratory studies have shown that low doses of certain POPs adversely affect some organ systems and aspects of development. Studies also have shown that chronic exposure to low doses of certain POPs can result in reproductive and immune system deficits. Exposure to high levels of certain POPs chemicals—higher than normally encountered by humans and wildlife—can cause serious damage or death.*

This is *really* important to understand: most of us aren't exposed to high levels of any *one* of these chemicals, but instead we are exposed to many tiny exposures, day after day. So, we don't even realize it's happening. That's what the EPA means by *"chronic exposure to low doses."*

Some of the chemicals we come in contact with regularly belong to specific categories, such as *endocrine disruptors* or *obesogens*. Let's take some time to learn what these are and what they may do within our bodies.

ENDOCRINE DISRUPTORS

Our endocrine system is made up of a series of glands (including the thyroid, pancreas, hypothalamus, pituitary, adrenal, reproductive glands, etc.). These glands produce and secrete hormones that are sent into the bloodstream and to various tissues of the body, coordinating complex processes like growth, metabolism, and fertility. Hormones influence the function of the immune system and even alter our behavior.

Think of hormones as *chemical messengers*. We rely on the correct messages getting to the right place so that our bodies' processes can work as they are designed to.

Unfortunately, many of the chemicals we are exposed to are known as *endocrine disruptors*. That means that they interfere in some way with the hormone-signaling pathways in our bodies.

Some of them are hormone *mimics*, which means they bind to a hormone receptor and send a false signal that confuses the body. One example is something called a *xenoestrogen*. Xenoestrogens are substances that are close enough in molecular structure to estrogen that they therefore have the potential to bind to an estrogen receptor.[18]

Other endocrine disruptors block the action of a hormone by preventing the hormones themselves from binding to the target receptors. Still others may affect the amounts of hormones produced.

The results? A wide range of problems within the brain and the body.

The problem is so serious that the Endocrine Society released a report in 2009 that said:[19]

We present the evidence that endocrine disruptors have effects on male and female reproduction, breast development and cancer, prostate cancer, neuroendocrinology, thyroid, metabolism and obesity, and cardiovascular endocrinology. Results from animal models, human clinical observations, and epidemiological studies converge to implicate EDCs as a significant concern to human health.

Where are these endocrine-disrupting chemicals found? All over the place. Here are some common endocrine disruptors that you likely come in contact with on a regular basis:

Endocrine Disruptor	What Is It?	Where You May Be Exposed
Bisphenol A (BPA)	Polycarbonate plastics and epoxy resins	Plastic products and food storage containers
Dioxins	Environmental pollutants, generally by-products of a wide range of manufacturing processes	Throughout the environment, and they accumulate in the fatty tissues of animals, soils, plants, water, and air
Perchlorate	A biproduct of the aerospace, weapon, and pharmaceutical industries	Drinking water, bottled water
Phthalates	Used to make plastics more flexible	Food packaging, cosmetics, children's toys, medical devices
Triclosan	An antimicrobial	Personal care products, such as soap, body wash, toothpaste, and cosmetics

As you see, these potentially endocrine-disrupting compounds are around us everywhere we go.[20]

OBESOGENS

Many of the endocrine disruptors we are exposed to are considered to be *obesogens*.[21] We are exposed to a variety of these obesogens through the foods we eat, through the packaging our food comes in, from our cookware, from our personal care and household products, and also through the environment.

Most of us think of our fat cells in a very simple way—as the places where our bodies store excess energy; but actually, that's far from the whole story. In fact, our fat stores are now considered to be an active endocrine organ, participating in the body's feedback systems involved in appetite and many of the body's metabolic processes. Obesogens disrupt these activities.

Obesogens are defined as *"chemical agents that inappropriately regulate and promote lipid accumulation and adipogenesis."*[22]

This means that these chemicals lead to not only more fat storage, but they also promote formation of new fat cells that are waiting to be filled.

Scientists studying obesogens believe that these chemicals affect fat cell function, fat accumulation, metabolic setpoints, energy balance, and the regulation of appetite and satiety—actually making you *hungrier.*[23] Certain environmental toxins act in our hypothalamus to change metabolic regulation. Others may disturb insulin pathways, which may affect the body's ability to access stored fat (insulin is *antilipolytic,* meaning that it inhibits fat burning), among other things.

In a 2010 study, scientists found that exposure to low doses of POPs (similar to the amount commonly found within food chains) led to *"severe impairment of whole-body insulin action and contributed to the development of abdominal obesity and hepatosteatosis."*[24]

In that 2010 study, they found that an increase in POP exposure raises the risk of developing both insulin resistance and metabolic disorder, which also led to the development of hepatosteatosis (which is the official name for fatty liver disease) and increased abdominal obesity.

Research into the effects of obesogens on our bodies is ongoing, and scientists still don't fully understand all the mechanisms of action. That last sentence speaks volumes: scientists are pretty sure that this *is* happening but can't fully explain *how* it happens.[25] Even so, according to the evidence, there's enough for these scientists to conclude that *"global environmental pollution contributes to the epidemic of insulin resistance–associated metabolic diseases."*[26]

In a 2019 review article, two of the scientists who study obesogens summarized the current thinking in this way:[27]

There was wide agreement on the following points:

- *The increase in obesity over the last 50+ years cannot be accounted for by genetic factors alone.*

- *Obesity has genetic, epigenetic and environmental components.*

- *The environmental component is multifactorial and includes environmental chemicals.*

- *Susceptibility to obesity is at least in part "programmed" during development by environmental factors broadly defined including stress, drugs, nutrition, microbiome, exercise and environmental chemicals.*

- *Altered programming may alter brain appetite and satiety centers, fat cell numbers, size and function, as well as effects on muscle, GI tract, pancreas and liver.*

It was estimated with confidence that:

- *Effects of obesogens will be due to "multiple hits" across the lifespan and generations.*

- *There will be multiple specific windows of enhanced sensitivity across the lifespan including preconception, in utero, neonatal, prepuberty and aging.*

- *The effects of obesogens will be sexually dimorphic.*

- *Obesogens must be studied along with nutrition, activity, stress, infections, microbiome etc. in order to accurately assess the effects of environment on obesity.*

- *Some obesogens will act transgenerationally requiring a multigenerational approach.*

- *The current approach of testing one chemical at a time at one window of exposure is almost certainly underestimating the importance of obesogens.*

Wow.

WHAT HAPPENS AS EXPOSURE TO TOXINS INCREASES?

To put it simply: **As the volume of toxins in your system goes up, your body can't keep pace.**

My favorite analogy for this concept is a scene from the classic TV show *I Love Lucy*. In the 1952 episode "Job Switching," Lucy and Ethel are hired as new workers in a chocolate factory. As they start their work, they face a slow-moving conveyer belt, and they are expected to wrap each piece of chocolate as it goes by. At first, they are able to keep up with the work, and everything flows smoothly. "This is easy!" Lucy says. "Yeah, we can handle this okay," replies Ethel.

Then, as the conveyer belt speeds up, they have to work faster. If they can't keep up, they know they will get fired. They start grabbing the pieces of candy off the conveyer belt as it speeds by, and it piles up in front of them. Eventually, they start eating the chocolate frantically, stuffing it into their mouths. "I think we are fighting a losing game," exclaims Lucy.

The next step is to cram the extra pieces into their hats, down their shirts, and wherever they can hide it away, as their supervisor comes back in to check on them. As their boss enters the room, the viewer can see that both Lucy's and Ethel's cheeks are puffed out from the chocolate in their mouths, their hats are sagging under the weight of the candy, and their midsections are bulging with the excess stashed in their clothes.

Our bodies do something very similar to Lucy and Ethel when

overloaded with toxins that are coming in faster than the body systems can process them. When these chemicals enter your body and your liver is dealing with more toxins than it can handle, one solution is that your body finds a fat cell to dump the toxic garbage into. And the more of these chemicals you ingest (or absorb), the more your body has to stash away.[28] Just like Lucy and Ethel, your body sticks the excess anywhere that's available.

Yes, our fat cells become a dumping ground for environmental pollutants over time. And most of us are accumulating fat cells at an alarming rate. As I mentioned in the introduction, obesity is now epidemic, if not pandemic. Some estimate that we are experiencing the first known generation of kids whose life span is expected to be shorter than that of their parents, due to the increase in obesity-related diseases. How is this related to the increase of toxins within our fat cells?

First of all, we already learned that certain toxins are linked to increased fat storage and decreased fat burning, which isn't helping.[29]

In addition, scientists have realized that adipose tissues (our network of fat cells) are more than just a passive storage depot for excess energy and toxins.[30] In fact, as I already mentioned, we have evidence that our adipose tissues actually play a role in both metabolic and endocrine (or hormonal) functions. Adipocytes, the fancy name for fat cells, secrete hormones such as leptin (important in body weight regulation and appetite)[31] and adiponectin (involved in regulating glucose levels as well as fatty acid breakdown), among other things.[32] When the cells are also packed full of toxins, this disrupts the functions the cells are designed to perform. The more packed-full of toxins our fat cells become, the higher our body burdens, and the more our bodies' natural processes become disrupted.

TOXIC LOAD, OR BODY BURDEN: THE BUCKET EFFECT

What is our "body burden"? Thanks to all these chemicals that we are exposed to on a daily basis, we all face an increasingly high *toxic load,* also known as our *body burden.* These miscellaneous toxins and disruptive chemicals in our bodies come from the environment, the foods we eat, the beverages we drink, and the personal care and household products we use, as well as the other items that we come in contact with throughout the day.

It's important to remember that toxins build up in our bodies over time. I already used the word *bioaccumulation,* and this is an illustration of that concept.

We know that tiny exposures don't seem like a big deal, especially because we don't even know they are happening. Even so, now we understand that these tiny (and seemingly invisible) exposures continue to build up over time, bit by bit, without us even knowing it.

Over ten years ago, when we were dealing with our younger son's chemical sensitivities, I read a wonderful analogy that helped me understand how our bodies become overloaded and what happens when they do.

Picture a bucket placed under a small leak in the roof. Drip, drip, drip.

Drop by drop, tiny amounts of water plunk into that bucket. Eventually, the bucket is full. Once it is, the very next drop sends water spilling over the bucket's edge. From that point on, the water can no longer be contained in the bucket.

In our analogy, your body is the bucket, and the dripping water represents the toxins coming in. Every drop is adding to your toxic load, accumulating over time: drip, drip, drip.

In the case of a roof leak dripping into a bucket, as long as that water leak is contained in the bucket, our house is fine, and no damage occurs. Some of us may have access to a small bucket to contain the water, while others are fortunate enough to have a larger bucket. But no matter the size of our individual buckets, if water keeps dripping in, the bucket will eventually overflow.

Once the bucket overflows, the problems begin.

This is what happens in your body. As long as your "bucket" can hold the "water," meaning as long as your body can manage your toxic load, you appear to be fine. But once your "bucket overflows" and can no longer manage your body's burden, you experience symptoms.

When exactly does your bucket overflow? The answer is that it's going to be different for everyone, and it depends on your "bucket size" as well as your own personal cocktail of chemical exposures (plus your overall health, genetic factors, etc.).

Once your toxic load gets to a certain point, your personal bucket overflows. This can manifest as a wide variety of symptoms, such as:

- Excess weight that you just can't seem to lose

- Unexplained tiredness

- Brain fog

- Insomnia

- Headaches

- Mood swings

- Aches and pains

- Chemical sensitivities

- Skin reactions

- Constipation

- Unusual body odor

- Hormonal issues

Now let's return to the roof leak analogy. You are home, and you see that the bucket is getting full, so you empty out some of the water. The bucket doesn't overflow, because you removed some of the water.

The good news is that our bodies are designed to "empty our buckets" through various self-cleaning pathways and also with the help of the food that we eat. More about both of those concepts in upcoming chapters.

Even so, isn't it better to fix the hole in the roof, so water stops dripping in? That's where getting clean(ish) can help.

FAT CAN BE PROTECTIVE, BUT . . . THERE'S A FLIP SIDE

As a part of understanding what's going on in our bodies when our toxic loads increase, studies performed on various animal species through the 1980s and 1990s found a correlation between POP toxicity and overall fat mass. When the animals had more body fat, they were actually more resistant to the negative effects from the POPs.

Think about it this way: The animals managed the excess POP exposure by stashing the toxic POPs in fat cells, which kept the toxins out of circulation. That's a positive: their bodies *resisted the negative effects* of the POPs by sequestering the toxins in their fat cells. The fat protected them.[33]

On the flip side of this, studies also show that these chemicals are released from fat cells back into circulation during the fat-loss process. This is something to keep in mind as someone is losing weight.

In a 2011 study, scientists followed seventy-one obese subjects who underwent bariatric surgery. They were compared to a group of eighteen lean women. Before surgery, the obese subjects had higher levels of leptin, fasting glucose, insulin, and inflammatory markers than the lean subjects.

At the beginning of the study, the scientists calculated the total POP body burden for each participant and found that it was *two to three times higher* for the obese subjects than the lean women.

Here's where it gets a little alarming. During the initial weight-loss phase, the participants had an *increase* in circulating POPs, as these chemicals were released from the fat cells.

Also, they found that the positive effects of the weight loss seemed

> to be *"slowed down or decreased by higher POP levels."* This means
> that the body had to deal with the increased levels of toxins in the
> blood as they were released from the fat cells before other health
> markers could show improvement.
>
> The good news is that within six to twelve months, the partici-
> pants had a 15 percent decrease in their overall body burdens, which
> is significant.[34]

Overall, this had a positive long-term effect: even though toxins
were released from the fat cells during the fat-loss process, the participants decreased their overall body burden over time. The fat loss
lowered their overall toxic load and partially "emptied their buckets."

FOOD CONTACT CHEMICALS: ADDING TO OUR BODY BURDENS

What else adds to our overall toxic loads? Something known as *food
contact chemicals*. In an article from 2020 published in *Environmental Health*, scientists from a variety of backgrounds came together
and published a paper called "Impacts of food contact chemicals on
human health: A consensus statement."[35] Here are a few quotes from
their paper.

First, who are these scientists?

> *We, as scientists working on developmental biology, endocrinology,
> epidemiology, toxicology, and environmental and public health, are
> concerned that public health is currently insufficiently protected from
> harmful exposures to food contact chemicals (FCCs).*

I find it to be meaningful that these scientists come from a wide
range of scientific disciplines. Together, they have the diverse background to understand the many factors that come into play.

They went on to say:

Importantly, exposures to harmful FCCs are avoidable.

And:

Food contact chemicals (FCCs) are the chemical constituents of food contact materials and finished food contact articles, including food packaging, food storage containers, food processing equipment, and kitchen- and tableware.

And:

It is clearly established by empirical data that FCCs can migrate from food contact materials and articles into food, indicating a high probability that a large majority of the human population is exposed to some or many of these chemicals. Indeed, for some FCCs there is evidence for human exposure from biomonitoring, although some FCCs may have multiple uses and also non-food contact exposure pathways.

And one more quote that reiterates the point I have made throughout this chapter:

When food contact material regulations were first developed, it had been generally assumed that low-level chemical exposures, i.e. exposures below the toxicologically established no-effect level, pose negligible risks to consumers, except for carcinogens. However, more recent scientific information demonstrates that this assumption is not generally valid, with the available evidence showing that exposure to low levels of endocrine disrupting chemicals can contribute to adverse health effects. In addition, chemical mixtures can play a role in the development of adverse effects, and human exposure to chemical mixtures is the norm but currently not considered when assessing health impacts of FCCs. The timing of exposures during fetal and child development is another critical aspect for understanding development of chronic disease. Currently, these new and important insights are still insufficiently considered in the risk assessment of chemicals in general, and of FCCs in particular.

WOW.

Just as I already explained, it can be easy to shrug off tiny exposures as irrelevant, but in the case of FCCs, these scientists emphasize that despite past assumptions, low levels of exposure *do* contribute to adverse health effects. They also mention the role of "chemical mixtures" and their contribution to overall adverse effects, which is what I referred to earlier when I used the words *chemical soup*.

While the context of this particular paper is "food contact chemicals" (food packaging, storage containers, and cookware), the concepts can apply to all the various chemicals that drip into our buckets: small exposures add up, they are coming at us from everywhere we turn, and we have to consider the overall combination of chemicals that make up our rising toxic loads.

SOUNDING THE ALARM: NEWBORNS

It's not surprising that adults have large toxic loads, because we have been around for decades: eating, drinking, breathing, and absorbing. But what about babies? Is there anything purer or more pristine than a newborn baby?

Unfortunately, babies in the modern world are not as pure and pristine as they should be.

As babies develop in utero, they receive nutrients from their mothers through their umbilical cords. These nutrients are not the only things being passed along, however. We are discovering that even before birth, our kids are exposed to hundreds of chemicals that could harm their health and affect their development.

You may have learned that the placenta acts as a filter, preventing toxins from being passed on to the growing baby. Unfortunately, the placenta doesn't filter out many of the things that we don't want to get to the baby. Alcohol, nicotine, drugs ... we all know about the negative effects these substances have on a developing fetus, and most of us would never dream of drinking alcohol, smoking, or taking drugs during pregnancy. But is avoiding these usual suspects enough? The answer is no.

In a 2009 study, scientists found that most of the toxic metals they measured crossed the placental barrier, and in fact, the mercury levels found within cord blood were almost *double* those found within the mother.[36] That's alarming on its own, but there's more.

In a 2015 review article, scientists combed the literature and found that we are right to be concerned when it comes to not only what mothers are passing on to their babies but also about the cumulative effects of chemicals.

Here is a summary of what they found when they surveyed the literature:

Chemical Class and Detection Frequency	Potential Health Concerns	Are These Chemicals Persistent, Meaning They Stick Around in the Body?
Phthalates Found in 90–100% of the mothers and 90–100% of the babies	Allergies, cognitive and behavioral development, altered male reproductive development, endocrine disruption, preterm birth	No
Phenols Found in 80–100% of the mothers and 40–60% of the babies	Asthma, cognitive and behavioral development, cardiometabolic disorders, endocrine disruption	No

PFCs (perfluorinated compounds) Found in 90–100% of the mothers and 90–100% of the babies	Endocrine disruption, reduced fetal growth	Yes
Flame retardants Found in 90–100% of the mothers and 70–100% of the babies	Cognitive and behavioral development, thyroid hormone disruption	Yes
PCBs (polychlorinated biphenyls) Found in 80–100% of the mothers and 90–100% of the babies	Cognitive and behavioral development, thyroid hormone disruption, reduced fetal growth	Yes
OCs (organochlorine pesticides) Found in 90–100% of the mothers and 90–100% of the babies	Cognitive and behavioral development, endocrine disruption, immune suppression	Yes

As you can see, these six classes of chemicals are all linked to a variety of health concerns, such as cognitive and behavioral developmental issues, endocrine disruption, thyroid hormone disruption, immune suppression, reduced fetal growth, preterm birth, and cardiometabolic disorders. This list, as scary as it is, is likely not all-inclusive, but simply a survey of what we believe to be true based on some of the research that has been done.[37]

Think of all the research that has **not yet been done.**

In addition to that data, the Environmental Working Group (EWG) conducted a small study of their own in 2004. They collected umbilical cord blood from newborns and found an average of *two hundred industrial chemicals and pollutants* in the babies they tested. That is the *average,* not the total. To read their report, go to www.ewg.org and search using the key words "Body Burden: The Pollution in Newborns."[38]

The chemicals they found come from a wide variety of sources, such as:

- Pesticides

- Stain- and grease-resistant coatings for food wrap, carpets, and furniture

- Electric insulators

- Industrial chemicals such as flame retardants

- Waste by-products (garbage incineration and plastic production wastes)

- Car emissions and fossil fuel combustion

- Power plants

Solving this problem is as easy as riding a bike. Except the bike is on fire, and you're on fire. And everything is on fire. I didn't make up this fiery-bike analogy, but it feels somewhat applicable here, am I right?

I just threw a bunch of scary words, facts, and figures at you.

Gulp.

Yes, we are inundated with chemicals in today's modern world, and exposure begins from our time in the womb. Some of these toxins are unavoidable because they are "out there" already, and we come in contact with them just by living our lives. Short of living in a bubble (which we can't do), what do we do now?

Don't panic. That won't help.

The first step is understanding that *Houston, we have a problem.* Our toxic loads are higher than ever before in human history, our buckets are full, and our bodies are straining under this burden.

Knowledge is power, though. Never forget that.

If only we could snap our fingers and eliminate all the PBTs and POPs that are already in the environment. Well, we can't do that. (Though we *can* work together to make a difference in what happens going forward.)

Because our buckets are more full than ever thanks to the pervasive nature of chemicals, especially those that are persistent and accumulate in our environments (and our bodies), it's even more essential in today's world to make sure we control *what else gets into our bodies.* Those are things we *can* control.

While we may not be able to do anything right now about the state of the world in general, in the next three chapters, I'm going to go through some of the toxins that we *can* immediately do something about. I'm going to teach you about some of the toxins in our cleaning products and personal care products, and also the ones within our foods. We are absolutely in control of what we buy and the foods and products we choose.

The good news is that when we become clean(ish), we slow the speed of the drip, drip, drip into our personal buckets.

REFLECT: HOW FULL IS YOUR BUCKET?

Use your Clean(ish) Journal (or the worksheets available at ginstephens.com/cleanish) to complete these end-of-chapter prompts.

- Had you heard the phrase "better living through chemistry" before? What did it mean to you before reading this chapter, and what does it mean to you now?

- Did anything surprise, shock, or even upset you as you read this chapter?

- Reread the list on page 50. Are you experiencing any of the signs of a full-to-overflowing bucket? If so, which ones?

TAKE ACTION: MAKE A DIFFERENCE

Use your Clean(ish) Journal (or the worksheets available at ginstephens.com/cleanish) to complete these end-of-chapter activities.

Remember what I said in my author's note at the beginning of the book:

> Let's come together as citizens of the world to insist that we have cleaner and safer foods, personal care products, and household cleaners, as well as a cleaner and safer environment in general. Becoming clean(ish) doesn't just help us individually, but it can help us all.
>
> Clean(ish) living is not about partisan politics, but you may feel like getting a little vocal after reading this book. No matter who you vote for or whichever side of the political aisle you embrace, I know we can agree that every human on earth deserves to live a healthy life. It should not be dependent upon socioeconomic status, disposable income, or zip code, either. I believe that health is our birthright, not just a political talking point. We have the power to vote with our wallets, and as we make changes to what we buy and which companies we support, the current trends toward a larger selection of cleaner and safer options will continue, and these options will become more affordable over time. That's already happening.
>
> One by one, we can join together to demand that we head toward a safer and cleaner future that we envision together. Our planet, our kids, and our grandkids depend on us.

You may be someone who has never considered getting involved in environmental issues; however, now you're concerned. You want to do something, but you don't know *what*. You may also feel like any type of "activism" isn't for you, because it feels like something that other people do . . . other people who are different from you.

The key is to educate yourself and speak the truth as you see it, and don't be afraid of speaking up when it comes to issues that are important to you. Every single one of us, completely unrelated to political affiliation, should be alarmed by the information that I have shared in this chapter, and I only shared the tip of the iceberg.

Get involved: Find organizations you can support that are working on making a difference. Decide what is most important to you and start there.

What does this look like for me? One of the organizations I support is the Environmental Working Group (EWG). They are by no means the only organization doing this work, but the key is to start somewhere, with an organization that has a mission matching your personal goals.

Their mission statement:

> *Our mission is simple: To empower you with breakthrough research to make informed choices and live a healthy life in a healthy environment.*

If you visit www.ewg.org/take-action, you can see all the ways you can support the work the EWG is doing and also how they recommend that you take action, right from your home and every time you shop.

Visit the Environmental Working Group's website (ewg.org) and take a look around, particularly the "Take Action" page.

Do some searching on the web to find other organizations besides EWG with missions that match your personal goals. Create pages in your journal to take notes about the organizations you find.

In your Clean(ish) Journal, your notes might look like this:

Name of organization / website: _____

_____

Mission: _____

_____

How I can get involved: _____

_____

_____

_____

_____

HOUSEHOLD CLEANING PRODUCTS: WHAT'S IN YOUR BUCKET?

After reading the previous chapter, you understand that our toxic loads increase over time based on chemicals that we come in contact with as we live our lives, and these all add up to increase our overall body burdens. Our rising body burdens are illustrated by visualizing rising levels in our personal "toxic load" buckets.

Now it's time to discover where these and other chemicals are found in the products we buy so we can begin to avoid them, slowing the overall drips into our buckets. While it's impossible to avoid all exposure in our lives, we absolutely can make decisions that make a difference in both *what* and *how much* we are exposed to by making safer and cleaner choices.

BEWARE OF DIHYDROGEN MONOXIDE: CHEMICALS ARE SCARY

Before I get into that, I want to give you a very important warning.

What if I told you that there is one chemical that you come in contact with daily, and in fact, your body is absolutely saturated with it at all times? This chemical can be downright dangerous:

- If this chemical gets into your lungs, it interferes with breathing. Oxygen can no longer be delivered to the heart. The body shuts down. Death occurs.

- If you overconsume this chemical, symptoms may include confusion, disorientation, nausea, and vomiting. In rare cases, you may experience swelling in the brain, which can be fatal.

- This chemical can be corrosive, and metal exposed to it for long periods of time will form iron oxide hydrate and experience a weakened structure.

- This chemical is the major component of acid rain.

These are just a few of the dangers of dihydrogen monoxide, so we need to band together to ensure that it is banned before more damage is done.

After reading this list, you are either:

1. Really worried about this dangerous chemical and hoping that I am going to tell you how to avoid it in the future.
2. Laughing, because you get the joke.

What is dihydrogen monoxide? It's the chemical name of water . . . two hydrogen atoms (di-hydrogen) and one oxygen atom (mono-oxide).

Everything I just said about it is true. Your body is about 60 percent water. And, yes—water comes with dangers. Yes, if you inhale water into your lungs, you drown and die. Yes, you can experience something called *water intoxication* if you drink too much water, and it is dangerous to do so. Yes, water is part of the rusting process. Yes, acid rain is mostly water.

I wish I could take credit for the origination of the concept of "beware of dihydrogen monoxide." If you google those words, you can find a wide variety of sources for and versions of this classic parody (one version or another has been around since at least 1983).

The reason I began this chapter with the dihydrogen monoxide parody is to point out a real limitation, and it's the real "warning" I want to communicate in this section: we can't tell just from reading the name of a chemical whether it is dangerous. Any advice you may have heard to read labels and avoid things with long, confusing names on the product list is clearly insufficient.

A second limitation is that even something as benign as water *can* be dangerous, but that doesn't mean water is something we should ban or avoid. It would be impossible to do either of those things and stay alive . . . Banning or avoiding dihydrogen monoxide is more dangerous than exposure to it, am I right?

LABELS ARE CONFUSING (BUT THAT'S NOT ALL!)

When we read product labels, we see all sorts of words we can't identify. Many of them might have hard-to-read, polysyllabic names, such as the example of dihydrogen monoxide from the previous section.

Since we can't tell if a chemical is safe just by reading its name, it's important that we have other sources of information to decide whether the ingredients in a product are safe. But to do that, we need to know what's actually *in* each product we buy. Can't we trust the labels on our products to identify everything that is inside?

Unfortunately, the answer is no. Shockingly, there are loopholes in labeling laws, which means that companies are not required to list all the ingredients (or their concentrations) on the label. One example is the way personal care products are not required to identify what chemicals are part of the innocent-sounding word *fragrance*. I'll talk more about this in the next chapter.

So, not only can we not determine if a chemical is safe based on the simplicity or complexity of its name, we also can't be sure what's actually in the products due to the way manufacturers are allowed to hide ingredients behind innocent sounding names such as *fragrance*.

For those reasons, many of us rely on other words on the labels to help us make decisions about the products we buy. We have become accustomed to looking for words on product labels that communicate the overall safety or purity of the products we buy: *Natural! Eco-friendly! Biodegradable!* Are these words meaningful? Do they really indicate that those products are the better choices? The answer is: not always.

"GREENWASHING" IN THE HOUSEHOLD PRODUCTS INDUSTRY

Welcome to the practice known as *greenwashing*. Often, manufacturers use words that sound fancy and make us think that a product is safe. The words sound "green" to us (hence the term *greenwashing*), but actually, the words they use are often meaningless and amount to nothing more than marketing-speak.

Personally, I'm a little embarrassed to admit how much I fell for this tactic. When I took a closer look at what products I gravitated toward in the stores, I realized that I have been duped by these fancy words many times over the years.

I bet you'll find the same to be true for you when you start looking more closely at your shopping habits.

Here are a few examples of how words on labels make a product (or its packaging) sound better, but actually don't indicate anything about the product's ingredients or safety:

What They Say	What It Actually Means
Natural	This implies that the ingredients come from natural sources. Well, so does arsenic. *Natural* doesn't necessarily mean "safe." And while these products may contain natural *ingredients,* they may also include other ingredients that are not natural, such as synthetic dyes and fragrances. "Made from natural ingredients" basically means nothing when you understand that point.
Nontoxic	When a product claims to be nontoxic, is it true? Well, even water and oxygen can be "toxic" to the body at certain doses, so there goes that idea.

	Nontoxic simply means the product doesn't contain ingredients that have been linked to toxic responses (like hormone disruption, cancer, etc.) in humans. Also keep in mind that any terminology you see on a product label is only as good as the regulations that back it up. There are no regulations defining what makes a product "nontoxic."
Eco-friendly or environmentally friendly	There are also no guidelines or benchmarks that a product must pass to call itself *eco-friendly* or *environmentally friendly*. While these words sound great, what about the products make them eco- [or environmentally friendly? If you see these words on a product label, it's important to look closer for information that explains exactly how or why they consider their product to be safer for the environment.
Unscented	If a product is marketed as *unscented,* that means that the product may actually have added chemicals that are there as "masking scents." Masking scents are added to cover up odors that would otherwise be apparent. So, the product would normally have a bad stench that they have covered up with masking agents? Um, no, thank you. On the flip side, some products are labeled as *fragrance-free,* which actually means something. When a label says a product is "fragrance-free," it means that no scented artificial ingredients or masking scents were added.[1]
Biodegradable	The term *biodegradable* might be applied to the product itself or to the packaging. The term means that a product or substance is naturally broken down when it's exposed to air, moisture, or organisms such as bacteria and fungi. When it comes to packaging, one factor that affects the rate of degradation is the availability of oxygen, and landfills tend to have little to no airflow. This means that even if a product package is biodegradable in optimal conditions, it may not actually biodegrade in a meaningful length of time in practice. Instead of *biodegradable,* the word *compostable* is much more meaningful.

WHAT'S IN OUR HOUSEHOLD PRODUCTS?

According to the EPA, the pollution inside our homes may be worse than the air outside. Much of this is related to the products we use to clean. Oh, the irony: by trying to keep our homes clean, we are actually making things worse

Cleaning supplies, personal care products such as our cosmetics, deodorants, and lotions, laundry detergents, plastic containers, paint, home, and garden supplies . . . The list goes on and on.

There are a lot of chemicals in the products within our homes. Which are safe? Which are dangerous? We don't always know, because many of them have not been tested for safety. As I already mentioned, the government doesn't even require that all the chemicals be listed on the labels, such as with the innocuous term *fragrance*. Sounds innocent, right? What does it even mean? In all honesty, it could mean almost anything.

Consider that "clean" has no smell. You may think of the pine scent of Pine-Sol (*that smell always meant my grandmother's house had been freshly cleaned*) or the "fresh" clean-clothes smell (*of the laundry detergent that your mom used*) as indications of "clean," when really, that smell indicates anything *but* "clean." What you are smelling is the chemicals within those products. When you think about it that way, that's not very *clean,* is it?

Let's examine some of the products that most of us have in our homes right now:

Room of House	Common Products	What Might Be in These Products?
Bathroom	Air fresheners Toilet cleaners Mold and mildew removers Drain cleaners Aerosols	Aerosol propellants, alkyl ammonium chlorides, bleach, dichlorobenzene, formaldehyde, hydrochloric acid, lye, naphthalene, p-dichlorobenzene, petroleum distillates, phenols, phthalates, sulfuric acid, terpenes, toluene
Kitchen	Insect sprays/baits All-purpose cleaners Glass and window cleaners Antibacterial cleaners Dishwasher detergent Oven cleaners Carpet cleaners Floor and furniture polish	Abamectin, ammonia, boric acid, chlorpyrifos, detergents, diazinon, disinfectants, ethylene formaldehyde, ethylene glycol, fragrance, grease-cutting agents, isopropanol, lye, naphtha, naphthalene, permethrin, phenolic compounds, phosphates, phthalates, propoxur, quaternary ammonium, phosphoric acid, silica, sodium hypochlorite, (chlorine bleach) solvents, sulfluramid, sulfuric acid, surfactants, trichlorfon, trisodium triclosan, tripolyphosphate

	Scouring powders and cleansers	
	Metal polishes	
Laundry	Laundry detergent	A-terpineol, benzyl acetate, benzyl alcohol, fragrance, sodium hypo-chlorite (chlorine bleach), styrene, toluene, trimethylbenzene
	Chlorine bleach	
	Fabric softeners	
	Dryer sheets	
Garage	Wood stains	Ethylene glycol, formaldehyde, mineral spirits, other petroleum distillate solvents, toluene, xylene
	Paint	
	Antifreeze	

Those chemical names in our common household products certainly *sound* alarming. But so did *dihydrogen monoxide,* and that is just water. So, are they dangerous?[2]

Here is a sampling of the warnings that are associated with these common chemicals in our household products:

- *May irritate the skin, eyes, nose, mouth, and throat.*

- *Can be highly poisonous / fatal if swallowed.*

- *May aggravate asthma.*

- *Linked to reproductive problems and liver and kidney damage.*

- *Exposure during pregnancy may lead to an increased risk of birth defects, low birth weight, and fetal death.*

- *Exposure in childhood has been linked to attention and learning problems, as well as cancer.*

- *Possible carcinogen.*

- *Caustic.*

- *Releases dangerous fumes.*

- *May cause blindness.*

- *May cause breathing problems.*

- *May increase the resistance of some bacteria to antibiotics.*

- *Fumes may cause kidney and liver damage.*

- *Damaging to central nervous system.*

- *Vapor may damage respiratory tract, aggravate asthma, emphysema, bronchitis, and other respiratory conditions.*

- *May cause headaches.*

- *May cause damage to internal organs through skin absorption.*

Even though the words *may, can,* or *possible* are used throughout that list, it sounds like a lot of potential risk to be taking to me.

What's under your cabinets may even be considered to be "household hazardous waste" by the EPA. What is hazardous waste? It's trash that contains chemicals that have been identified as toxic to fish, wildlife, plants, or humans. Hazardous waste requires special handling and disposal . . . yet we are using these products to clean our homes?[3]

It's easy when your products say *poison* or when they have warnings right there on the labels. Those are easy to identify. But keep in mind what we have already learned: drop by drop, the chemicals we are exposed to add to the levels in our personal buckets.

WHAT WE USE AT HOME DOESN'T STAY AT HOME

Cleaning products don't just affect us at the point of use. We wash these products down the drain, and residues end up in our streams, rivers, lakes, and oceans. One example? Dangerous levels of dioxin were found in San Francisco Bay. The EPA identified the source:

municipal gray water that contained chemical residue from laundry bleach.[4] The U.S. Geological Survey found all sorts of chemical residues in 80 percent of streams tested. These included residues from insect repellent, triclosan, fire retardants, detergents, and plasticizers.[5]

It really is true: these cleaning products are leaving behind a real mess that itself needs to be cleaned up.

WHAT DO WE DO NOW?

The good news is that we can trade out almost every potentially problematic product (or food storage container / cookware) in our homes with safer options. More about that in part 3, where we will design our personal plans to live (mainly) clean.

REFLECT AND TAKE ACTION: WHAT'S IN YOUR CABINETS?

Use your Clean(ish) Journal (or the worksheets available at ginstephens.com/cleanish) to complete these end-of-chapter prompts and activities.

Have you been fooled by greenwashing on cleaning product labels? Time to take a look!

1. Pull out some of the cleaning products you've been using that you chose because they seemed like "cleaner" options.
2. Download the Environmental Working Group's app. It's called EWG Healthy Living.
3. Use the search feature to check some of the products that you've been using.

GIN'S PERSONAL APPLICATION: DISH SOAP

There's a brand of cleaning products that I've used for years, assuming that they were a safer alternative because they have done a great job marketing their entire product line as natural and better for the environment. This is greenwashing in action. Well, they may be a better choice than many other conventional products that are out there, but I was shocked at what I found out when I took a closer look.

The dish soap I had been choosing, believing it was a great choice? It got a **D** ranking in the Environmental Working Group's EWG Healthy Living app. One of their scents actually gets an **F**.

Here's what was so surprising to me. One of the dish soaps I would never have considered to be "clean" (a major brand that is blue and we've seen it in the stores for years) has a foam version that ranks as a **C**.

All these years, I avoided the big-name blue brand and chose the "better" option, when actually the big-name brand would have been a better choice.

When I browse through the "Hand Washing Detergent Cleaners" list in the EWG Healthy Living app, sorted from best to worst, there's a long list of options that are available to me that score an **A** or a **B**. On the date that I wrote this, there are twenty-two different brands that have an **A** ranking, and so I know I have plenty of options to choose from. While I have said goodbye to the brand I thought was a good choice, the switch to cleaner options was painless. The dish soap I chose as a replacement? It has the same overall scent as the one I used to use, so other than knowing that it has fewer questionable chemicals, I can't tell there is a difference when I am using it. It was a painless swap to make.

Time to analyze your cleaning products.

Create a section in your journal to take a closer look at a few of your favorites. Create these tables in your journal, adding as many rows as you need.

My products and their ratings/concerns on the Environmental Working Group (EWG Healthy Living) app:

PRODUCT List items that I use frequently	PRODUCT RATING (from 1–10 or A–F)	INGREDIENT CONCERNS Which ingredients are identified as ones I should be concerned about?

When I analyze the information I just learned about my household cleaning products:

Products with scores that greatly concern me: it's time to consider alternatives	Products that I'm iffy about	Products that I couldn't find in the database	Products that have a green rating (1–2 or A–B), so I know they are safe

Based on what I learned, I can make these easy changes today:

PERSONAL CARE PRODUCTS: ADDING TO YOUR BUCKET

Toxins can enter the body through multiple pathways. We all understand that our health is affected by what we eat, but it's also affected by what we put *on* our bodies. Our skin is our largest organ, and chemicals that come in contact with our skin are absorbed and then can enter our bloodstreams. We are all familiar with transdermal medication applications, such as a patch delivery system for nicotine or birth control. With that in mind, you understand why it's important to consider what we come in contact with: if therapeutic doses of medications and hormones can enter through our skin, then so can toxins and other harmful chemicals.

Many of the ingredients used in conventional cosmetics and personal care products are toxic, especially in combination and over time. Molecule by molecule, they go into your bucket. It may not seem like much, but as I already said, small exposures add up: never forget that many drops of water ultimately flow together to form the oceans.

Cosmetics and personal care products touch every part of our bodies. A recent survey of 2,300 people found that most Americans use an average of nine products per day, and more than a quarter of women use at least fifteen. These products have at least 126 unique ingredients when combined. This would include things like shampoo and conditioner, toothpaste, mouthwash, deodorant, makeup, lip balm, lotion, sunscreen, hair spray, shaving cream, perfume, and soap. And it's not just women. Men use a lot of products these days, and there's a whole different set of products that are marketed as just for kids.[1]

According to the Environmental Working Group, our personal care products are manufactured with at least 10,500 unique ingredients, and most have not gone through any required safety testing. Shocking, but true. In general, the United States' cosmetics industry is poorly regulated. The FDA provides much less oversight than you would expect, meaning the ingredients don't have to go through a rigorous testing process for safety before being used. We all assume that if chemicals are in our shampoo bottle that they must be safe. Otherwise, the government wouldn't allow them to be sold in our stores, right? Wrong.

While this may change in the future (and I hope that it does), as of early 2021, the U.S. government hadn't passed a federal law that regulates the cosmetics industry since 1938. That's shocking. Think of how many new chemicals have been introduced since 1938. Also consider how much our scientific understanding has increased since then.

From the FDA's own website:[2]

> Companies and individuals who manufacture or market cosmetics have a legal responsibility to ensure the safety of their products. Neither the law nor FDA regulations require specific tests to demonstrate the safety of individual products or ingredients. The law also does not require cosmetic companies to share their safety information with FDA.

Yes, you are reading that correctly: there are no required tests for whether either the *products* or *ingredients* are safe. And the cosmetic companies don't even have to share their safety information *with* the FDA.

Some of the products contain ingredients that are regarded as safe by the government and industry, but there may still be troubling study results related to these chemicals. Parabens are one example. They are used as preservatives and are found in a wide variety of personal care products such as lotions. The problem is that parabens are generally considered to be endocrine disruptors, and they are known to bioaccumulate.[3] They have even been detected in human breast tumors.[4] We have widespread exposure to parabens: in one study from 2006, parabens were found in the urine of 96 percent of those tested.[5]

The personal care industry would tell you that you don't need to worry about the ingredients in your products. *"Trust us!"* they say. After all, these ingredients are present in such small amounts. But when you remember that you are probably using somewhere between nine and fifteen different personal care products on your body every day, every tiny exposure really adds up. Keep in mind that most safety analyses of individual ingredients are conducted as if you're exposed one chemical at a time, which isn't at all what happens in the real world.

As I already mentioned, it is difficult to come to 100 percent consensus about the link between these chemicals and specific health disorders. Even if these chemicals are safe in isolation or in small doses, the issue is that we don't use these chemicals in isolation, and even small doses are likely to add up over time and add to the loads within our buckets.

Just now, I paused from writing and went into my bathroom to take inventory of just how many products I use every day. If I were going on vacation, what would I pack to take with me? I consider those to be the essentials.

I pulled everything out and lined it all up on my counter, and then I counted to see the number of personal care products I use as a part of my combined morning and evening routines. Keep in mind that I didn't count *all* the items in my bathroom drawers and cabinets, only the ones I use daily.

Before doing this experiment, I would have told you I'm a pretty simple person. But I counted TWENTY-SIX different products that

I use daily. I can't even imagine how many individual ingredients are within those twenty-six different products. If I'm using twenty-six different products on my body each day, I want to know that they are all safe. Don't you?

It's a lot easier in other parts of the world. The European Commission, which is the governing body of the European Union, takes a much more cautious stance than the U.S.'s FDA.[6] Unlike in the U.S., European cosmetic products must undergo safety testing before they hit the market.[7] That makes a lot more sense to me.

FRAGRANCE: THAT STINKS!

Just as is the case with household cleaning products, one of the most innocent-sounding ingredients in our personal care products is *fragrance*. What could be wrong with that? Lots, actually.

Unfortunately for us, fragrances have been identified as a trigger for asthma, allergies, and migraines.[8] They are also a common cause of contact dermatitis.[9]

There are thousands of chemicals that make up the fragrances used in cosmetics and skin care products, and they are used to either add a scent or to cover up a foul-smelling product. (Can we all just say *yuck* at the sound of that?) What's surprising is that manufacturers are not required to list the ingredients used in any "fragrance." Thanks to a legal loophole, the mix of ingredients in anything considered to be a fragrance is a trade secret. This law was written to protect major perfume brands and is part of the Fair Packaging and Labeling Act of 1966. It is estimated that 80 percent of ingredients in fragrances are not tested for human safety.[10] That really stinks. (*Sorry, I had to.*)

Here's something else that is shocking. A product can be labeled as "paraben-free" or "phthalate-free" but could actually contain parabens or phthalates hidden within the fragrance mixture.

The takeaway here is this: when you see the word *fragrance* on any product label, you now understand this is likely code for "we are using mystery chemicals and we don't even have to tell you what they are." These mystery chemicals may or may not be harmless.

WHAT'S IN YOUR PERSONAL CARE PRODUCTS?

This table only contains a small sampling of some of the chemicals you might find in your medicine cabinet or bathroom.[11]

Category	Common Products	What Might Be in These Products?
Hair care products	Shampoo and conditioner Hair color Hair spray Gels, mousse, etc. Hair dyes	Ammonia, aronopol, diethanolamine, DMDM hydantoin, diazolidinyl urea, formaldehyde, fragrance, imidazolidinyl urea, various petrochemicals, miscellaneous preservatives, peroxide, p-phenylenediamine, quaternium-15, sodium laureth sulfate, sodium lauryl sulfate, triethanolamine
Makeup	Lipstick Mascara Eyeliner Foundations Eyeshadow Blush	Bismuth oxychloride, butylated compounds (BHT, BHA), carbon black, dibutyl and diethylhexyl phthalates, formaldehyde, fragrance, isobutyl and isopropyl p-phenylenediamine, parabens, lead, methylene glycol, octinoxate, polyethylene glycols, quaternium-15, siloxanes, talc
Skin care	Moisturizers Sunscreen Firming lotions Antiaging lotions Cleansers Makeup removers	Avobenzone, DEA, fragrance, homosalate, hydroquinone, imidazolindinyl urea, octinoxate, octisalate, octocrylene, oxybenzone, parabens, petroleum distillates, propylene glycol, quaternium-15, retinol, retinyl acetate, retinyl linoleate, retinyl palmitate, sodium lauryl sulfate

Other products that we use on our skin	Antiperspirants	Aluminum chlorohydrate, aluminum zirconium, butyl acetate, dibutyl phthalate, ethyl acetate, formaldehyde resin, fragrance, isopropyl alcohol, phthalates, toluene, toluene sulfon-amide, triclosan
	Deodorants	
	Fragrances/Perfume	
	Nail Polish/Remover	
	Shaving cream	
	Lotion	
Dental hygiene products	Toothpaste	Artificial sweeteners, dyes, para-bens, perfluorohexane sulfonic acid, propylene glycol, sodium lauryl sulfate, triclosan
	Mouthwash	
	Dental floss	
Feminine hygiene products	Tampons	Chlorine dioxide, dioxins, fragrance, parabens, phthalates, sodium lauryl sulfate,
	Pads	
	Feminine washes	

As I already mentioned, we can't tell whether a chemical is safe or dangerous simply because it has a scary-sounding name. However, many of the chemicals in the list above are chemicals of concern.

Here is a sampling of the warnings that are associated with chemicals found in our personal care products:

- *Linked to increased occurrence of breast cancer, kidney disease, bladder cancer, leukemia, ovarian cancer, or Alzheimer's.*

- *Linked to neurotoxicity.*

- *May irritate the skin, eyes, nose, mouth, and throat.*

- *Can be highly poisonous / fatal if swallowed.*

- *May aggravate asthma.*

- *Linked to reproductive problems and liver and kidney damage.*

- *Exposure during pregnancy may lead to an increased risk of birth defects, low birth weight, and fetal death.*

- *Exposure in childhood has been linked to attention and learning problems, as well as cancer.*

- *Possible carcinogen.*

- *Caustic.*

- *Releases dangerous fumes.*

- *May cause blindness.*

- *May cause breathing problems.*

- *May increase the resistance of some bacteria to antibiotics.*

- *Fumes may cause kidney and liver damage.*

- *Damaging to central nervous system.*

- *Vapor may damage respiratory tract, aggravate asthma, emphysema, bronchitis, and other respiratory conditions.*

- *May cause headaches.*

- *May cause damage to internal organs through skin absorption.*

- *May speed the development of skin tumors and lesions when applied to the skin in the presence of sunlight.*

- *May cause liver damage, brittle nails, hair loss, and osteoporosis and hip fractures in older adults.*

Again, even though the words *may, can be,* or *possible* are found throughout the list, the possibility of these effects is very concerning to me.

GREENWASHING IN THE PERSONAL CARE INDUSTRY

Some of the words used on personal care product labels make us think that these products are safer options. This is another example of greenwashing. As I mentioned in the last chapter, these terms— such as *natural*—may steer you toward certain products, but they are basically meaningless.

In the personal care product world, here are a few terms that you may think are an indication of safety but are actually more examples of greenwashing:

What They Say	What It Actually Means
Hypoallergenic	This is a marketing claim, pure and simple. But it doesn't mean the actual *product* is really "pure" or "simple." According to the FDA: "*There are no Federal standards or definitions that govern the use of the term 'hypoallergenic.' The term means whatever a particular company wants it to mean. Manufacturers of cosmetics labeled as hypoallergenic are not required to submit substantiation of their hypallergenicity claims to FDA.*"[12]
Noncomedogenic	We've seen this term on many of our products, but what does it mean? *Noncomedogenic* products are less likely to cause skin pore blockages or acne. The term is completely unregulated, and therefore these products may actually *cause* you to have pore blockages or acne.
Cruelty-free or not tested on animals	I never want to think that I'm doing anything that would be cruel to animals, and I am sure you feel the same way. For that reason, this is a popular labeling claim. But does it mean anything? According to the FDA: "*Many raw materials, used in cosmetics, were tested on animals years ago when they were first introduced. A cosmetic manufacturer might only use those raw materials and base their 'cruelty-free'*

	claims on the fact that the materials or products are *not* currently *tested on animals*."[13] Oops.
Dermatologist-approved	It's true that a dermatologist may approve a product, especially if the company pays them to do so. That being said, the wording does *not* mean that a product has necessarily been evaluated for either short- or long-term safety. While it's likely that products with this labeling may be less likely to irritate your skin, that doesn't mean that these products couldn't have chemicals within them that are endocrine disruptors or linked to cancer, for example.
Chemical-free	Water is technically a chemical. The air you breathe is a mixture of chemicals. In fact, everything is made of chemicals at the molecular level. It is impossible, therefore, to buy *any* product that is chemical-free. Nice try, beauty industry, nice try.

REFLECT AND TAKE ACTION: WHAT ARE YOU USING?

Use your Clean(ish) Journal (or the worksheets available at ginstephens.com/cleanish) to complete these end-of-chapter prompts and activities.

In this chapter, I told you about my experiment: I went into my bathroom and imagined that I was going on a trip. I pulled out all the products that I would take with me on the trip, because those are the ones that I use every day. I counted twenty-six different cosmetic and personal care items that I considered to be essential enough to pack for my imaginary trip.

Now, it's your turn.

1. Go into your bathroom and pull out everything you consider to be a daily essential, something that you use every day. What is your count? Are you within the average (nine to fifteen items), or are you more like me (remember that I counted twenty-six)? Or is your number even higher?

2. Download the Environmental Working Group's app, if you haven't already done so. It's called EWG Healthy Living.

3. Use the search feature to check some of your staple products. It can be especially interesting to check things that you think are "safer" options, as you did in the last chapter.

4. Complete the activity to determine the safety rankings of your key products.

GIN'S PERSONAL APPLICATION: MOUTHWASH

One day, I used the EWG app to check a mouthwash that my husband purchased. The name of the product has *natural* in it, and the label also uses the word *healthy*. It contains aloe vera, and that's featured prominently on the label, as well. It's a product you'll find in health food stores or in the natural section of a regular grocery store. It claims to be formulated by a dentist and seemed like an excellent option to me. Who wouldn't choose a "natural" and "healthy" mouthwash with aloe vera in it that was formulated by a dentist? Thanks, greenwashing!

In the app, however, EWG scores it at a 3, indicating it has "limited" hazards. Since products get a score from 1–10, that's not bad at all, but that puts it into the yellow ("caution") rating area rather than in the green zone.

Why did this item get a 3? First, it has unspecified *flavors*. Just as manufacturers can hide behind the word *fragrance*, they also hide all sorts of ingredients using the word *flavors,* and *natural flavors* aren't necessarily any better than *flavors*. It also has an ingredient called polysorbate 80, which EWG considers to be low risk but still a concern due to what they call *data gaps*—meaning we don't have enough data to be completely sure.

After realizing that this specific mouthwash was a 3, I checked the EWG database for other mouthwash options, and I decided to make a simple swap based on the data I could find in the app.

I typed in the word *mouthwash* and then sorted based on the filter "best score." There were only three mouthwashes with a rating of 1: two were spearmint flavor, and I don't like spearmint, and one of them was a tablet. I have no desire to use a mouthwash tablet, so that one was out. Because I am clean(ish), I always choose the safest option that both fits my preferences and is readily available to me. I can live with a 2 rating over a 1 rating, as both are in the green rating category.

I moved on to the 2-scoring section of the list. To my surprise, Listerine Original was the second choice in the 2 section. It actually had a higher score than many options from what most of us would consider to be a natural or more healthy-focused brand, many of which scored a 3, 4, or even a 5. (Side note: Yes, I know that 3, 4, and 5 are mathematically "higher" numbers than 2. But I am considering 1 to be the "top," and through that particular lens, 2 is "higher" than 3, 4, or 5.)

Listerine Original it is! I didn't select a mouthwash option with a formulation or flavor I don't like simply because it ranked higher. I'm clean(ish), and 2 is just fine with me.

What does my example illustrate? It shows that just because a product is in the natural section of the store and says *natural* and *healthy* on the label doesn't mean it's automatically a better choice. It also shows that products that we may perceive as "less healthy," such as a major brand name with no clean or natural claims on the label, may actually be a smarter choice.

One other interesting realization: this is the exact brand and flavor that my grandmother used. So, I feel a little nostalgic every time I use it.

Time to analyze what's in your bathroom.

Create a section in your Clean(ish) Journal to take a closer look at your favorite products. Create these sections/tables in your journal, adding as many rows as you need.

Date: _____ Number of personal care items I use daily:_____

The average number of personal care items used per day is around nine to fifteen. My average is:

Lower than the average of nine to fifteen _____

Within the average of nine to fifteen _____

Like Gin's, higher than the average of nine to fifteen _____

My products and their r≠atings/concerns on the Environmental Working Group (EWG Healthy Living) app:

PRODUCT *List items that I use frequently*	PRODUCT RATING *(from 1–10 or A–F)*	INGREDIENT CONCERNS *Which ingredients are identified as ones I should be concerned about?*

When I analyze the information I just learned about my personal care products:

Products with scores that greatly concern me: it's time to consider alternatives	Products that I'm iffy about	Products that I couldn't find in the database	Products that have a green rating (1–2 or A–B), so I know they are safe

Based on what I learned, I can make these easy changes today:

FOOD, GLORIOUS FOOD

We've just spent a few chapters learning that potentially harmful chemicals are everywhere, including within our overall environment and in both our household cleaners and personal care products. Funky modern chemicals are also in most of the "food products" we buy in the grocery store.

Why did I write "food products" in quotation marks? This begs the question:

What *is* food?

And a follow-up question: What is *not food*?

Just because we can eat it or they sell it in the grocery store, does that make it *food*? Why or why not? And why is this so complicated?

Twenty-four-seven, thousands of chemical reactions are taking place within our bodies. These chemical reactions take place in every single one of our cells. The food we eat provides chemical support to our cells as they do their important tasks.

Well, that's how it is supposed to work.

What happens when the "food" we are eating is made up of chemicals that are not supposed to be there? What if the nutrients our bodies need are absent from our food? What if the entire industrial farming industry that solved society's food supply issues are creating new problems?

I think most of us understand this to be true:

Food is different now.

Why? I'll explain over the next couple of chapters.

Rather than providing chemical support to the body, what we eat may actually add to our overall toxic load and become a burden on our bodies rather than an essential support. When we are hoping to lower our overall toxic loads, the last thing we want to do is choose food products that *add to* our overall body burdens.

Within the past century, we have increasingly turned away from growing, harvesting, and preparing our own foods and instead become consumers of food and food-like *products*. Instead of being directly responsible for obtaining our food from nature, we buy it at the store.

Let me take a moment to celebrate that, actually. And I am not being sarcastic or tongue-in-cheek here. I am grateful for many things about our modern food system:

- I am *so grateful* that I don't have to personally hunt to find meat or grow all my own fruits and vegetables.

- I am grateful that we can transport food long distances, meaning I can enjoy juicy oranges in the winter months or have fresh avocado whenever I want it.

- I am grateful for innovations in food manufacturing that ensure my food is safe from pathogens.

- I am grateful that there is sufficient food production that I have access to more food than I could ever eat.

- I am grateful that when I want bread, I can go buy it . . . or I can mill wheat berries into flour and make my own bread if I want.

- I am grateful for the fact that there are options and choices available to me in the marketplace.

That being said, I want to make sure that all the food I eat is nourishing my body and supporting vibrant health. The bad news is that most of what is sold in today's grocery store is not actually *food*. It's what I call *not-food*.

It comes in boxes, bags, and packages. It's full of artificial flavors, colors, and preservatives. It's more flavorful, colorful, and long-lasting than anything we've ever experienced from nature, actually.

Most of those boxes, bags, and packages contain very little in the way of actual *food*.

This leads me to one more important concept that I want to get out of the way now. There is no "good" food and "bad" food. We don't have "clean" food and "dirty" food. (Unless you drop your food in the dirt. That's dirty food.)

No, what we have is "Hey—that's food!" and "Oops . . . that's *not* food."

Let's define the two categories:

Food: Nourishes our bodies, providing all the building blocks we need. Our bodies know what to do with food.

Not-food: An empty source of energy, and it won't sustain a healthy body and its many functions. We consume a large amount of chemicals in our not-foods: preservatives, artificial sweeteners, flavoring agents, emulsifiers . . . yikes! Not only are these chemicals affecting us (and adding to the overall toxic load within our buckets), they also affect the health of our gut microbiomes. We rely on a healthy gut microbiome to be healthy ourselves. More about that coming up in a later chapter.

So, why are we eating so much *not-food*? Where is all this processed food *coming from*? Also, why is it missing so many necessary nutrients? Those are interesting questions, indeed.

To understand the scope of the problem, let's do a little backtracking and examine how we got here.

In this chapter, I'll go into details that explain why modern farming practices lead to many of the problems we face with today's food supply. Then, in the next chapter, I'll go into more details about issues related to ultra-processed foods and the many problems they bring to our table.

THE PROBLEM WITH COMMODITY CROPS

Have you heard of "commodity crops"? This is a foundational topic in the quest to fully understand why our modern food landscape is increasingly barren.

Back in the 1930s, as a part of FDR's New Deal, the farm commodity program was born. Back then, farming was a risky business, and most farmers were poor. Not only that, but they depended on both nature and the market for their survival. When they had a bad year (due to a *poor* growing season) or prices fell (due to overproduction from a really *good* growing season), they risked losing everything. It's as if they couldn't win, so the federal government got involved, and in a big way. Not only did the government control the supply of certain crops (by storing the surplus, therefore taking it off the market), they also controlled the prices farmers received.

This only worked with crops that could be stored long term, such as corn, wheat, and soybeans.[1] Those specific commodity crops became heavily subsidized, and this practice continues to incentivize farmers to grow these crops to the exclusion of nonsubsidized crops, such as other vegetables or fruits. In the year 2020, approximately 40 percent of farmers' income came directly from the federal government, to the tune of about $46.5 billion. Typically, corn production receives the highest subsidies, followed by soybeans, sugar, cotton, and wheat.[2]

This begets another problem: now we have an overabundance of these commodity crops, and we have to do something with them. The good news is that Americans are creative.

Also, the *bad news* is that Americans are creative. What to do with this excess corn and soybeans? Corn syrup! Corn starch! Soy protein! Corn oils! Soybean oils! And let's put those ingredients in *everything*! Yep. These ingredients are in almost every processed food product on the grocery store shelves.[3]

Note: I want to emphasize that I am not demonizing corn here. Fresh organic corn on the cob with butter and salt? Amazing. Corn is a whole food. What big industrial food has done with corn is the problem, not corn grown and eaten as nature intended.

Once the government got involved, suddenly farming and food production was big business.

BIG FOOD = BIG BUSINESS

Did you know that there are a handful of companies that control almost all the food and beverage products you buy in the store? According to an annual report released by *Food Engineering* magazine, the top fifteen food and beverage companies for 2020 were:[4]

Rank	Company	Familiar Brands and/or Products They Sell
		Note: This is not a complete list of all the brands or products from each company but is instead just a sampling of a few of their most recognizable brands and products
1	Nestlé	Gerber, Poland Springs, both Perrier *and* San Pellegrino, Nescafé, Nespresso, Stouffer's, Lean Cuisine, Carnation, Coffeemate, Dreyer's, Häagen-Dazs, and a large number of pet food brands, such as Alpo, Purina, and Fancy Feast
2	Pepsico	Pepsi, Frito-Lay, Gatorade, Tropicana, Quaker Foods, Starbucks, Aquafina, Lipton
3	Anheuser-Busch	Budweiser, Bud Light, Busch, Stella Artois, Landshark, Hoegaarden, Shock Top, Ritas, Hiball energy
		Did you know they also have a "Brewers Collective" that is considered their "craft unit"? So, that "craft beer" you are enjoying may be Anheuser-Busch after all. Examples include Kona Brewing Co., Breckenridge Brewery, Blue Point Brewing Company, and Golden Road Brewing.

4	JBS	They call themselves the "largest animal protein company in the world." Much of the world's beef comes from them (5 Star Beef, Grass Run Farms, Chef's Exclusive), as well as poultry (Pilgrim's) and pork (Swift Premium).
5	Tyson Foods	Tyson, Jimmy Dean, Hillshire Farms, Sara Lee, Nature Raised Farms, Ball Park, Bryan Foods
6	Mars	Ben's Original (rice products), Altoids, M&Ms, Life Savers, Wrigley's, Dove, Combos, Mars, Skittles, Starburst, Twix, and a variety of pet products such as Sheba, Temptations, Cesar, and Eukanuba
7	The Coca-Cola Company	Coca-Cola, Fanta, Dasani, Smartwater, Minute Maid, Simply juice and drinks, Fuze Tea, Honest, Honest Kids, Powerade, Topo Chico, Fairlife
8	Archer Daniels Midland Company (ADM)	ADM doesn't sell food products directly to *you*, but they do sell "food and beverage solutions" to the companies that make many of the foods you buy. They sell things like "bases, seasonings, & powders," "colors," "emulsifiers and stabilizers," "fibers," "flavors, extracts, and distillates," "edible oils," and "sweetening solutions."
9	Cargill	Cargill doesn't feed *you*, they actually feed your *food* by supplying "animal feed and nutrition products."
10	Danone	Dannon yogurt, Oikos, Silk, Activia, International Delight, Evian, Volvic
11	Heineken	Heineken, Tecate, Amstel, Dos Equis, Strongbow, Red Stripe
12	Mondelēz International	Oreo, Nutter Butter, Chips Ahoy!, Newtons, Wheat Thins, Ritz, Nabisco, Honey Maid, Trident, Dentyne, Sour Patch Kids, Halls, Toblerone
13	Kraft Heinz Company	Kraft, Heinz, Ore-Ida, Classico, Velveeta, Capri Sun, Kool-Aid, Jell-O, Philadelphia, Lunchables, Planters, Maxwell House, Grey Poupon, Cracker Barrel cheeses, Crystal Light, Oscar Mayer
14	Smithfield Foods	Smithfield, Eckrich, and Nathan's brands of hot dogs, bacon, pork, hams, lunch meat, sausage, and breakfast sandwiches
15	Unilever	This company sells a wide variety of cleaning/beauty/personal care products in addition to foods: Breyers, Ben & Jerry's, Klondike, Magnum, Hellmann's, Knorr, Lipton, Pure Leaf, Cup-a-Soup, Popsicle

When I am working on projects (such as writing this book), I like to follow my husband around the house and tell him things. (*Do you ever do that? Follow your partner or close friends around chattering excitedly because you're so full of information? Or is it just me?*)

Today when he came home for lunch, I couldn't stop talking about what I had discovered. First of all, I told him about Kona Brewing, because our son Cal went to their brewery in Hawaii when he was there (and Chad loves to wear the T-shirt he sent home to us). I asked him if he was surprised that they were owned by Anheuser-Busch, and he was. Then I mentioned Ben & Jerry's, which I remember visiting when I was in Vermont in 1989, and that they are now owned by the megacorporation Unilever. I always picture them as a small business and not part of a top food conglomerate. It really surprised me how many brands I think of as niche or a small business are actually no longer independently owned companies. Am I saying that Kona Brewing and Ben & Jerry's are bad choices because they were acquired by large companies? Of course not. What I am saying, however, is that brands are not always what we think they are. The two childhood friends Ben and Jerry no longer develop their flavors at a little shop in Vermont, for example. That doesn't stop me from buying their ice cream, but it does affect my perception of the company overall.

I next told him about Archer Daniels Midland, the number-eight-largest food company on the list, and how most of what they sell isn't even identifiable as actual *food*. "Bases, seasonings, and powders"? Yum?

He said, "What's your point?"

I promise I have one, and I am getting to it.

You may also be wondering *what's my point* and what I want you to take away from this list.

Well, we have learned from this list that we buy a lot of beer and other beverages (#2, #3, #7, and #11 on the list sell mostly beverages, and #1, #10, #13, and #15 sell some beverages). Also, we *really* like snack foods and packaged products. And, the number six company, Mars, sells mainly *candy*.

Beer. Beverages. Snack foods. Packaged foods. Candy. That's most of what the world's top fifteen food companies are selling to us, along with meat, food-like ingredients, and pet foods.

I also want you to consider the proliferation of food-like products within the brands identified on this list, and if you have any of the products from these brands in your cabinets, take a moment to look at the ingredients.

Recall that the top five subsidized crops are corn, soy, cotton, sugar, and wheat. (*You may be surprised to learn that cotton isn't just for T-shirts. Did you know that 65 percent of conventional cotton products end up in our food chain either directly or indirectly? It's true: animals are fed cottonseed meal and cotton by-products. I told you that Americans are creative!*)[5]

I would be willing to make a bet with you that almost 100 percent of the foods/beverages from these top fifteen food and beverage companies are made using ingredients derived from at least one of these top five subsidized crops. Even the meat products and pet/livestock foods on this list are impacted; the livestock feed and pet food are full of these commodity crop products and by-products. (Approximately 98 percent of soybean meal is used in livestock feed, for example.)[6]

So, most of the products on the grocery store shelves (and in our pantries) are produced by the big food companies, and they are full of the top commodity crops that we now produce in abundance.

Because these companies want to produce more-more-more of these profitable crops, agricultural scientists have gotten creative in finding ways to increase yield even more. Enter GMOs.

WHAT ARE GMOS?

Modern genetically modified organisms, better known as *GMOs,* have been engineered by changing an organism's genetic code. This is done by adding genetic material from a different organism. Think of it like loading new software onto your computer. In the United States, there are five common crops that have undergone genetic modification: corn, cotton, soy, sugar beets, and canola. According to the FDA,[7]

Up to:

- 92 percent of corn

- 94 percent of cotton

- 94 percent of soybeans

- 99.9 percent of sugar beets, and

- 95 percent of canola

are genetically modified. I also read an estimate that said GMO ingredients are in at least 75 percent of processed foods.[8]

Did you notice that of those top five GMO crops, I've already mentioned four of them (corn, cotton, sugar, and soybeans) as top commodity crops? Well, canola is also a heavily subsidized commodity crop. And again, we have already seen that these ingredients are in almost everything you buy.

So, what's the risk with GMO ingredients? Is there one? Or, as with dihydrogen monoxide, do they just *sound* scary?

First, let's understand why these plants were modified. One reason is so they will become herbicide tolerant. As an example, these crops have been genetically engineered to be "Roundup Ready," meaning that they can withstand what would normally be a lethal dose of the herbicide Roundup, which is a glyphosate-based herbicide. Thanks to the genetic modifications, the entire field can be sprayed with the herbicide, and everything is killed except for the crop itself. This leads to increased yields, which is a positive outcome. The question remains, though: Are these genetically modified crops safe for consumption by humans and/or livestock?

If you ask random people on the street, you'll get a varied response, ranging from: GMOs are perfectly safe, GMOs are killing us and ruining the earth, and there will also be some who prefer the classic Pontiac GTO to the GMO (*sorry, bad joke*). People on the street definitely won't all agree on this topic, which is true for most topics. But what happens if you ask scientists? Shouldn't all scientists agree?

In an open-access article in a European scientific journal, over three hundred independent researchers published a joint statement with the title "No Scientific Consensus on GMO Safety." You can google the title and read the statement in its entirety, and I would encourage you to do so.[9] But in the meantime, I want to summarize what they are (and aren't) saying.

It's important to understand that these scientists *aren't* saying that GMOs are *safe*, but they also *aren't* saying that GMOs are *unsafe*. What they *do* say is summarized in several key points:

1. *There is no consensus on GM food safety*

2. *There are no epidemiological studies investigating potential effects of GM food consumption on human health*

3. *Claims that scientific and governmental bodies endorse GMO safety are exaggerated or inaccurate*

4. *EU research project does not provide reliable evidence of GM food safety*

5. *List of several hundred studies does not show GM food safety*

6. *There is no consensus on the environmental risks of GM crops*

7. *International agreements show widespread recognition of risks posed by GM foods and crops*

In the conclusion, they state that "the totality of scientific research outcomes in the field of GM crop safety is nuanced; complex; often contradictory or inconclusive; confounded by researchers' choices, assumptions, and funding sources; and, in general, has raised more questions than it has currently answered."

Let me put that in easy-speak: "*We just don't know.*"

For me, that's enough to give me pause.

Even if the genetically modified foods *themselves* pose no risk (which we now understand that we don't know for sure, one way or the other), there's a separate issue: we do know that eating these foods adds to our overall toxic load.

The Environmental Working Group commissioned independent labs to conduct three separate rounds of tests on common oat-based breakfast foods, because oats are often sprayed with glyphosate right before harvest.[10] According to EWG, "*Almost all of the products had levels of glyphosate above 160 parts per billion, which is our health benchmark for glyphosate in oats.*" This means that when you eat these oat products, you are ingesting glyphosate. This same result (high levels of glyphosate) has been found in hummus,[11] wheat-based products,[12] as well as in corn and soy products.[13]

So, for me, the safest option is to avoid GMO foods and other foods that are likely to be contaminated with glyphosate. Even if the GMO foods themselves are safe, I don't want to add to my body burden by consuming small amounts of herbicide in every bite I take. And rest assured, if you are purchasing the standard brand-name products in the grocery story, that's exactly what you're getting: an (un)healthy dose of chemicals along with your (possibly unsafe on their own) GMO ingredients. To be on the safe side, look for the Non-GMO Project Verified label on the foods you purchase. I'll explain what that label means in a moment.

Other than looking for the Non-GMO Project Verified label, how else can we avoid foods that have been genetically modified (or coated in herbicides such as glyphosate)? We can choose organic foods and look for the USDA Organic label. That label distinction has stricter guidelines than the Non-GMO Project Verified label.

CHEMICALS, CHEMICALS, EVERYWHERE

Besides issues related to genetic modification, industrial crops (both plants and livestock) are inundated with chemicals at every step along the way, from germination (or gestation) to packaging. They are bathed in chemicals that kill things, such as pesticides, herbicides, and fungicides. They are bombarded by chemicals like fertilizers, antibiotics, and growth hormones that make things grow more quickly (or grow larger). When they are prepared and packaged, they are also combined with chemicals that make them last longer, look better, and taste differently from how they normally would, such as preservatives, artificial colors and flavors, and other additives.

Let's look into each of these categories briefly and see where the concerns might lie.

Chemicals that kill things	Pesticides are linked to a whole host of negative effects. They have been shown to have negative effects on many of our bodies' systems, including the gastrointestinal, neurological, respiratory, and reproductive systems. Many are carcinogenic and/or endocrine disruptors.
Pesticides, herbicides, fungicides	Residues of pesticides are found in many of our foods and beverages, and washing and peeling cannot completely remove these residues. While it's true that most concentrations don't exceed the legislatively determined safe levels, concerns remain that what's "safe" doesn't consider exposure to multiple chemicals at once or the effect of repeated exposure over time.[14]
	One of the most widely used herbicides is glyphosate, commonly known as Roundup, which I already mentioned. It's a suspected carcinogen, and also suspected to negatively affect our microbiomes and work in our bodies as an endocrine disruptor.[15]
	Residues of glyphosate are found in many of our foods, such as sugar, corn, soy, canola, alfalfa, and wheat.[16]

Chemicals that make things grow more quickly or grow larger	The use of synthetic fertilizers leads to environmental pollution, lowers the overall diversity of life within the soil itself, and produces crops that have fewer nutrients.[17,18,19]
Fertilizers, antibiotics, growth hormones	Scientists believe that this widespread use of antibiotics leads to an increase in the number of antibiotic-resistant bacteria.[20]
	Hormonal residues in the meats we eat may have hormonal effects within our own bodies.[21]
Chemicals that make things last longer, look better, and taste differently from what they normally would	Preservatives such as nitrates and nitrites are linked to neurological conditions and certain types of cancers.[22] Other preservatives such as sulphites may contribute to chronic skin and respiratory symptoms.[23]
Preservatives, artificial colors and flavors, other additives	Artificial colors are linked to organ damage, cancer, birth defects, and allergic reactions, and are suspected to have behavioral effects in children, particularly when used in combination.[24]
	Artificial flavors lead to increased palatability (science-speak for "they make the foods taste extra-amazing"), which has been shown to lead in turn to overeating.[25] The long-term safety of artificial flavors is also not well understood.
	Artificial sweeteners may alter the gut microbiome in a way that leads to negative metabolic changes. One review article put it this way: "While the data are controversial, mounting evidence suggests that low calorie sweeteners should not be dismissed as inert in the gut environment."[26] What does that mean? Basically, they are saying, "We just really don't know yet, but it might be a problem."[27,28]
	Artificial sweeteners are all chemically different, and therefore, they act differently in the body, but many are suspected of having specific negative effects. As an example, aspartame has been linked to behavioral and cognitive problems, such as learning difficulties, headaches, seizures, irritability, anxiety, depression, and insomnia. Consuming aspartame can elevate the levels of phenylalanine and aspartic acid in the brain, which can affect the synthesis and release of key neurotransmitters, such as dopamine, norepinephrine, and serotonin.[29]

As you can see, there's a lot going on along the way. All throughout the food production channels, chemicals are being added at every step. Let's examine a few of these issues more closely.

WE ARE WHAT OUR *FOOD* ATE

I'm sure you've heard the saying, "You are what you eat," and it is true. Taking it a step further, you are very much what your *food* ate.

Animals all naturally eat different things. Some animals are grazers, others hunt, and still others are more opportunistic eaters, and so they may be herbivores, carnivores, or omnivores. What's important is that each is perfectly suited for the style of eating that is natural for their bodies.

What happens when we feed animals in a different way from what nature intended, and why would we do it?

Let's learn about the common cow. Cows are ruminants, meaning they are uniquely suited to digest grass and other foliage. They have a compartment within their stomach called the *rumen,* and it's where microbes assist in the digestion of their food, breaking down the fiber in these foods to assist with overall nutrient absorption.

Corn is now the primary feed grain used in the U.S., and we feed it to most cattle as the last stage of the growth process.[30] Cows are moved to a feedlot to be "finished" on corn, and they gain weight quickly when they are fed grains—up to four pounds per day.[31] Unfortunately, because their bodies are not well suited for digesting corn, many of the cows get sick. Eating corn or other grains disrupts the cows' normal digestive processes, which in turn encourages the growth of harmful microorganisms, including dangerous strains of *E. coli.*[32]

Despite this, corn-fed beef is delicious. When cows eat corn instead of grass, they grow larger and have a higher fat content than grass-fed cows, which adds flavor and also makes the meat more tender. What can be wrong with that?

While flavor matters, and I definitely want to always eat food that is delicious, I also want to get the most nutrients possible from my food. Nutritionally, there is a difference between grass-fed and corn-fed beef. Grass-fed beef is lower in overall fat, but higher in beneficial omega-3s, as well as vitamins, minerals, and antioxidants. These antioxidants can help protect *us* after we consume the meats, but they also protect the meat itself, reducing perishability/spoilage before it ever gets to your plate.

Now that we have learned about cows, let's talk about another of our favorite sources of meat: the chicken. What about chickens? Is the way they are fed important? The answer is yes.

Chickens who are considered to be "free-range" are allowed to spend their time poking around in the dirt just as nature intended. They eat bugs, greens, seeds . . . whatever they can scrounge up. When *Mother Earth News* tested the eggs from free-range chickens and compared them to those from typical commercial eggs, they found that the eggs from free-range chickens have lower levels of cholesterol and saturated fat, and higher levels of vitamins A and E, beta-carotene, and polyunsaturated omega-3 fatty acids.[33]

What about the meat? Several studies show that free-range chicken simply tastes better.[34] It also may be more nutritious, containing higher levels of protein, iron, zinc, and collagen.[35,36,37]

There's another issue related to how animals are raised, and that is how certain practices in the agricultural industry are linked to increased antibiotic resistance in humans. Cattle, hogs, and chickens are often raised in factory farm environments. Because of close quarters, the animals tend to get sick more often, and that leads to widespread antibiotic use on these farms.

According to a 2019 FDA report:[38]

More than 6.1 million kilograms of medically important antibiotics were sold to U.S. farmers in 2019, and of those, an estimated:

- 41 percent were intended for use in cattle

- 42 percent in swine

- 10 percent in turkeys, and

- 3 percent in chickens.

> The most frequently sold class of medically important antibiotics in 2019 for use in livestock were:
>
> • tetracyclines, accounting for 67 percent of all sales
>
> • penicillins accounted for 12 percent of sales, and
>
> • macrolides for 8 percent.
>
> The vast majority of antibiotics sold were for use in:
>
> • animal feed (65 percent) and
>
> • water (29 percent).
>
> *Note: "Medically important" means these antibiotics are also used in humans.*

While some sources claim that the antibiotics we give to animals don't affect the quality of the meat, recent evidence says otherwise. Antibiotic residues have been found in the tissues of both beef and chicken, and that means that when we eat that meat, we take in those residues. Based on that, concerns have been raised as to whether this is partly responsible for the increase in antibiotic resistance in humans.[39] Many scientists believe the answer to that question is yes.[40] Overall, consensus is rising that this widespread use of antibiotics does, indeed, lead to an increase in the number of antibiotic-resistant bacteria.[41] The World Health Organization (WHO) recommends that farmers stop using antibiotics preventatively, acknowledging that this practice is linked to the spread of antibiotic resistance globally.[42]

There are also other issues I didn't talk about yet, such as the practice of feeding hormones to animals to make them grow faster or produce more milk. Just as residues of antibiotics remain in the foods, so do hormonal residues. Can these hormonal residues affect our own hormone function? Well, if there is a possibility that the answer is yes, do you really want to risk it? I don't.

In this section, I talked primarily about only two of the animals that are among our main sources of meat (cows and chickens), and

I also focused on just a few of the issues that surround the topic of what our food eats (including the medications and hormones they are given). I could keep going, but I'm sure you get the main point I am making here: there are many reasons why we should choose animal products that are sourced from animals raised eating foods they are biologically suited to eat, without the use of antibiotics or hormones. Not just when it comes to cows and chickens: this applies to pigs and seafood as well, and really to any animal product you can think of.

The good news is that we have a choice. When you choose animal products identified as "organic," they must be raised according to stringent USDA standards.

> Organic livestock must be fed 100 percent organic feed or grass that is grown without pesticides or harmful fertilizers. The use of antibiotics or hormones is strictly forbidden. Livestock must be treated humanely and given access to both the outdoors and uncrowded living conditions.

You can also look for the Certified Humane label on your meat, poultry, egg, and dairy products. Visit certifiedhumane.org to learn more about their independent verification process. They also have a free mobile app that can help you shop.

ARE THERE BENEFITS TO ORGANIC FOODS?

Short answer: yes. For the long answer, keep reading.

Looking for the USDA Organic label is a reliable way to be sure that our foods are GMO-free. According to the USDA,[43]

> *The use of genetic engineering, or genetically modified organisms (GMOs), is prohibited in organic products. This means an organic*

> farmer can't plant GMO seeds, an organic cow can't eat GMO alfalfa
> or corn, and an organic soup producer can't use any GMO ingredi-
> ents. To meet the USDA organic regulations, farmers and processors
> must show they aren't using GMOs and that they are protecting their
> products from contact with prohibited substances, such as GMOs,
> from farm to table.

Based on that information alone, if you have ever wondered whether the USDA Organic label means something, you can be assured that it most certainly does.

Besides helping us avoid GMOs and glyphosate, the USDA certification program also protects us (and the environment) from dangers such as other common herbicides, pesticides, and fertilizers, and even heavy metals such as cadmium and uranium, which can be found in phosphate fertilizers.[44,45]

Why are we concerned about herbicides, pesticides, and fertilizers, not to mention heavy metals? Not only do those chemicals affect us (by adding to our body burdens), they run off into woodlands and streams, where they have an impact on a wide variety of plants, wildlife, and humans. They also accumulate in the soil and kill the microorganisms that live there, which affects the level of nutrients within the soil.

Why do we care about the level of nutrients within the soil? Because that's where the *plants* get their nutrients. When we eat plants grown in nutrient-depleted soil, we are eating nutrient-depleted *food*. One review article from 2010 reports:[46]

> Reviews of multiple studies show that organic varieties do provide
> significantly greater levels of vitamin C, iron, magnesium, and phos-
> phorus than non-organic varieties of the same foods. While being
> higher in these nutrients, they are also significantly lower in nitrates
> and pesticide residues. In addition, with the exception of wheat, oats,
> and wine, organic foods typically provide greater levels of a number of

important antioxidant phytochemicals (anthocyanins, flavonoids, and carotenoids).

This indicates that organic foods contain more nutrients and phytochemicals (that's good for us) and also fewer toxins (that's *also* good for us). More of what we want, and less of what we don't. Even if amounts are small, remember that small amounts add up over time.

Another review article, this one from 2019, found:[47]

Significant positive outcomes were seen in longitudinal studies where increased organic intake was associated with reduced incidence of infertility, birth defects, allergic sensitization, otitis media, pre-eclampsia, metabolic syndrome, high BMI, and non-Hodgkin lymphoma.

That's really exciting news because these studies indicate that the more organic foods we choose, the better our overall health may be over time. Also, they reported that the organic foods had *higher* antioxidant concentrations (particularly polyphenols) and *lower* levels of toxins such as those from synthetic fertilizers and pesticides. This is similar to the earlier review article from 2010.

One study compared participants who ate a diet of less than 10 percent coming from organic foods to those who ate a diet of greater than 50 percent coming from organic foods, and they found that there were significant differences in various nutritional biomarkers between the two groups: the participants who ate more organic foods had higher concentrations of a variety of nutrients that we need for vibrant health.

It all makes sense: when the *soil* has more nutrients, the *plants* have more nutrients, and thus the *animals* who eat those plants have more nutrients, and the *people* who eat those plants (and those animals) will receive more nutrients.[48]

So, as we can see, plants grown in organic soils have higher levels of minerals, more phytochemicals . . . but did you know that they also have a lower *yield*? Think about that for a minute. If we have a finite "pool" of nutrients available to the plants growing in a field, and if we breed those plants to grow bigger and faster (giving us that higher yield we are looking for), then the nutrients are going to have to stretch further. We actually have research showing this.

If you want to read more about it, google to find a very informative 2007 report called "Still No Free Lunch: Nutrient levels in US food supply eroded by pursuit of high yields" by Brian Halweil. This report is available for free and in pdf form through the Organic Center website.[49] Actually, that website (www.organic-center.org) is a veritable gold mine of resources that you can explore.

So, you can see: we are what *we* eat, what the *animals* eat, and what the *plants* eat.

Here's another factor that means a lot to me, as someone who loves good food. Not only is much of our food now less nutritious because of the way it's been grown or bred, it's also less delicious, whether we are talking about tomatoes or chickens. You know what I mean if you have ever had a tomato fresh out of a backyard garden. It's a far cry from a watery and tasteless grocery store tomato.

As we can see, there's a lot of evidence supporting the idea that choosing organic foods whenever possible makes sense. Not only is it good for the environment, but it is also likely to be beneficial to us. And the food simply tastes better.

Now that we know why it matters, how do we know which foods to buy when we are shopping?

WHAT DO OTHER LABEL DESIGNATIONS MEAN?

Product labels can be confusing, as I mentioned in an earlier chapter. We have already learned how manufacturers use *greenwashing* to make cleaning and personal care products seem healthier or safer than they actually are. This also happens on food labels.

Examples of greenwashing on food labels include:

What They Say	What It Actually Means
All-natural	According to the FDA, *natural* means that nothing artificial or synthetic has been included in, or added to, that food. That doesn't mean that pesticides weren't used in the growing process. Also, these foods may still contain residues from antibiotics, growth hormones, and so on.
Hormone-free or no hormones added	The USDA doesn't allow hormones to be used with any pork or poultry, so all of it can technically be sold as "hormone-free." It sounds better, but it isn't. The distinction is more meaningful when you see it on beef or dairy products.
Cage-free or free-range	When a product is labeled *cage-free* or *free-range,* the animals must be allowed to roam and forage freely over an area of open land. However, the wording is loosely regulated. It's possible that producers may have the animals closely confined but still be able to use the label since they technically aren't in cages.
Locally grown	That sounds nice, doesn't it? You imagine that the produce is fresh out of a local farmer's field. Unfortunately, there is no regulated definition or independent verification of this term. *All* produce is local to somewhere, am I right? So you can't be sure that this label means locally grown to *you.*
Grass-fed	This can be misleading because all cows (even those finished on a feedlot) spend part of their lives grazing on grass. So, not all beef identified as grass-fed had a full grass-fed diet, and they may have been finished on grains. Also, a grass-fed cow may not have been raised on a pasture. Grass-finished cows, on the other hand, didn't have grain finishing. 100 percent grass-fed or 100 percent grass-fed and grass-finished is what you're looking for.
Farm fresh	This distinction sounds great, but means nothing at all.

This is just a small sampling of some of the misleading, confusing, or meaningless wording that you might see on a food label. There are many more examples of greenwashing out there. The moral of the story is this: don't trust every label designation you see on food products.

The good news is that certain label designations *can* be trusted. Here are some examples of meaningful product labels:[50]

Label Designation, Image, or Wording	What Does This Designation, Image, or Wording Actually Mean?
Non-GMO Project Verified NON GMO Project VERIFIED	The Non-GMO Project is a nonprofit organization that offers a rigorous third-party product-verification program. This verification process ensures that all products with this label have been verified to avoid GMOs through all aspects of production, from farming to processing. This process is not overseen by the federal government, but it's still a great way to avoid GMOs.[51]
USDA Certified Organic USDA ORGANIC	This labeling system is regulated by federal law, so all products must meet strict guidelines to qualify.[52] As with the Non-GMO Project Verified label, all products certified as USDA Organic are prohibited from using GMOs in all aspects of farming and processing. In addition, regulations: prohibit the use of chemical/synthetic fertilizers and pesticides; prohibit antibiotic and synthetic hormone use for animals; prohibit artificial coloring, flavoring, and preservatives; and require that animals eat only organic feed and pasture.
100% Organic	When a product falls into this category: ALL ingredients must be certified organic; any processing aids must be organic; and the USDA Organic Seal may be used.

Organic	When a product falls into this category:
	all agricultural ingredients must be certified organic;
	nonorganic ingredients are allowed, up to a combined total of 5 percent of nonorganic content; and
	the USDA Organic Seal may be used.
Made from Organic Ingredients	This category refers to products that meet these criteria:
	At least 70 percent of the product must be certified organic
	Any other ingredients aren't required to be organic, but must be produced without certain excluded methods
	USDA Organic Seal *may not* be used on these products
Specific Organic Ingredients	Manufacturers who don't meet the guidelines above (at least 70 percent of the product is certified as organic) are allowed to identify which ingredients are organic, but can't use the USDA Organic Seal or use the word *organic* on the primary product label display panel.

REFLECT AND TAKE ACTION:
WHAT'S IN YOUR KITCHEN?

Use your Clean(ish) Journal (or the worksheets available at ginstephens .com/cleanish) to complete these end-of-chapter prompts and activities.

It's time to take stock of what is in your kitchen pantry and fridge. How many of the packaged foods you have on hand are made with at least one ingredient from the most common GMO commodity crops? How many foods do you have from the big fifteen?

Re-create this chart in your Clean(ish) Journal to record what you find.

Packaged food item in my pantry or fridge	Does it contain ingredients from one of the major GMO crops? How many of those ingredients are in it? *Look for ingredients derived from corn, soy, sugar, canola oil, cotton (such as cottonseed oil)*	Is it a brand produced by one of the big fifteen companies? *Look for: Nestle, PepsiCo, Anheuser-Busch, JBS, Tyson, Mars, Coca-Cola, Danone, Heineken, Mondelēz International, Kraft Heinz, Smithfield, Unilever (Note: a product could include ingredients from Archer Daniels Midland and Cargill without being noted on the label)*

Look back over that list. Are you surprised at what you've found? Write about it in your Clean(ish) Journal.

Now that you have taken the time to read a few of the labels and identify what's in your kitchen pantry and fridge, think about what you can do about it.

Based on what I learned, I can make these easy changes today:

TAKE A BREAK FROM FAKE: PROBLEMS WITH ULTRA-PROCESSED FOODS

In previous chapters, we learned about the rise of chemicals within our foods due to modern farming practices, food packaging, and food additives. Besides just avoiding these chemicals that might be harmful, however, when becoming clean(ish), it's important to make sure that we are eating mostly *food* rather than *not-food*. Even organic highly processed products may fall under the category of *not-food*.

Remember what I said in the last chapter:

Food: Nourishes our bodies, providing all the building blocks we need. Our bodies know what to do with food.

Not-food: An empty source of energy, and it won't sustain a healthy body and its many functions.

It's important for us to make sure that we are choosing mostly food rather than not-food to give our bodies what they need to thrive. In today's modern food environment, we are increasingly **overfed and undernourished.** I didn't make up that phrase, but the first time I heard it, though I can't remember when or where that was, it immediately rang true. Now, it's a phrase you hear more and more people using.

I have already talked about how obesity is rampant these days (which is a constant visual reminder of how we are "overfed" as a society), yet as many as 60 percent of those classified as obese are also considered to be malnourished, meaning that their bodies do not receive the nutrition required to sustain a healthy body and its important functions. One editorial from a 2015 edition of *Critical Care Medicine* proclaimed in its title: "The True Obesity Paradox: Obese and Malnourished?"[1] In a recent study, researchers found that as many as 60 percent of the obese patients studied suffered from malnutrition.

> It is interesting to note that the prevalence of nutrient deficiency is higher in overweight, obese, and morbidly obese compared to normal weight patients, suggesting that obese patients may consume an excess of dietary energy, but they may not meet their entire essential nutrient needs.[2]

One explanation could be that those who are obese lack the ability to absorb nutrients from their foods somehow, and that would mean that the malnutrition is an effect of this inability to absorb the nutrients. This would mean there's an underlying condition related to obesity that causes the malnutrition to occur.

Another explanation, and one I find to be more plausible, is that a malnourished body is an unsatisfied body, and so hunger goes into overdrive. The body is in search of nutrients, yet the food provided isn't meeting those important nutritional needs. The drive to eat—your appetite—is ramped up, and yet nutrition never arrives. In that situation, you can eat and eat and never be fully satisfied because the food doesn't contain the nutrients the body craves. What's even worse is that we feel guilty for overeating, even though we are driven to do so thanks to the increased signals from our bodies to eat-eat-eat. I remember being 210 pounds, obese, and always hungry. The amount of guilt I felt was overwhelming. We are made to feel like something is wrong with us, when really, it's what we are eating that is to blame.

I know that when I was obese, I most definitely made food choices that didn't nourish my body. I am certain that my body was crying out for nutrients.

> The cause of these nutritional deficiencies in overweight and obese individuals is not completely known, but in large part is likely due to higher intake of higher-calorie processed foods associated with poor nutritional quality, particularly in highly developed countries in which there is an abundance of relatively cheap, energy-dense, but nutrient-poor food.[3]

A recent study provides some clues as to what is going on in the body when we eat this type of nutrient-poor diet. In a 2019 study, scientists took twenty adults, admitted them to the Metabolic Clinical Research Unit at the National Institutes of Health, and kept them there for four weeks.[4] They were randomly assigned to either an ultra-processed or unprocessed diet for the first two weeks, and then they followed the alternate diet for the next two weeks. Participants were provided with all their food (three meals per day plus snacks) and instructed to eat as much or as little as they wanted.

If you're wondering what exactly I mean by "ultra-processed diet," I am going to fully explain that in a few pages. Stick with me and I'll get to it in a minute.

The unprocessed and ultra-processed diets that were presented to the participants were matched as closely as possible for total number of calories, sugar, fat, fiber, and macronutrients. What we don't have is information about the micronutrient (i.e., vitamin and mineral) content of each diet. Based on other studies, however, we know that ultra-processed diets are generally significantly lower in nutrients, such as vitamins A, B$_{12}$, C, D, and E, niacin, iron, zinc, potassium, copper, phosphorus, magnesium, selenium, and calcium.[5,6]

Results were fascinating. When eating the ultra-processed diet, participants ate approximately five hundred calories more per day of the foods offered to them than when eating the unprocessed diet. They gained, on average, about two pounds during the two weeks of ultra-processed eating, and body fat went up; they lost an average of about two pounds during the two weeks of unprocessed eating, and body fat went down.

Here's what was even more fascinating. Appetite-*suppressing* hormones went *up* during the weeks eating the unprocessed diet and went *down* during the weeks eating the ultra-processed diet.

So, to summarize: when eating an ultra-processed diet, participants had an increased appetite, they ate a larger quantity of food, and they gained weight. And, on the flip side, when eating an unprocessed diet, their appetites decreased naturally, they ate less food, and they lost weight.

Why? If we go back to the nutrient-hypothesis and the idea that our bodies respond to lack of nourishment by increasing our drive to eat so that we will take in the nutrients our bodies desperately need, we can see that what happened in this study fits the hypothesis nicely. The ultra-processed diet didn't provide sufficient nutrients, so the participants had an increased appetite, and they consumed more food, leading to weight gain.

Our bodies are very skilled at seeking just the right nutrients that we need when we are eating high-quality, unprocessed foods. In a very interesting (and old) study that was published in 1939, a pediatrician named Dr. Clara Davis did an experiment with fifteen children.[7] She took custody of them when they were babies, between the ages of six and eleven months, and kept them in her care for anywhere between six months and four and a half years. She called it the "self-selection of diet experiment," and the goal was to find out what would happen if these children were allowed to eat entirely according to their own preferences with no interference from adults.

She ensured that the foods offered made up an overall healthy diet, providing all vitamins, minerals, and nutrients required for health. To do that, she came up with a list of thirty-four different food items. Not all the foods she selected would be found in the modern pantry, that's for sure.

This is the list, as written in the 1939 publication. I'm not even sure what "sour (lactic) milk" is, are you?

Water	Sweet milk	Sour (lactic) milk	Sea salt	Apples
Bananas	Orange juice	Fresh pineapple	Peaches	Tomatoes
Beets	Carrots	Peas	Turnips	Cauliflower
Cabbage	Spinach	Potatoes	Lettuce	Oatmeal
Wheat	Cornmeal	Barley	Ry-Krisp	Beef
Lamb	Bone marrow	Chicken	Sweetbreads	Brains
Liver	Kidneys	Fish (haddock)		

I think back to 1999, when my older son, Cal, was a toddler. I remember joking that he only ate things that were beige (chicken nuggets, vanilla pudding, crackers, applesauce, yogurt, french fries, etc.). Looking at this list, I can't find a lot of things that I had on hand to feed him. Brains? Liver? Kidneys? Sweetbreads, which is a lovely sounding name for the thymus or pancreas? Um, no, no, no, and lordy, no. I definitely wasn't offering those tidbits to my picky toddler.

In Dr. Davis's study, the babies were offered a variety of foods at each meal: both kinds of milk, two kinds of cereals, some sort of animal protein, and either fruits or vegetables. Each item (even the salt) was served in a separate dish, and portions were weighed and measured before and after the meal to determine the portions consumed. Nurses assisted with the feedings but were not allowed to comment on the infants' choices or steer them toward any particular foods.

Results were interesting. In the narrative section of her publication, she discusses one particular child who came into their care suffering from rickets, which is caused by a severe vitamin D deficiency.

They offered cod liver oil on his feeding tray, and he helped himself over a period of time until his rickets were completely healed. Then he never selected it again.

Over time, this is what is most striking about this experiment: the children constructed unique and extremely personal diets that varied from meal to meal.

Dr. Davis says:

> Within a reasonable time the nutrition of all, checked as it was at regular and frequent intervals by physical examinations, urine analyses, blood counts, hemoglobin estimations and roentgenograms of bones, came up to the standard of optimal so far as could be discovered by examinations.

Overall, the children's feeding behavior illustrates that when offered a variety of nutritious foods, they were mini master nutritionists. Their bodies directed them to precisely the right mixture of nutrients that they needed to grow and thrive. Those (like the boy with rickets) that began with nutritional deficiencies selected the foods their bodies needed to correct those deficiencies.

The kids ate their foods until they were satisfied, and then they stopped. None of them overate (or underate). Not one of them became a "picky eater" who only ate beige foods like my son.

When left to their own devices, these kids instinctively *knew* what to eat. They were offered a wide variety of real foods, full of nutrients and building blocks for healthy bodies, and their instinct guided them to select a well-balanced diet that was right for their needs.

What do we learn from this experiment? These kids were able to construct a healthy diet by following their bodies' instincts. So can we. But when we *don't* eat foods that provide sufficient nutrients, we are more likely to overeat, searching for nutrients that never arrive.

Besides the search for nutrients, there are other reasons why we overeat ultra-processed foods. Eating is supposed to be pleasurable, but the ultra-processed foods we buy are actually *too* pleasurable. They are considered to be "hyper-palatable," and the characteristics that make them so delicious drive us to overeat when we consume them.[8] That's by design.

CAN FOOD HAVE TOO *MUCH* FLAVOR?

According to Mark Schatzker, author of *The Dorito Effect*, the answer to that question is yes.

Instead of appreciating the subtleties and nuances of the flavors found in real foods, scientists have created chemical versions of these flavors in labs, and these chemicals are added to almost all the processed foods in modern grocery stores.

Today, there are more than 2,200 different varieties of man-made flavors. These flavors are *like* nature's flavors, only turbo-charged. The more flavors industry adds, the more we want to eat the foods containing these flavors . . . and the more we crave the artificial hits of super-flavor rather than the subtler flavors found in real foods.

Not to mention, there's one more problem. The increased yields we have bred into our crops didn't simply dilute the nutrients found within them. They also diluted the *flavors*. Recall that watery tomato from the grocery store, which is a far cry from a freshly grown organic tomato picked from your backyard garden. They taste nothing alike.

Schatzker puts it this way:[9]

The food problem is a flavor problem. For half a century, we've been making the stuff people should eat—fruits, vegetables, whole grains, unprocessed meats—incrementally less delicious. Meanwhile, we've been making the food people shouldn't eat—chips, fast food, soft drinks, crackers—taste ever more exciting. The result is exactly what you'd expect.

It all boils down to what I will call the Rules of Flavor:

1. Humans are flavor-seeking animals. The pleasure provided by food, which we experience as flavor, is so powerful that only the most strong-willed among us can resist it.

2. In nature, there is an intimate connection between flavor and nutrition.

3. Synthetic flavor technology not only breaks that connection, it also confounds it.

We are hardwired to seek pleasure from eating, and these hyper-palatable foods are expertly designed, with manufacturer's manipulating these flavors in foods to get us to eat more and more. As they told us in the commercial, "You can't eat just one!"

Never mind the idea that these flavors are linked to overeating—are these flavors *safe*? Maybe. Maybe not.

Just as the word *fragrance* can be used to hide all sorts of unknown chemicals, the word *flavor* on a food label could really be almost anything. Artificial flavor ingredients may be any of approximately two thousand chemicals regulated by the Flavor and Extract Manufacturers Association of the United States. What are those two thousand chemicals, and what effects do they have on our bodies? Your guess is as good as mine. *Natural flavor* doesn't mean it's safer, by the way.

These foods that are hyper-palatable and full of flavors that make us eat more-more-more are examples of ultra-processed foods. Let's learn how to identify these not-foods.

WHAT ARE ULTRA-PROCESSED FOODS?
USING THE NOVA FOOD CLASSIFICATION SYSTEM

Sometimes when people talk about food, they may put it into two main categories: when we do that, everything we eat is either a "whole food" or a "processed food."

Whole foods are usually thought of as foods that have not been processed, refined, or had ingredients added to them. Let's say you go out to the field and pick an ear of corn. That's a whole food.

"Processed," however, gets a lot trickier to define. Technically, "processed food" includes any food that has been cooked, canned, frozen, packaged, preserved, or prepared. So, any time we cook, bake, or do something with a whole food, we're processing food.

That ear of corn straight out of the field? It's a whole food. The minute I shuck it, cook it, slice it off the cob . . . technically, it's been processed. But nothing I did to it made it less nutritious or "worse" for me. I wouldn't have been able to eat it in the state it came in fresh from the field. I *needed* to process it to make it edible.

Milk is another example of a whole food. If I went out and milked a cow, the milk is a whole food. But if I churn it into butter, or make cheese, it's now been processed.

Wheat harvested from the field is another whole food, but we can't eat it in its raw form. We have to process it before we can consume it.

So, whole foods are actually tricky to define, aren't they? If we used the definition of whole foods as foods that haven't been processed, refined, or had ingredients added to them, what are we supposed to eat? I don't want to eat unshucked raw corn or raw wheat kernels.

There tends to be a train of thought that sounds very simple:

Whole foods: GOOD.   **Processed foods: BAD.**

Unfortunately, though, we now see that is *way too simple*. No, it's not as simple as thinking of food as either one or the other. Instead, think of foods as falling somewhere along a continuum.

The continuum has whole foods on one end, and ultra-processed foods on the other.

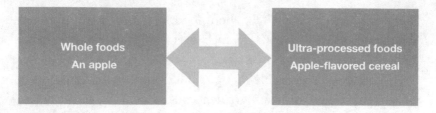

Whole foods
An apple

Ultra-processed foods
Apple-flavored cereal

In between the apple (a whole food) and apple-flavored cereal (an ultra-processed food), there are a wide variety of apple-foods you might prepare at home or purchase from the store.

Homemade applesauce is closer to the whole foods side of the continuum, whereas a packaged applesauce made with added sweeteners would be closer to the ultra-processed foods side. The strawberry-flavored applesauce I used to buy my kids? It did have apples, but also included high fructose corn syrup, natural flavors, and Red 40 to make it so cheerfully *red*. That's an ultra-processed food.

What are ultra-processed foods by definition? According to the UN's Global Panel on Agriculture and Food Systems for Nutrition:[10]

The term "ultra-processed" was coined to refer to industrial formulations manufactured from substances derived from foods or synthesized from other organic sources. They typically contain little or no whole foods, are ready-to-consume or heat up, and are fatty, salty, or sugary and depleted in dietary fibre, protein, various micronutrients and other bioactive compounds. Examples include: sweet, fatty, or salty packaged snack products, ice cream, sugar-sweetened beverages, chocolates, confectionery, French fries, burgers and hot dogs, and poultry and fish nuggets.

Even though that may be the official definition, I am going to take issue with two of the foods they listed as ultra-processed: "French fries" and "burgers." Yes, fries and burgers can be ultra-processed foods if you get them from a typical fast-food establishment, but they can also be prepared in a way that moves them closer to the whole foods side of the continuum.

If I slice up a raw potato, toss it in olive oil, and bake it in the oven, I'll have french fries that aren't ultra-processed. The same is true for a burger; if I take some grass-fed and grass-finished ground beef and make it into a patty, cook it, and then put it on a homemade whole wheat bun with high-quality cheese, lettuce, and tomatoes, it's nothing like a fast-food burger. Quality matters.

So, how do we know where foods fall along this continuum? Fortunately, leading voices in the nutrition field developed something called the NOVA food classification system to help us figure this complicated question out.[11,12]

	Group 1 UNPRO-CESSED OR MINIMALLY PROCESSED FOODS	Group 2 PROCESSED CULINARY INGREDI-ENTS	Group 3 PROCESSED FOODS	Group 4 ULTRA-PROCESSED FOODS
What are they?	These foods are fresh foods that come from plants or animals with little processing.	These are ingredients that we use in our cooking.	These are foods made from a combination of foods from group 1 and group 2.	These are products made with little to no fresh foods, with a large quantity of refined and processed additives.
Description	• Edible parts of plants and fungi/algae (seeds, fruits, leaves, stems, roots).	• Substances obtained from group 1 foods or from nature through processes such as pressing, refining, grinding, milling, or drying.	• Created by adding sugar, oil, salt, or other group 2 ingredients to group 1 foods.	• Formulations made either mostly or entirely from substances derived from foods.

• Edible parts of animals (muscle, organ meat, eggs, milk). • Inedible or unwanted parts have been removed. • May have been crushed or dried for preservation, storage, or to make them safe or edible.	• These items are rarely consumed alone and are generally meant to be combined with foods from group 1. • Some of these items may be combinations of 2 group items or may contain additives used as preservatives.	• Processed through preservation, cooking, and/or fermentation. • Most of these foods have two or three ingredients, including recognizable foods from group 1. • These foods may contain additives used as preservatives.	• Usually include chemical additives. • Contain very little actual food. • Usually have preservatives, stabilizers, dyes, artificial flavors, etc.
Examples			
All fruits and vegetables, milk, eggs, meats, fish, grains, legumes, nuts, rice.	Salt, sugar, molasses, honey, syrup, vegetable oils, butter, lard.	Canned vegetables, fruits, or legumes, salted or sugared nuts, cheese, fresh bread, canned fish, alcoholic drinks such as beer, cider, or wine.	Carbonated drinks, most packaged beverages, snacks, ice cream, candy, packaged breads, margarines and spreads, breakfast cereals, bars, meat products, most packaged and canned foods, frozen meals.

When I examine the homemade fries and burger meal I described before, using the criteria from the chart, it seems to me that it's clearly in the "processed foods" category rather than the "ultra-processed" category.

So, are processed foods clean(ish)? Yes. Can you eat ultra-processed foods and still be clean(ish)? Also a yes. We aren't aiming for an unattainable level of perfection with every bite we eat. That being said, there are many reasons why you want to limit or avoid ultra-processed foods and stick to foods from groups 1–3 most of the time.

ULTRA-PROCESSED FOODS ARE LINKED
TO MANY POOR HEALTH OUTCOMES

Now that scientists have begun to examine the effects of ultra-processed diets, more and more research is coming out about how our health is being affected. Do you want to hear a shocking statistic? In one study, they reported that ultra-processed foods "account for slightly more than half of US adults' daily total calories."[13] Wow. The average adult in the U.S. is consuming more ultra-processed foods than *any other foods*.

When we begin to understand how this is affecting our health, we should become alarmed.

Here is a sampling of recent research:

Year	Title of Study	What They Found
2018	Consumption of ultra-processed foods and cancer risk: Results from NutriNet-Santé prospective cohort[14]	They found that there was an association between ultra-processed food intake and overall risk of cancer in general, as well as an overall risk of breast, prostate, and colorectal cancer. They report that a 10 percent increase in the proportion of ultra-processed foods within the participants' diets was linked to an increase they call significant—greater than 10 percent *more* risk of developing cancer.
2019	Dietary share of ultra-processed foods and metabolic syndrome in the US adult population[15]	They found that participants that consumed the highest amount of ultra-processed foods (those who ate more than 70 percent ultra-processed foods) had a 28 percent higher prevalence of metabolic syndrome than participants who ate fewer than 40 percent of calories from ultra-processed foods.
2020	Ultra-processed foods and health outcomes: a narrative review[16]	This was a review paper, and the authors examined all the evidence to make some general statements about how ultra-processed foods may affect our health. What they found was so important that I am going to include a direct quote: "*Of 43 studies reviewed, 37 found dietary UPF [ultra-processed food] exposure associated with at least one adverse health outcome. Among adults, these included overweight, obesity and cardio-metabolic risks; cancer, type-2 diabetes and cardiovascular diseases; irritable bowel syndrome, depression and frailty conditions; and all-cause mortality. Among children and adolescents, these included cardio-metabolic risks and asthma.*"

		No study reported an association between UPF [ultra-processed food] and beneficial health outcomes." Wow. Read that again if you need to, especially that last sentence.
2020	Ultra-processed food consumption and the risk of short telomeres in an elderly population of the Seguimiento Universidad de Navarra (SUN) Project[17]	What are telomeres? They are an essential part of human cells that affect how our cells age, and therefore affect how *we* age.[18] Shorter telomeres = an *increased* incidence of diseases and *decreased* longevity. In the study, they found that participants with the highest consumption of ultra-processed foods had almost twice the odds of having short telomeres when compared to participants with the lowest consumption of ultra-processed foods.
2021	Association between ultra-processed food intake and cardio-vascular health in US adults: a cross-sectional analysis of the NHANES 2011–2016[19]	They found that as percentage of calories from ultra-processed foods went *up,* overall cardiovascular health went *down,* and risk factors went *up.*

If you want to keep up on the latest research for yourself, you can go to PubMed online and use the search term *ultra-processed* to see all the studies in their entirety, including new ones that come out. Expect to see more and more of them over time.

What are some of the very worst ingredients found in ultra-processed foods that you won't find in foods from the other categories? I've made a list for you here:

Toxic oils and highly pro-cessed fats	If you listen to *The Intermittent Fasting Podcast* with cohost Melanie Avalon, you have probably heard her talk about the dangers of modern industrial seed oils, such as soybean, canola, sunflower, safflower, cottonseed, and corn oils (*there are some of those commodity crops again!*). Because I take a clean(ish) approach, I ignored what she was saying about these oils for a long time. I was clean(ish) enough already, thank you very much. Unfortunately for me (and for all of us), I have realized she is right.[20]

In traditional diets, most of the fat they consume is either saturated or mono-unsaturated and comes from traditional sources: butter, lard, coconut oil, or olive oil. Today, however, most of the fats in our diet are polyunsaturated: vegetable oils derived from soy, corn, safflower, and canola. Our modern diets may contain as much as 30 percent of our calories from polyunsaturated oils, whereas in traditional diets (where polyunsaturated fats are only found naturally in small amounts from real food sources), the percentage is more like 4 percent. We have been told these oils are "heart healthy." But are they?

No. At least not at the levels we're taking them in these days.

We need some PUFAs in our diets, as they have important functions in our bodies. For example, omega-3 is generally beneficial. Two types of omega-3s—EPA and DHA—help reduce inflammation and may help lower the risk of certain chronic health conditions. Omega-6 in high levels, however, is not beneficial. Even though *low* levels of omega-6 are helpful for brain function, metabolism, growth, and overall development, high levels of omega-6 PU-FAs are linked to chronic inflammatory diseases, such as nonalcoholic fatty liver disease (NAFLD), cardiovascular disease, obesity, inflammatory bowel disease (IBD), rheumatoid arthritis, and Alzheimer's disease (AD).[21]

Chronic inflammatory disorders are increasing in today's society, and many in the health and wellness community are sounding that alarm that one cause of increased inflammation is the PUFAs that are in almost all processed foods. As an example, inflammatory bowel disease (IBD) is on the rise, and studies show that an increase in dietary PUFAs leads to an increased risk of IBD.[22] In general, many believe that eliminating high-PUFA seed oils may be one of the best things you can do to promote good health. As the use of vegetable seed oils (canola, corn, cottonseed, soy, sunflower, safflower, and grapeseed) have gone up, health has gone down. Can we say that one directly causes the other? Not necessarily, but it's definitely a red flag in general.

One issue is that these seed oils are chemically unstable, and therefore, they oxidize easily, especially when exposed to heat—which is what we do when we cook with them: we expose them to heat. The harmful by-products of this process promote aging and also lead to the development of chronic diseases, such as high blood pressure, heart disease, and both intestinal and liver damage.[23] Turns out, this is just another example of what happens when we take foods from their natural state and overly refine them. Natural foods with small amounts of omega-6: beneficial. Ultra-processed foods with overly concentrated forms of omega-6: harmful.

Take a look at the ultra-processed foods you have in your cabinets, and I bet you'll find that most of them are full of these types of ultra-processed oils.

| MSG | Monosodium glutamate (MSG) is used as a flavor enhancer, and it is common in many packaged foods. MSG has been shown in studies to affect the regulation of appetite and satiety.[24] |
| | Researchers believe it plays a role in a variety of neurodegenerative brain diseases, such as Alzheimer's, Parkinson's, and Huntington's disease. It stimulates appetite and leads to overeating. It has also been linked to headaches, nausea, mood swings, insomnia, seizures, and digestive issues. |

Glutamate itself is naturally occurring in foods, and it's essential for a healthy brain. But when we have excess glutamate, it overstimulates brain cells, even overstimulating them to the point of death.

MSG is often hidden in the product label under various names, such as glutamic acid, yeast extract, autolyzed yeast, calcium caseinate, soy protein isolate/concentrate, hydrolyzed protein, plant protein extract, whey protein/concentrate/isolate, sodium caseinate, textured protein, malt extract, autolyzed plant protein, hydrolyzed oat flour, textured protein, sodium caseinate, and calcium caseinate. It may also be hiding under natural-sounding names, such as *natural flavors, bouillon, broth,* or *stock.*

Highly refined grains	Refined grains have been stripped of their essential nutrients. They are missing vitamins, minerals, fiber, and other important factors. They are so devoid of nutrients that manufacturers have to *add certain vitamins back in.* "Enriched." How dumb is this? We take the good stuff out, processing it away, and then add synthetic vitamins to make up for it.[25] Enrichment doesn't replace all of that very good stuff that processors took out, however. Each whole wheat kernel contains bran (the outer skin, containing important antioxidants, B vitamins, and fiber), the germ (which is the plant's embryo, containing B vitamins, protein, minerals, and fats), and the endosperm (the new plant's food supply, containing carbohydrates, proteins, and a few vitamins and minerals). When the whole wheat is refined, the bran and germ are both removed, along with 25 percent of the grain's protein and at least seventeen key nutrients. Enriching can't make up for all of that missing good stuff.[26]
Sugar	Is sugar a healthy food? I think we can all agree that the answer is no. Is an increased consumption of sugar linked to negative health outcomes in general? No question. Can it be addictive for some people? Absolutely. Where does sugar fit into *your* life? That is something for you to figure out for yourself as you become clean(ish). Is sugar a toxin? Not in the sense of the word, no—it's not literally poison, though you will read opinions that it *should be* considered a toxin due to the overall effects it has on our bodies, especially as consumption increases. For now, though, we need to answer this question: Is sugar prevalent in ultra-processed foods? Yes. The amount of added sugars in ultra-processed foods (a whopping 21.1 percent of calories) is eight times higher than the amount found in processed foods (2.4 percent of calories) and five times higher than found in the unprocessed/minimally processed foods and processed culinary ingredients categories when they are grouped together (3.7 percent of calories).[27] So, when we limit our intake of ultra-processed foods, we naturally limit our intake of sugar, without even trying.

High fructose corn syrup	In the last chapter, we learned about commodity crops, and corn is a big one. Much of the billions of bushels of corn grown in the U.S. is turned into corn syrup. It's cheap. It's easy to work with. And it's everywhere.
	Corn syrup is thought to act as an obesogen by affecting appetite control, metabolic function, insulin sensitivity, and signaling between our adipose tissue and the hypothalamus.[28] It also seems to be a major contributor to the development of fatty liver disease. Long-term use is associated with obesity and general metabolic risk.[29]
Artificial sweeteners	Artificial sweeteners have been controversial as long as I can remember. I remember back in my childhood when suddenly saccharin was under the microscope, and a warning label was added to all foods containing saccharin. Prior to that, my grandmother always added a saccharin tablet to her unsweetened tea, but she made the switch to first the little blue envelopes and later to the yellow ones. Her sweetener of choice may have gone from pink to blue to yellow packets over the years, but she still stuck to artificial sweeteners, believing them to be "better" for her. I remember going with her to the hair salon as a child and then a teen. In early years, she would drink Tab. Then she switched to Diet Coke. There was always a diet soda of one kind or another next to her during the day, and her artificially sweetened tea was always on the table at lunch and dinner. As an adult, she developed Parkinson's disease and suffered from dementia at the time of her death in 2007 at the age of eighty-one. Are the two related? I don't know. The answer could be yes.
	Overall, the evidence against artificial sweeteners indicates that use may contribute to metabolic syndrome and the obesity epidemic. These sweeteners tend to lead to negative microbiome changes, decreased satiety, blood glucose control, and are generally associated with *increased* caloric consumption and weight gain rather than an overall decrease in consumption.[30,31]
	But what about neurological health? Could artificial sweeteners have caused my grandmother's health conditions? Of course, we will never know for certain.
	In a 2017 study called "Neurophysiological symptoms and aspartame: What is the connection?" researchers tell us: "*Possible neurophysiological symptoms include learning problems, headache, seizure, migraines, irritable moods, anxiety, depression, and insomnia. The consumption of aspartame, unlike dietary protein, can elevate the levels of phenylalanine and aspartic acid in the brain. These compounds can inhibit the synthesis and release of neurotransmitters, dopamine, norepinephrine, and serotonin, which are known regulators of neurophysiological activity.*" None of that sounds good to me, how about you?[32]
	In mice, there does seem to be a link between aspartame consumption and increased degeneration of the type that is related to Parkinson's disease.[33]

| Other food additives | There are so many funky food additives out there (emulsifiers, preservatives, artificial flavors, and the like) that it would take a great deal of time to discuss each one individually. In general, however, we can say this: ultra-processed foods have more of these types of additives than any other category of foods. The more ultra-processed foods we eat, the more additives we consume. |
| | One concern is the way these additives influence the health of our gut microbiomes. Evidence is accumulating that tells us that an increased consumption of food additives in general promotes damaging inflammatory responses within our bodies, which in turn damages our tissues and also disrupts gut health.[34] |

Overall, this evidence paints a pretty clear picture. We know that the more ultra-processed foods we consume, the more of these types of potentially harmful ingredients we ingest. While it's difficult to say, *"This is the one! This is the one thing you need to avoid to be healthy!"* I think we *can* say that it's really an accumulation of these various chemical concoctions that add up over time and prove to be detrimental in the long run.

You can experiment and see how you feel when you choose fewer ultra-processed foods. Here's an example from my personal life. Recently, I joined an online marketplace that sells a wider variety of organic and natural foods than my local stores. I was excited to order a number of ultra-processed snacks. Remember: I'm clean(*ish*). Emphasis on the -*ish*. I still eat ultra-processed foods, and I was choosing organic options.

Because all these options were either organic or Non-GMO verified, I enjoyed them with less moderation than usual, and as the days went on, my face got puffier and puffier. It also showed up on my scale. Even though I haven't weighed myself using a traditional scale for years, I have a scale that doesn't show your actual weight. Instead, it gives you a daily color to indicate what your overall weight trend is doing. As time went on, my weight-trend color turned to gray (indicating that my weight was trending upward). My scale also gives you an "age" based on your body composition, and my age went up from day-to-day as I increased my snacking on those tasty treats. I could absolutely tell that those organic and Non-GMO Verified ultra-processed foods were increasing inflammation in my body, which showed up as weight gain on the scale. So, I cut back. Did I throw them in the trash? No. I will still eat them, just not with the intensity that I was eating them over that period of time. I'm clean(ish), and these ultra-processed foods are still on my menu, just not as something I need to eat every day. Even though they were organic, they were still ultra-processed. Here is the ingredients list from one of them:

> Black Beans, Navy Beans, Brown Rice, Safflower or Sunflower Oil, Seasoning Blend (Tapioca Maltodextrin, Salt, Jalapeno Pepper, Tomato Powder, Sugar, Onion Powder, Yeast Extract, Dehydrated Red and Green Bell Pepper, Natural Flavors, Paprika, Extractives of Annatto, Lactic Acid, Grill Flavor from Sunflower Oil)

Can you even tell what that product was, based on those ingredients? It was a tortilla chip made from beans. They were delicious. And they have all the can't-eat-just-one flavor characteristics of most ultra-processed foods, including some of the code words for MSG (*yeast extract, natural flavors*) and also at least one of the highly refined oils I prefer to avoid.

This makes me think of something else, and it's how confused we tend to be as a society about food. So often, I'll hear someone say something like, "I need to eat fewer carbs. Carbs don't work well for me." I always ask them to clarify. They say something like: "You know, cookies, pizza, chips, fries. Carbs."

Let's consider each of those foods. Are they "carbs"? Actually, they *have* carbs, but they are really a combination of carbs and fat (among other things) all mixed together in a super-palatable and ultra-processed package. They are both high carb *and* high fat and also all have a very low nutrient density. I have a hunch that many people who think "carbs don't work well for me" or "I have to eat low carb to lose weight" are really people who have realized that ultra-processed foods don't work well for their bodies. News flash: they don't work well for *any* of our bodies. Ultra-processed foods are solidly in the not-food category. So, maybe it's not the "carbs" that are the problem. There's a huge difference between an apple and a Cheeto.

Side note: I want to clarify here that I am not saying that all bodies do well with the same ratio of carbohydrates within our diets. I am a big believer in bio-individuality, and we all have differences when it comes to what foods work for us. As an example of this, a recent study illustrates that about 50 percent of us have a gene variant that helps our bodies regulate blood glucose, which means we are physically adapted to a higher carb intake.[35] On the flip side, that would mean that the other 50 percent of us do not have that gene variant, and so a higher-carb diet might not work as well. The theory is that our ancestors developed this gene variant in response to the agricultural revolution.

WHAT ABOUT VITAMINS AND OTHER SUPPLEMENTS? ARE THEY HEALTHY? DO WE *NEED* THEM?

Supplements have such a healthy sheen, don't they? But have you ever thought that they may just be the ultimate example of ultra-processed foods?

When scientists first began isolating the chemicals found within foods, they discovered a wide variety of phytochemicals within them. There are thousands of these types of chemicals within the fruits and vegetables we eat. With great excitement, companies began producing individual supplements based on these isolated phytochemicals.

Our bodies are not designed to take in nutrients in this way. Remember that thousands of nutrients are found in foods, and we don't even know what they all *are*. Does it make sense that we can isolate the important chemicals in a lab, produce them synthetically in a factory, and then expect them to provide the same benefits as the thousands of phytochemicals in our foods? The answer is no. According to one science researcher: "History indicates that single-nutrient approaches often fail and on occasion are harmful."[36] One example is what happened with the trials of beta-carotene, which were expected to reduce lung cancer risk but did not yield expected results.[37]

> The observation that fruits and vegetables may reduce lung cancer risk led to implementation of 2 large, randomized clinical trials in which high doses of ß-carotene were used: the Beta-Carotene And Retinol Efficacy Trial (CARET) in the United States and the Alpha-Tocopherol, Beta-Carotene Cancer Prevention (ATBC) trial in Finland. The CARET intervention tested the efficacy of 30 mg of ß-carotene plus 25,000 IU of retinyl palmitate daily in male and female heavy smokers and in men exposed to asbestos. The ATBC trial tested 20 mg of ß-carotene plus 50 IU of vitamin E daily in male heavy smokers. Both trials found that ß-carotene, alone or in combination with vitamin E or retinyl palmitate, increased the incidence of lung cancers by 36% (in CARET) and 16% (in the ATBC trial) compared with placebo.

According to these researchers, the beta-carotene supplementation *increased* the incidence of lung cancers by 16–36 percent rather than *decreasing* it. Ouch.

These researchers went on to say:

> These results also led to concern about the millions of Americans using supplements, because the doses of ß-carotene and other carotenoids in dietary supplements are much higher than would typically be acquired from diet.

What they are saying is this: when we take supplements, we take in much more of a compound than we would normally consume by eating actual food sources of these compounds, and the effects of a dose this large may be harmful rather than good for us. Have you ever heard the saying "The dose makes the poison"? This is an example of that.

One other elephant in the room (and it's a BIG one) is that dietary supplements are poorly regulated by the FDA. This means that most of the supplements you can find on the shelf (or through your favorite online retailers) have not been evaluated for either safety *or* whether they actually contain what the label *claims* is in the bottle. One recent governmental report found that when three memory supplement products were tested in a lab, all of which were marketed as ginkgo biloba supplements, they weren't as expected. According to the analysis:[38]

> We found that two of the three memory supplement products tested either did not contain their stated ingredients or did not contain the ingredient quantity stated on the label. The *Ginkgo biloba* single-ingredient product we had tested was determined by laboratory scientists to contain no *Ginkgo biloba,* and was found to be adulterated with one or more substitute ingredients.

So, one of the three samples tested had *no ginkgo biloba at all.* Instead, it had "substitute ingredients." What are these substitute ingredients? Are they good for us or dangerous? Who knows. That certainly gives me pause when it comes to trusting supplement labels.

It gets worse than that. According to an article published by Harvard Medical School:[39]

> Another, much larger study, finds that the problem of tainted supplements—and lack of oversight—is widespread. Researchers analyzed warnings issued by the US Food and Drug Administration (FDA) between 2007 and 2016. These included 776 dietary supplements that contained contaminants, including

- a prescription drug, sildenafil (Viagra), in supplements sold for sexual enhancement.

- sibutramine (Meridia), found in weight-loss supplements. This drug was approved in 1997 for weight loss but was taken off the market in 2010 when studies linked it to heart attacks and stroke.

- steroids or drugs with steroid effects in supplements marketed as muscle builders.

About 20% of the contaminated supplements contained more than one unapproved ingredient. In more recent analyses, more than one-third of the contaminated supplements were found by sampling products ordered online, and another third arrived by international mail delivery.

Unfortunately, the FDA announced voluntary recalls for less than half of these tainted supplements.

As we can see, they found that some of the tested supplements were contaminated with actual prescription drugs such as Viagra, or even dangerous drugs such as Meridia, which had been taken off the market due to serious side effects.

It is shocking to see that approximately 20 percent of those contaminated supplements tested had *more than one unapproved ingredient.*

In summary, when it comes to supplements, even if the capsules or pills *do* contain what they claim to contain, those supplements may be harmful rather than helpful, as in the case of beta-carotene. Even worse, they might contain dangerous substances such as prescription drugs you aren't counting on. What happens when a medication you are taking by prescription has an interaction with a medication you are *accidentally* taking because it is hidden illegally in your supplements?

Personally, I'll just stick with real food whenever I can. I know that whatever is in my organic tomato, it's supposed to be there, with no ingredient label required.

NOW WHAT?

Eating clean(ish) is about a lot more than what food-like products we want to *avoid*. It's also very much about what we need to put *into* our bodies to properly fuel us throughout the day and make sure we are taking in essential nutrients. We very much are what we eat, and so quality building blocks matter.

And here's something else that I've heard from people over and over again:

> The more real food you eat, the better real food tastes and the worse artificial food tastes.

That's what we will talk about in the next chapter: the power of *real food*.

REFLECT AND TAKE ACTION: FINDING FOOD

Use your Clean(ish) Journal (or the worksheets available at ginstephens .com/cleanish) to complete these end-of-chapter prompts and activities.

- What do the words *overfed* and *undernourished* mean to you? Do you suspect you may be either *overfed* or *undernourished*? Explain.

Take stock of what is in your pantry and fridge. How much of it is actually food versus not-food?

Recall the continuum that has whole foods on one end and ultra-processed foods on the other.

Whole foods	Ultra-processed foods
An apple	Apple-flavored cereal

While you probably don't want to take the time to list everything in your kitchen, choose a few things that you eat frequently and consider where they would fall along the continuum. Create a table like this one, with as many rows as you need.

Closer to the "Whole Food" Side	Closer to the "Ultra-Processed Food" Side	Which Problematic Ingredients Are in It?
Items that would fit in groups 1, 2, or 3 on the NOVA Food Classification System	*Items that would fit in group 4 on the NOVA Food Classification System*	*Look for refined/enriched grains, sugar, corn syrup, artificial sweeteners, emulsifiers, preservatives, artificial flavors, highly processed oils,* or MSG** (either obvious or hidden)*

* Highly processed oils might include soy, canola, sunflower, safflower, corn, cottonseed.

** MSG may be hidden using the *words glutamic acid, yeast extract, autolyzed yeast, calcium caseinate, soy protein isolate/concentrate, hydrolyzed protein, plant protein extract, whey protein/concentrate/isolate, sodium caseinate, textured protein, malt extract, autolyzed plant protein, hydrolyzed oat flour, textured protein, sodium caseinate, calcium caseinate, natural flavors, bouillon, broth,* or *stock.*

How are you doing? Based on your kitchen analysis, are you eating more ultra-processed foods than you realized? Which of your favorite foods may be problematic? Write about it in your Clean(ish) Journal.

Based on what I learned, I can make these easy changes today:

WHAT'S A HEALTHY DIET?
AND HOW DO WE KNOW?

The foods we put into our bodies can either nourish us or add to our toxic loads. Our best bet, therefore, is to stick to high-quality real foods (rather than ultra-processed foods) as a basis for our overall diets. But even within the category of real foods, there is a lot of confusion about what to include. When you do an internet search using the term *clean eating,* you realize that there are so many definitions of what it means to "eat clean" that you don't know where to begin. Should you include dairy? Meat? Grains? What about fat? Or carbs?

What the heck is "clean eating"?

Before we make a concrete plan for becoming clean(ish), we first need to cut through the confusion about food.

In my book *Fast. Feast. Repeat.,* I have a chapter about a concept I call *diet brain.* In that chapter, I explain that you suffer from *diet brain* when you no longer feel confident in making any food choices because you're confused by all the conflicting information out there.

Why are we so confused?

Much of our confusion stems from the way the media reports medical/nutrition studies, and recently, I have become aware of just how widespread this problem actually is. I am subscribed to a weekly email list from the National Obesity Research Center that summarizes all the latest research within the nutrition and obesity fields and gives links to the studies that came out in the past week. The summary always has a section called "Headline vs. Study," and it is almost comical to compare the two. (It *would* be funny if it were not such a huge problem that affects our whole society negatively.) It turns out that a large number of the claims made in the headlines are not at all what the study discovered.

Other confusion comes from the huge array of diet books on the shelves. It seems that for every diet book, there is at least one that recommends the exact opposite approach. At one point over the past year, you could look at the bestseller list within the "weight loss" category for a major online book retailer and see both a carnivore diet book (*eat only meat and other animal products and avoid foods that originate from plants*) and a plant-based diet book (*eat only foods that originate from plants and avoid meat or animal products*). There was also a book that recommended "*eat a lot of plants except for certain plants, which you shouldn't ever eat.*" I'm confused just typing that, actually.

Dear diet industry:

We are tired.

Yes, we are bone-weary from constantly being told how to eat.

We are tired of giving up whole food groups. We want to eat carbs. And fats. And we want to eat them together in one meal.

We don't want to do a math problem every time we want to eat.

We don't think that food and eating should be so complicated.

When we get right to the heart of the matter, eating should be simple. And maybe it is.

Let me begin this chapter with the words of Michael Pollan from his important book *In Defense of Food*:[1]

> *Most of what we need to know about how to eat we already know, or once did until we allowed the nutrition experts and the advertisers to shake our confidence in common sense, tradition, the testimony of our senses, and the wisdom of our mothers and grandmothers.*

That's pretty simple, yes? But he makes it even simpler with his recommendation:

> *Eat food. Mostly plants. Not too much.*

According to Dr. Tim Spector, a professor, physician, and award-winning expert in personalized medicine and the gut microbiome:[2]

> *My scientific research has focused increasingly on nutrition and food-related questions in recent years. I have been astonished to discover how much of what we are told about food is at best misleading, and at worst, downright wrong and dangerous to our health . . . this is true whether the advice comes from dieticians, doctors, government guidelines, science reporting or anecdotally through friends and family. How did we get into this mess where unqualified people dictate the best ways for us to eat? This situation is unique in the field of medicine and science. There are many reasons for this, but I would pinpoint three major obstacles to better understanding about food and nutrition: bad science, misunderstanding of the results, and the food industry. Diet is the most important medicine we all possess. We urgently need to learn how best to use it.*

Irony alert: I am actually one of those "unqualified people" he describes. As you read this book (or any of my books), keep in mind that I am not a nutrition researcher, doctor, or nutritionist. I am a teacher. But also keep in mind that I am doing what teachers always do: we gather resources, study multiple sources, and redeliver content to others. I am also going to do another thing that teachers do: I'll point you to the primary sources and the research so you can go more deeply into the science where it interests you. Check the endnotes for all my sources, and go straight to them for more information.

There are many nonscientists who are credible when it comes to reporting nutrition information in a way that stands up to scrutiny. Michael Pollan is a journalist, and he began his work as a quest to uncover the truth about food. The same is true for Dan Buettner, whose investigative work led to the research about the Blue Zones. More about the Blue Zones research later in this chapter.

Both Michael Pollan and Dan Buettner came to very similar conclusions, though their journalistic research took them down different paths to get there.

What about me? As I already explained, I'm a teacher turned writer and podcaster. In my intermittent fasting communities and podcasts, questions about what we are "supposed to" eat come up . . . *a lot*.

Because of that, I've read a lot of books and research studies over the years in search of the answers. As I already mentioned, I was inspired to do much of this research in 2017 when I wrote my second book, *Feast Without Fear*. And when digging into the research, I've ended up with similar conclusions to those of both Michael Pollan and Dan Buettner.

WHO SHOULD WE TRUST?
IGNORE THE FRINGE AND FOLLOW THE CROWD

What do I mean by "follow the crowd"? I am referring to seeking out and listening to the recommendations that are based on decades of evidence from the fields of medical and nutritional research.

Reading all the conflicting theories about foods and health might make you think that there is no agreement about what we should be eating, but actually, there is solid consensus among most doctors, nutritionists, and nutrition researchers about what should form the basis of a healthy diet. Keep reading—I'm going to offer some of the strongest evidence here within this chapter.

Many of us love a good story of intrigue, and nutritional recommendations have their share of twists and turns over the decades (and even a conspiracy theory here and there). Maybe some of those conspiracy theories are grounded in truth, but we can all agree there have been many examples of contradictory information about what to eat over the years. Eggs are a great example of this confusion. Eggs have been "good," "bad," "good," and I think they may be "bad" again. That's okay. They will be "good" again tomorrow. (I'll wait and eat an egg tomorrow, just to be safe.)

Much of the advice is later recanted (*Oops! We were wrong . . . again!*) and this has made us jaded. We begin to distrust *all* mainstream dietary advice as if it is part of a giant master plan to keep us sick and unhealthy.

Much of the confusion originates from:

- **Studies funded by industry.** These studies almost always have findings that support the industry that funded them. (To learn more about this topic and fully understand the impact of these types of studies on food policy and recommendations, read *Unsavory Truth: How Food Companies Skew the Science of What We Eat* by Dr. Marion Nestle), or

- **Studies that have focused on "reductionist" views of foods.** This happens when we reduce foods into their parts (giving each *part* emphasis) rather than considering that every food is actually the *sum of its parts*. The components within our meals work *together* synergistically. We don't eat foods in isolation, so studying the most basic components of foods in isolation means we miss the big picture: both foods and our bodies are *systems* that cannot be isolated in a lab.[3]

Despite these two major problems, we do have *a great deal of evidence* for what types of foods form the foundation of a healthy diet for humans. While it's true that there has been some bad advice over the years, that doesn't mean that *all* mainstream recommendations are incorrect, and I am going to get into that in a minute.

Before I do, I want to explain what I meant when I said, "Ignore the fringe." When someone has a novel theory that certain whole foods should be avoided by every human alive, we should be very cautious about jumping on board such a restrictive plan long term.

Because of the poor state of health that's widespread in today's modern world in general, there's been a recent rise in alarming recommendations designed around statements such as "People aren't designed to eat grains" or "Beans are bad for our gut lining." An overwhelming majority of evidence supports the opposite of those two statements, actually. There is a *mountain of evidence* supporting the benefits of diets full of a wide variety of plant foods—and yes, that includes grains and beans. Does that mean that grains and beans work well for every person's body? No, and especially not if your gut health is poor. The key is that a *healthy gut* is able to tolerate a wide variety of whole foods—and these foods help us thrive.

When you read one of the high-profile books that cautions you to avoid grains forever, or never eat beans, or *only* eat meat and animal products and skip fruits and vegetables long term, or (*insert new and restrictive theory here*), they are pretty convincing. Suddenly, you begin to doubt what you have always been told about veggies or whole grains being good for you. Was that just another piece of bad info? Vegetables and other foods from plants begin to sound scary, and you start eyeing the meat counter in a new way. Diet brain kicks in.

While it can be tempting to think that someone has made an *amazing new discovery!* that goes against the way humans have eaten for all of human existence, do you really think that is likely? Let's dig into some of the evidence.

Before we do, there's one important caveat for what I just said, and it's that not all bodies react the same way to the same foods.

Some people *do* need to restrict certain foods, and for very good reason. Someone with celiac disease needs to avoid gluten, as an example. Those with food allergies to things such as eggs or shellfish should avoid eggs or shellfish. Does that mean that everyone should avoid the foods that are problematic for others? Of course not.

If you have food sensitivities in general or if your gut health is poor and your body doesn't tolerate many plant foods *right now,* you may need to temporarily make changes in what you are eating. In that case, a restrictive elimination diet can help you in the short term with symptoms you're experiencing, or guide you toward finding the foods that make you feel your best. Never forget that it's important to work with your body in the condition that it is in, whatever that may be.

And now, let's examine some of the evidence.

WHAT WESTON PRICE DISCOVERED

Who was Weston Price? He was a dentist from Ohio who traveled the world in the 1930s searching for the cause of dental disease. In his practice, he noticed that his patients suffered from many cavities, physical degeneration, crowded, crooked teeth, and dental arch deformities. As he traveled, however, he noticed that people who lived in nonindustrialized areas didn't seem to suffer the same types of dental issues as his patients. He went to remote villages in Switzerland and the Outer Hebrides, visited Native American populations throughout North America, and also traveled extensively among the Melanesian and Polynesian South Sea Islanders, African tribes, Australian Aborigines, New Zealand Maori, and the Indians of South America.[4]

Dr. Price reported that whenever he found a population eating a traditional diet (rather than the Western diet of the U.S.), they had straight teeth, no decay, and seemed to be in overall better physical health in general. The more Westernized the diet, the worse their health. His theory became that the dental malformations and health conditions so prevalent in the Western world are a result of nutritional deficiencies caused by the modern refined diet.

Dr. Price is not the only early-twentieth-century researcher to draw the same conclusions. Other researchers found the same thing as they traveled the world and spent time among populations eating traditional diets: Albert Schweitzer and Denis P. Burkitt (Africa), Robert McCarrison (India), Samuel Hutton (Labrador), and Aleš Hrdlička (Native Americans).

Here's a summary of what they all found: the native populations they studied had very low levels of modern-lifestyle diseases, such as heart disease, diabetes, cancer, obesity, hypertension, and stroke. They also were less likely to suffer from other health ailments, such as ulcers, hemorrhoids, and diverticulitis, and even their teeth were healthier.

Just as Dr. Price found, these other researchers noted that as these populations moved away from the way they traditionally ate and adopted more Western diets, they all began to find the same lifestyle diseases start to pop up within their populations. The term *Western diseases* was coined at that time because of the connection between those of us in the West and the constellation of lifestyle diseases and health issues that are connected to the Western diet.

What is important is that no two of the populations studied had the exact same diets. They ate what was available to them locally. (This gives "eat local" a whole new meaning . . . It really is how we are designed to live.) Some of them ate a lot of seafood, while others ate no seafood. Others included a great deal of dairy, while others ate no dairy. They all ate the plant foods that were in season and the animal foods that were available to them, including all the organ meat.

The commonality was this: real foods from nature, grown and raised in harmony with nature itself, rooted in soils that were rich in nutrients, and completely without modern chemicals, additives, and industrial processing.

Rather than trying to find the magical macronutrient ratio found in these traditional diets (especially since they are all different when it comes to their ratios), it boils down to this: eat anything at all *other than a Western diet of nutritionally devoid foods* and your health will likely improve.

WHAT WE'VE LEARNED FROM THE BLUE ZONES

According to Dan Buettner, there are five places in our modern-day world that help us decipher the secrets of a long and healthy life, and the five longevity hot spots they identified have been named the *Blue Zones*.[5]

The five Blue Zones are located in Ikaria, Greece; Sardinia, Italy; Okinawa, Japan; the Nicoya Peninsula in Costa Rica; and Loma Linda, California. In all five areas, researchers from the National Geographic Society found people live well into their nineties and even past the age of one hundred. Not only are they living longer, but they are healthy and thriving as they age.

Unlike many of us who follow a Western diet, those in the Blue Zones don't count calories or macros. They also don't stress about what they eat or feel guilt about enjoying their food. They eat. They enjoy their lives. They celebrate together.

So, what do all these populations have in common when it comes to what they eat? They are all eating real food, and it's the food their ancestors ate. They aren't eating many (if any) ultra-processed foods. They all eat a variety of foods from plants, including both grains and starchy vegetables, such as potatoes, sweet potatoes, and yams. While they all eat meat, it isn't a main focus of their meals. Most have a moderate alcohol intake.

What the residents of the Blue Zones are eating sounds a lot like what the populations studied by Dr. Price and the other early-twentieth-century researchers ate.

WHAT WE LEARNED FROM PREDIMED

In a study (PREDIMED) that took place from 2003 to 2010, scientists in Spain investigated the effects of a Mediterranean diet on a variety of health outcomes.[6] This type of eating pattern is generally high in fruits and vegetables and also includes plenty of legumes/beans, fish, whole grains, nuts and seeds, and olive oil. Those eating a Mediterranean diet consume moderate amounts of dairy products and wine, and a lower consumption of red/processed meats or foods with a high sugar content.

The Spanish scientists collaborated with researchers from Columbia University, Harvard University, and Loma Linda University. They enrolled 7,447 participants from the ages of fifty-five to eighty, all of whom were considered to be at high risk for cardiovascular disease, and assigned them to three groups: a Mediterranean diet with supplemental olive oil, a Mediterranean diet with supplemental nuts, and a control diet that was modeled after the American Heart Association's low-fat eating recommendations. The three groups were followed for about five years to access the effect of these dietary patterns on their overall health and specifically their cardiovascular outcomes. None of the participants were asked to limit their calorie intake or increase exercise.

What happened? The two Mediterranean diet groups had a 30 percent risk-reduction for cardiovascular events when compared to the control diet group. The two Mediterranean diet groups also had a lowered risk of stroke. They ended the trial early because the effects appeared to be so dramatic that they felt it was unethical to continue.[7]

There's one caveat when it comes to PREDIMED, and it may be a big one (or maybe not—I'll let you decide). When the data was examined later, it turns out that the participants weren't as "randomized" as the study claimed. These methodological flaws called all the results into question, though the lead researcher said that the problems with the study randomization were not clinically meaningful and that they didn't change the conclusions of the study. Still, critics may disagree. Scientific research about nutrition is very difficult to conduct in the real world with real people, particularly when it is of this magnitude, and this study is an example of that.

There are many other studies on the health outcomes of a Mediterranean diet, and a 2020 meta-analysis of twenty-nine studies (that all met stringent criteria for inclusion in the meta-analysis), found that overall, the higher the participants' adherence to a Mediterranean diet, the higher the reduction in the risk of all-cause mortality.[8]

If you've been paying attention, and I am sure you have, you may have noticed one thing: the types of foods featured in a Mediterranean diet are the same types of foods that the healthy Blue Zones residents consume, and they are also the types of foods eaten by the various populations in the early-twentieth-century studies.

WHAT WE ARE LEARNING FROM THE NUTRINET-SANTÉ STUDY

The NutriNet-Santé study launched in 2009 in France, and it's designed to study the relationship between overall nutrition and a variety of health outcomes. By 2021, they had regularly collected data from more than 171,000 people.[9]

They consider this to be a *web-based prospective cohort study,* and participants complete online questionnaires about their dietary intakes and other factors every six months. Data from the participants' medical and insurance records are linked with their self-reported data to give researchers an overall picture of their health and wellness. In addition, they have collected blood, urine, and stool samples from about twenty thousand of the participants.[10]

Data from the study show that as the level of ultra-processed foods in the diet goes up, so does the risk of cancer, cardiovascular disease, type 2 diabetes, depression, gastrointestinal disorders, and overall mortality. In addition, a higher consumption of ultra-processed foods has been associated with a significant increase of both overall cancer rates and breast cancer rates.[11]

Besides the negative impact of ultra-processed foods, we are also learning other things from the NutriNet-Santé data. For example, they have found positive associations between organic food and a variety of positive health outcomes: *higher* levels of organic foods are associated with *lower* concentrations of pesticides in participants' urine (which shouldn't surprise any of us), as well as a *lower* risk of breast cancer, lymphoma, obesity, and metabolic syndrome. While it's difficult to assume a cause-effect relationship from all this data (though it's safe to assume that the pesticide concentration is most likely cause-effect), it's still another piece of evidence encouraging us to choose organic foods.[12]

Data from the NutriNet-Santé studies have been used to create something called a Nutri-Score, which gives each product in the store a label with a score from A to E. A means the item is the healthiest, and E is the unhealthiest. In one study, participants' diets were ranked using data related to an overall dietary score based on the Nutri-Scores of what they were eating. The better the participants' overall score, the lower their overall levels of mortality for all causes and for cancer and diseases of the circulatory, respiratory, and digestive systems. Overall, over forty studies support the use of the Nutri-Score to guide food choices. Bottom line: when people ate foods with a better score, they were healthier.[13]

HOW DOES YOUR GUT MICROBIOME FACTOR IN?

Your gut microbiome is as unique as your fingerprint, and its composition is a major contributor to how the rest of your body functions. In 1996, scientists first began sequencing the organisms living within the gut microbiome, and in the relatively short time since, our understanding has increased exponentially.[14] It may surprise you to learn that it wasn't until 2005 that scientists first demonstrated that a change in diet could alter the activity of the microbiota.[15] So, in many ways, we are still in the early days when it comes to this field. The good news is that inquiry has continued at a rapid pace, and we are learning more and more each year.

The diversity within our gut microbiome is complex, and there are thousands of species that reside there. I read one estimate that says we each have about *50 trillion* individual microorganisms that live in our guts. To put that into perspective, there are only about 7.8 billion humans alive on the earth (as of 2021). That is seriously mind-boggling. You may think of your poop as being composed of waste products left over from your meals, but your fecal matter is actually about 60 percent bacteria.

Increasingly within the medical literature, a healthy gut microbiome is linked to positive health outcomes, and gut dysbiosis (a fancy word for an "unhealthy gut") is linked to negative health outcomes. If you have "good" guys living in your gut, and you feed them the types of food that make them thrive, they help you by releasing compounds that lower inflammation and promote good health. The bad news is that if you have an unhealthy community within your microbiome, they release compounds that actually lead to increased inflammation.

There is a great deal of evidence that many of the inflammatory conditions that are on the rise in the modern world have gut dysbiosis as a root cause. Examples would include, but not be limited to inflammatory bowel disease, multiple sclerosis, rheumatoid arthritis, lupus, and psoriasis/psoriatic arthritis. These are all examples of what are called *immune-mediated inflammatory diseases,* and the full list includes more than one hundred different clinical diseases. Science has also linked an unhealthy gut microbiome to many other health conditions, such as obesity, diabetes, kidney disease, and Alzheimer's disease, just to name a few.

What does a healthy gut do for us? Besides being essential for proper food digestion and linked to lower levels of inflammation within our bodies, the gut is a key player in our immune system function.[16]

Our gut microbiome differences explain much of our bio-individuality. What lives in *your* gut is different from what lives in *my* gut. And that means that what *you* consume will be processed differently from what *I* consume. This is true for the foods we eat as well as the medications we take.

Bottom line (pun intended):

A healthy gut = A healthy YOU

Our goal, then, is to feed our gut microbiome communities well. We want to take care of them, so they can take care of us.

WHAT FOODS FEED OUR GUTS WELL?

Throughout our lives, our gut microbiomes continue to develop and change in response to what's around us and what we eat. What we eat is incredibly important in developing a healthy microbiome, in fact.

It's important to understand that when you eat, you are not just feeding yourself. You are also feeding your gut community, and they are there to break down your food for you. The relationship has evolved to be beneficial to both us and to them. If you have "good" guys living in your gut, and you feed them the types of food that make them thrive, they help us by releasing compounds that lower inflammation and promote our health.

You're probably not surprised to hear that a diet high in ultra-processed foods is linked to an unhealthy gut microbiome composition, whereas a diet high in a variety of vegetables, fruits, and whole grains, along with probiotic foods such as yogurt and fermented foods like sauerkraut, kefir, and kimchi, is linked to a healthy gut microbiome composition.[17]

Plant foods are really important for gut health. There are many different types of fiber in the plants we eat, and when we eat a wide variety of fibrous plants, we feed the different strains of gut bacteria. They can't survive without it.

WHAT WE ARE LEARNING FROM
THE PREDICT STUDIES

Dr. Tim Spector is one of my favorite science researchers, and I have been a huge fan of his ever since I read his book *The Diet Myth* in 2016. His most recent work as a lead researcher on the PREDICT studies examines how we are all different when it comes to what foods work for our bodies and why.

In the original PREDICT study released in 2019, Spector and his team measured blood glucose, insulin levels, fat levels, and other blood markers in response to a variety of meals. They also collected data from the participants related to the composition of their gut microbiomes. They found that there is a wide variation among participants when it comes to how they respond to the exact same meals, and these differences are related to individual factors such as how quickly their bodies clear blood glucose or blood fat after a meal and also the composition of the inhabitants of their gut microbiomes. A great deal of the individual variability was related to the gut.[18]

According to Sarah Berry, one of the researchers involved in PREDICT, "Our study has found that the increase in fat and glucose in our blood after eating a meal initiates an inflammatory response which differs hugely between individuals. This meal-induced inflammatory response is largely dependent on the rise in blood fat after the meal. Dietary and lifestyle strategies to reduce prolonged elevations in blood fat and glucose may, therefore, be a useful target to reduce low-grade inflammation in preventative health."[19]

They have found that overall diet diversity is important, and gut health markers improve along with increased diversity in our diet.[20] Overall, what this means is that the higher the variety of plant food in the diet, the healthier the gut microbiome profile. While meat consumption was more likely to be linked with a negative gut microbiome profile, they found that as long as a participant's overall diet is healthy and diverse, there is no need to exclude meat. Other than plant foods, foods such as dark chocolate, yogurt, shellfish, oily fish, and eggs, as well as red wine, were all linked to a healthy microbiome.[21]

I was fortunate enough to participate in the PREDICT 3 study, and I learned that my body doesn't clear glucose or fat quickly after meals. I wasn't surprised to learn that about fat, as I never felt well when I attempted a high-fat diet, such as my very brief keto days of 2014. Not only did I not lose a pound for the entire summer that I went keto, but I felt inflamed and I was always hungry. Learning that my body doesn't clear fat well and that increased fat can lead to increased inflammation in my body absolutely matches my personal experiences. The PREDICT 3 study taught me that my body does best when I emphasize a wide variety of plant foods in my diet. When I got my results back, I committed to a period of time following their personalized recommendations for my body, many of which are designed to feed the "good" gut bugs that I have living within my microbiome. The overall goal is to choose foods that feed the population that we want to thrive and starve out the ones we don't want to promote, meaning we encourage proliferation of the bacteria that are linked to positive health outcomes in general. When I centered my meals around the dietary recommendations that were based on my personal blood and gut microbiome analysis and glucose/fat clearance levels, I could tell a difference in my energy levels . . . and after a few days, my husband asked me if I had lost weight. Because I am clean(ish) and at my ideal weight range, I don't always follow their recommendations these days, but when I do, I can feel the difference.

WHAT DOES ALL THIS EVIDENCE HAVE IN COMMON?

After looking at all the evidence from each of these sources and studies, we find that they all reached similar conclusions.

We can sum it up using the words of Michael Pollan that I shared at the beginning of the chapter:

Eat food. Mostly plants. Not too much.

SCIENTIFIC RESEARCH ABOUT NUTRITION HAS FLAWS

Before moving on, I want to talk about one thing: it is very difficult to conduct nutritional research of any kind using humans as subjects because we are both complicated organisms and also difficult to control. Mice in a lab? Fairly easy to control. People? Not so much.

Randomized controlled trials (RCTs) are considered to be the gold standard when it comes to nutritional research. In this type of study, participants are randomly assigned into either an experimental group or a control group. As the study is conducted, the researchers attempt to keep all variables equal except for the one outcome variable being studied. Over time, evidence-based dietary guidelines are developed based on systematic reviews and meta-analyses of these RCTs.[22]

In these studies, participants are assigned to different dietary treatment groups where they are expected to follow a prescribed dietary approach. One limitation to this type of research is that it can be difficult to determine whether participants in a study followed the dietary recommendations they are expected to follow. We have *all* probably tried to stick to a diet at one time of our lives and had a "fall off the wagon" moment . . . or *many* of those moments. If you are participating in a study, are you going to mention to the scientists that you had those *oops* moments? Maybe, but maybe not.

Some studies attempt to control for this by having participants reside in what's referred to as a *metabolic ward*. They are closely monitored by the researchers, and it is a lot easier to control the variables when the subjects are in the monitored environment. Because they are required to remain on-site, however, most of these studies are of short duration. We know that it can take years (or even decades) for the positive or negative effects of our diets to show up, so it's difficult to draw conclusions from some of these studies. As an example, let's think back to a study I mentioned in the "Better Living Through Chemistry" chapter that was not a metabolic ward study, meaning it could be continued for a longer duration.

In that 2011 study, scientists compared seventy-one obese subjects who went through bariatric surgery to eighteen lean women. During the initial weight-loss phase, the participants who had weight-loss surgery had an increase in their POP body burden. If this study had been of short duration, scientists could have concluded that bariatric surgery leads to an increase in your overall toxic load.

The good news is that this study continued over time, and within six to twelve months, the participants had a 15 percent overall decrease in their body burdens. Because the study continued long term, scientists saw the bigger picture—which was positive—rather than the short-term results, which may have been interpreted as negative. I can see the headlines now: WEIGHT-LOSS SURGERY INCREASES YOUR TOXIC LOAD! Well, that's what happened—in the short term. But not in the long run, which is what matters.

Keep in mind that study was not a metabolic ward study, but I think it illustrates the point: sometimes we experience short-term changes that may be negative, whereas the long-term effects may be positive . . . or vice versa.[23]

We see this concept play out every day in our intermittent fasting community. As I explain in my book *Fast. Feast. Repeat.*, when someone begins an intermittent fasting lifestyle, they often feel awful during the adjustment period as their bodies are learning how to tap into fat stores for fuel. If I designed an RCT for intermittent fasting and put people in a metabolic ward for three weeks, it wouldn't surprise me to see that they still haven't received any positive benefits by the end of the three weeks—their bodies are likely not metabolically adapted to the changes yet. However, six months later, it would be a completely different story.

It can take a lot more than three weeks to see measurable or lasting changes in our health markers, and I am sure you understand that. We don't develop high cholesterol, insulin resistance, gut dysbiosis, and the like in three weeks, and we don't correct them in three weeks, either. Instead, we need to rely on longer-term data to know what the long-term effects of certain eating patterns might be.

Even longer-term studies have limitations, however, and it is important to understand what these may be. Observational or longitudinal studies that follow large groups of people (such as the NutriNet-Santé studies) may last for many years, but most of them rely on the subjects to self-report and accurately remember—and report—what and how much they consume. Quick! Do you remember exactly what you ate one week ago today? I sure don't. If you asked me, I could come up with something that *might* be what I ate, but it would probably not be completely accurate. In these types of surveys, some people underreport what they are eating or don't share what they really ate, particularly if they feel that the foods are unhealthy.

Also, there is another flaw when it comes to research that leads to a great deal of confusion: much of the funding for *food research* is provided by the *food industry*. Often, this research can be spun two different ways: through studies that find certain chemicals or notfoods are "harmless," even though that may be far from the truth long term (especially when ingested or absorbed in quantities that build up over time) or when showing that a compound found in food in isolation is "dangerous" (particularly when consumed in quantities that are unlike those we would take in through a diet of real foods). When we have an agenda, we can find "evidence" to support almost any conclusion.

Even with all these "nutrition research is flawed" concepts in mind, when we look at all the evidence from Weston Price and the other researchers from the early twentieth century, the collection of what we have learned from the Blue Zones, from PREDIMED, PRE-DICT, and NutriNet-Santé, and also what we know about cultivating a healthy gut microbiome, we can see that they are all saying essentially the same things:

Eat real food.

I've also noticed a *good* trend within the restrictive dietary approach communities. Whether they are low-carb, low-fat, plant-based, Paleo, carnivore, or anything in between, while they completely disagree with exactly what should be on your plate, they increasingly agree with one concept:

Eat real food.

When this many sources agree, it gives me confidence that they are onto something.

So, what is "clean eating"? It's eating real food and limiting ultra-processed food. It really is as simple as that.

REFLECT AND TAKE ACTION:
EXAMINE THE DIET OF YOUR ANCESTORS

Use your Clean(ish) Journal (or the worksheets available at ginstephens .com/cleanish) to complete these end-of-chapter prompts and activities.

In the early-twentieth-century research done by Dr. Weston Price and others, and also in the work done by Dan Buettner within the Blue Zones, they all found that residents achieved excellent health by eating the foods that had been traditionally eaten in their regions for generations. They all ate local foods in season rather than the ultra-processed Western diet, and while what they ate varied widely from location to location, they all were thriving.

When we think of this from an evolutionary perspective, we understand that survival was linked to the ability to eat the foods that were available. Because of this, our ancestors' dietary patterns led to genetic adaptations that allowed them to thrive on the foods that were accessible to them within their environments.[24] As an example of this in action, only 35 percent of adults worldwide are genetically adapted to consuming dairy products into adulthood. This ability depends on whether you're *lactase-persistent* or not, and those who are lactase-persistent continue to produce lactase (an enzyme that allows for digestion of dairy) into adulthood. This genetic variation likely appeared in Europe as dairy became a part of the population's diet, and this enzyme is present in 89–96 percent of those with genetic roots in the British Isles and Scandinavia—though as few as 10 percent of the Asian population is genetically suited to digesting dairy.[25,26] Whether dairy works well for you (or not) depends very much on your genetics.

In another example, some populations adapted to a greater consumption of starchy foods, particularly when agriculture became a major part of their societies. These populations developed increased levels of amylase, a salivary enzyme required to break down starches. The more amylase, the more adapted the population was to consuming starchy foods.[27]

How can we use this information to help us figure out what foods may be ideal for us? Consider what your ancestors ate.

Experts used to suggest looking at what your grandparents ate, but my grandmother always had Bugles, Chicken in a Biskit crackers, and cans of Tab on hand. No, most of us need to go back further than our grandparents these days. We need to go *way* back.

Do you know your genetic heritage? Thanks to one of the mainstream DNA analysis sites, I learned that I am 99 percent of European descent, with 86.9 percent of my heritage originating from the British Isles, with a small percentage of ancestors that are French,

German, and Scandinavian, and around 1 percent of ancestors that are Western Asian and North African.

Because most of my ancestors are from the British Isles, I am more likely to be suited to eat foods that are traditionally eaten in that region. Dairy? Starchy foods? Yes and yes.

If you know your genetic heritage, take some time to learn about what foods are traditionally eaten in that region of the world.

- What did your ancestors eat?

Plan to try some traditional foods that were eaten by your ancestors.

Write down some of the recipes you want to try in your Clean(ish) Journal.

EXTRA CREDIT: SEQUENCE YOUR SQUAD

Oscillibacter sp. 57_20.
Clostridium sp. CAG:167.
Eubacterium eligens.
Faecalibacterium prausnitzii.

Am I suddenly speaking in a strange new language? Is this some kind of typo or printing error?

No, these are four of the inhabitants of my gut microbiome, whom researchers have nicknamed Oscar, Cheng, Euan, and Felicia. As I mentioned in this chapter, I took part in the PREDICT 3 study recently, and part of that study involved an analysis to determine my gut-dwellers.

I learned that certain foods act as "gut boosters" for me, and these include foods such as apples, broccoli, zucchini, lentils, spinach, and avocados. Other foods act as "gut suppressors" for my particular gut bugs, and these include foods such as: white bread, sausage, beef, and chocolate candy.

If you're interested in having this type of testing done, keep in mind that the field is evolving each year. As of the date that I am writing this, I have a link to the company that is linked to the PREDICT studies at ginstephens.com, and they offer a program you can purchase that includes not only the gut microbiome analysis but also a CGM (continuous glucose monitor) that allows them to see how your body reacts to the foods you eat in real time. Upon completion, you have personalized recommendations of what foods should work best for your unique body. You can find the link by going to ginstephens.com/cleanish. I'll update the website over time if my recommendations ever change.

You can also go to mymicrobiome.info to see recommendations from the American Gut Project researchers. These are also updated over time with their most up-to-date recommendations. Not all gut-testing companies are created equal, and your goal is to find the one that is using the most up-to-date science to make their recommendations.

PARALYSIS OF ANALYSIS: WHEN GETTING HEALTHY BECOMES AN OBSESSION

As we become clean(ish), we know that it's not only about what we *eat* (or don't eat). We also want to become clean(ish) when it comes to our personal care and cleaning products so we can lower our overall toxic loads and support vibrant health. In this chapter, however, I want to focus on clean(ish) eating and talk about what happens when we take a good thing too far.

When I scroll through my Instagram feed, I see a lot of posts about different eating styles. Instagram has figured out that I am interested in food and health, so it shows me post after post from health and wellness influencers.

In one post, a vegan tells us all how wrong it is for anyone to eat meat, and if we were truly animal lovers, we would never eat a steak, and it's actually exactly like eating your pets. (*Is it? Really? I look at my cat and she gives me the side-eye. Gulp. Wait, though. My cat eats meat. She gets me.*)

A proponent of the carnivore eating style shares a photo of a huge pile of nothing *but* steak and makes complete fun of plant eaters, as if they are somehow not as advanced in their thinking. "*Ha ha! Look at those poor plant eaters, destroying their health with every bite.*"

A keto-vangelist tries to sell me his own special blend of fat-magic. "*Buy my special bottled liquid fat and you will burn fat a-l-l day!*" The message: if you're not eating mostly fat at every meal, you must be a loser.

Post after post includes judgments about foods and entire macronutrient groups and also judgment about the people who might dare to eat them. Some of the Instagram posters are actually mean about it, as if their way makes them more enlightened than those "other people."

It feels almost like we are somehow looking for a new religion, and as we scroll, we are constantly searching for the cult of the most devout. Anyone who makes different choices has what must be "bad information," and they are clearly not as enlightened.

Can I make a confession? I'm over it. It stopped being funny a long time ago. Now I just find it to be sad.

My Instagram feed, however, teaches me something important. It shines a light on the dark side of the health and wellness movement.

Let's not be like that.

We are here to become clean(ish). But is the opposite of clean(ish) "dirty(ish)"? Absolutely not. It's time to remove all morality from how you live or eat. We also aren't going to judge the way other people live or eat.

And I mean that. Even though I think some of the more extreme ways of eating may have long-term consequences that the proponents don't yet understand, I 100 percent believe them when they say that they feel better when they eat that way. And if they feel better, I am certain that there is a biological reason why. Feeling great is usually a positive sign. And our bodies are all different. Saying mean things about people who choose to eat differently from how you do isn't helping anyone.

So, always remember this: you aren't a "better" person because you make different food or lifestyle choices from someone else. Everyone else isn't "deceived" or "bad."

You're simply someone who wants to live a healthy lifestyle overall, and you are learning how foods nourish your body and *not-foods* do not support overall health. You fine-tune what you are eating because you want to *feel great*. And you deserve to feel great! Becoming clean(ish) can most definitely help you feel great.

There's another consideration, however, and I want to talk about it now. One of the major criticisms of the clean-eating movement in general has been that it can lead to an unhealthy fixation on maintaining certain food standards. This is actually a valid concern. Will this happen as you become more clean(ish) yourself? Can a focus on health and wellness go too far? And how does it happen?

AVOIDING FEAR

One problem is that we can read books (or articles, blogs, wacky Instagram posts, etc.) that really scare us. The author uses words that make whatever they are warning us about sound really dangerous. And everything they say sounds plausible, especially because it's usually rooted in *just enough* science to ring true.

Let me use an example that will make sense: exercise. We all know that exercise helps us build larger and stronger muscles. And I am sure you also know that when you work out hard, you may feel some pain the next day. Even so, despite the pain, we all know that exercise is healthy and it's good for us.

What if I told you this, however:

> *NEVER exercise! It is dangerous. In fact, when you exercise, you will literally RIP YOUR MUSCLE FIBERS. You don't want to rip your muscle fibers, do you? You know this is dangerous because you're sore after a workout. Don't make this mistake. Keep your muscles intact. Sit on the couch and be safe.*

That sounds like nonsense, right? But isn't it exactly like some of the scare tactics you read in nutrition blogs and books?

It's *founded* on truth: when you exercise, you experience micro-tears in your muscle fibers. As the muscle heals post-workout, your body builds it back stronger than it was before.

So, these micro-tears are an important part of the muscle-growth process and not something to be scared of.

But that doesn't mean that I can't make it sound positively terrifying.

> Using the example of exercise, you see:
>
> • I can make exercise sound scary by describing the natural processes in an alarming way.
>
> Even though we actually know:
>
> • The right amount of exercise challenges our bodies in a good way and makes us stronger and healthier.

Even the book you are reading right now might make you feel scared as you read. I'm sure some of the preceding chapters have alarmed you in more ways than one. Who wants an increased toxic load? Not me. Who wants to be overfed and undernourished? Still not me. I'm sure you agree completely. You picked up this book because you want to make better choices. Yet, while reading, you may start to become so afraid that you begin to get obsessed.

WHEN FEAR BECOMES OBSESSION

What happens when we are so afraid that we become obsessed about what we eat? When we are judging ourselves with every decision we make? With every bite we take, we can become anxious:

> • Is this food good for me or bad for me?
>
> • Is this food damaging my gut or healing my gut?

- Now that I know ultra-processed foods aren't ideal, should I feel guilty for eating this food?

- What happens if I include some *not-food* into my life? Is it destroying my health? Did my bucket just fill completely up from this one meal?

- Even worse: Should I feel *guilty* for *enjoying* this?

Eating a varied diet made up of delicious foods (and some *not-foods*) that we enjoy is not something we should ever feel guilty about. Perfection is not required. Our goal is to have a healthy attitude toward food and eating, based on an understanding of nutrition in general but also with a confidence that we are looking for *balance*. A "healthy diet" refers to the overall pattern of what you eat over time. We prioritize eating a wide variety of foods and also can enjoy *not-foods* for the pleasure they bring to us. Pleasure is okay. It's *important*, in fact.

- Carbs are not "bad."

- Fat is not "bad."

- Protein is not "bad."

- Meat is not "bad."

- Vegetables are not "bad."

- Fruit is not "bad."

- Potatoes are not "bad."

- Grains are not "bad."

- Even Doritos . . . they are not "bad." (They're an example of *not-food*, but they are still not *bad*.)

- YOU are not "bad" if you eat any of the foods on this list or any other list.

"Bad" is a moral judgment. If we eat "bad foods," we must be "bad people." Cue the guilt.

Choosing to eat in an overall healthy manner is not about developing strict rules or living a life of deprivation. It's about making choices that support health, fuel our bodies, and promote nutritional balance.

There's that word again: *balance.*

The desire to eat healthy foods is *not* a problem. An absence of moderation, however, *is* a problem. "Clean eating" can turn into an obsession where you literally become scared of nourishment. That is not healthy. It can lead you down the path toward orthorexia.

Because this criticism of the clean-eating movement is valid, it's something we need to talk about so you understand what the warning signs are and how to get help if you need it.

The term *orthorexia nervosa* originates from the physician who first used it in 1997, Dr. Steven Bratman. *Ortho* means "right" or "correct," and *orexia* stems from the Greek word *orexis,* meaning "appetite" or "desire." So, *orthorexia* means "having the correct appetite." *Nervosa* means "obsession." Put that together and you have "obsession with eating correctly."

Dr. Bratman's book *Health Food Junkies* explains his personal journey into (and back out of) a life consumed by disordered eating thoughts, and in his book he teaches us how to identify when a focus on healthful eating takes a dangerous turn and becomes all-consuming.

In his book, Dr. Bratman tells a very poignant story.[1] I want to retell it here.

In 1975, he had some health-conscious friends over for a dinner party. One guest found a can of something called Nalley's Beef Stew in his cabinet and ridiculed his choice. Dr. Bratman realized: he had bought the "wrong" food! The good news is that his new friends were happy to help him clean out his cabinets and teach him about the *right* food. He replaced all the "wrong" food with beans, grains, seaweeds, and dried fruits.

He jumped right into his new lifestyle and took it one step further, becoming a raw food vegan. After living that way for a time, he made a new friend who explained that he was wrong to eat raw food. No, his new friend said, raw food is the "wrong" food. The *right* way to eat was to follow macrobiotics. Dr. Bratman began to eat only brown rice and lightly cooked vegetables. He felt virtuous and was proud of his excellent diet.

One day, a famous master of Chinese medicine came into town. He was said to have great wisdom, and Dr. Bratman asked for his help in solving a few health issues that had come up in his life recently. The master asked for a description of his diet.

Here's my favorite part of this whole story.

After Dr. Bratman described his pure macrobiotic diet, Dr. Bratman tells us that the master said: "*Very bad diet. Very bad way to eat. My opinion, you eat like a crazy man . . . You ever heard of Nalley's Beef Stew? Very good for you.*"

In his quest for dietary perfection, Dr. Bratman had come full circle.

The descent into disordered eating happens slowly for most people. The focus on food quality increases. Eating well is a virtue, and you feel pride in the choices you are making. Over time, you may develop a fear of eating food that is not "pure." You become obsessed with the rules that make up your diet and will go to great lengths to ensure that what you eat lives up to certain standards. The rules make you feel safe. You feel superior to others, because *you* are maximizing your health, and *they* are not.

If you notice that you begin to have more and more self-imposed dietary rules couched in "I'm doing this for my health," that begins to manifest as "I must stick to extreme dietary purity to be safe," that's when it's time to become concerned. The obsession grows, boundaries become smaller, and eating becomes more restrictive.

You stop eating foods that you don't prepare yourself. You can no longer go to a restaurant. There are fewer and fewer things that are "safe" for you to eat. If and when you "break the rules" (usually, self-imposed rules) you feel a deep sense of guilt or shame. Your dietary virtue has now crossed over to the dark side.[2]

Here is how Dr. Bratman explains it:

> Orthorexia is an emotionally disturbed, self-punishing relationship with food that involves a progressively shrinking universe of foods deemed acceptable. A gradual constriction of many other dimensions of life occurs so that thinking about healthy food can become the central theme of almost every moment of the day, the sword and shield against every kind of anxiety, and the primary source of self-esteem, value and meaning. This may result in social isolation, psychological disturbance and even, possibly, physical harm.[3]

On the flip side, Dr. Bratman tells us this:

> If you eat a healthy diet but don't obsess over it, if you follow dietary guidelines effortlessly and focus most of your energy on living life, you almost certainly don't have orthorexia. You just eat well. It's the forcefulness, the overdetermined nature of orthorexia, that constitutes an illness.[4]

HOW TO GET HELP

The first step is to determine whether or not you have a problem. If you recognize that you may have an obsession with healthy food, and you want to free yourself from this trap that you're stuck in, you've already made a positive step. Next, you may want to find a counselor who can help you work through it.

It's important to understand that orthorexia is not an officially recognized mental disorder, though it's getting attention in the field as occurrences of this condition increase. For a mental disorder to be officially recognized, it needs to be named in the *Diagnostic and Statistical Manual of Mental Disorders, Fifth Edition* (*DSM-5*), the gold-standard publication of the American Psychiatric Association, which is the guide for diagnosing psychiatric disorders.

Why does it matter if orthorexia isn't officially recognized? Well, it often determines whether you receive mental health treatment or not. In many instances, an official diagnosis (based on the criteria found within the *DSM-5*) is required for insurance to cover treatment. Until orthorexia is officially recognized, it's important to understand that you still may be able to get help if you need it.

Dr. Bratman and his colleague Thomas Dunn propose these as potential future diagnostic criteria for orthorexia:[5]

Criterion A: obsessive focus on "healthy" eating, as defined by a dietary theory or set of beliefs whose specific details may vary; marked by exaggerated emotional distress in relationship to food choices perceived as unhealthy; weight loss may ensue as a result of dietary choices, but this is not the primary goal. As evidenced by the following:

- A1. Compulsive behavior and/or mental preoccupation regarding affirmative and restrictive dietary practices believed by the individual to promote optimum health

- A2. Violation of self-imposed dietary rules causing exaggerated fear of disease, sense of personal impurity and/or negative physical sensations, accompanied by anxiety and shame

- A3. Dietary restrictions escalate over time, up till removing entire food groups, and involve progressively more frequent and/or severe "cleanses" (partial fasts) regarded as purifying or detoxifying. This escalation commonly leads to weight loss, but the desire to lose weight is absent, hidden or subordinated to ideation about healthy eating

Criterion B: the compulsive behavior and mental preoccupation becomes clinically impairing by any of the following:

- B1. Malnutrition, severe weight loss or other medical complications from restricted diet

- B2. Intrapersonal distress or impairment of social, academic or vocational functioning secondary to beliefs or behaviors about healthy diet

- B3. Positive body image, self-worth, identity and/or satisfaction excessively dependent on compliance with self-defined "healthy eating behavior"

Again, if you think that description sounds like you, it is likely time to get help. You can also go online to orthorexia.com and find Dr. Bratman's orthorexia self-test.

Never forget this: when we become clean(ish), our goal is to work toward a lifestyle that supports health and wellness but without developing fear or obsession.

REFLECT: AVOIDING AN UNHEALTHY OBSESSION WITH FOOD AND LIFESTYLE

Use your Clean(ish) Journal (or the worksheets available at ginstephens .com/cleanish) to complete these end-of-chapter prompts and activities.

- Are there any foods that you are currently afraid to eat? What are they, and why do you feel that way about them? Are they foods that would fit into groups 1–3 on the NOVA Food Classification Scale, or are they ultra-processed foods?

- Do you want to find a way to incorporate these foods back into your life? Why or why not?

It's important for us to understand these words from Dr. Bratman:[6]

> *Adopting a theory of healthy eating is NOT orthorexia. A theory may be conventional or unconventional, extreme or lax, sensible or totally wacky, but, regardless of the details, followers of the theory do not necessarily have orthorexia. They are simply adherents of a dietary theory. The term "orthorexia" only applies when an eating disorder develops around that theory.*

If you suspect that you may have a problem, please go to orthorexia .com and take the self-test. It's a simple test with only six questions, but after you take it, you should have an indication as to whether your "healthy eating habits" may be going too far.

- What did you learn about yourself by taking the self-test?

PART 2

WHAT COMES *OUT*: UNLOCK YOUR BODY'S SELF-CLEANING TOOLS

Our bodies have a remarkable capacity to heal . . . *if* we provide the right environment for health. Now that we have learned about the overwhelming onslaught of toxins in today's world, we need a plan to manage the overflow.

Our goal is to slow the speed of what's coming *in* and support our bodies as they work to take the junk *out*. The good news is that each of us is a living and breathing detoxification machine.

In this section of the book, we are going to learn about our bodies' amazing self-cleaning pathways and how we can support them through the foods that we eat, by eating less frequently, and by employing a variety of different tools—that we will actually enjoy using.

It's true! Everything we will learn how to do is enjoyable. Nothing should feel like a struggle, and you won't have to do a "cleanse" or order special supplements.

- We'll eat delicious (yet nutritious) foods that support our bodies' natural detoxification pathways.

- We'll take a break from eating from time to time in a way that feels natural rather than difficult.

- We'll add some focused movement to our days, choosing activities that we enjoy.

- We'll take some time for a variety of healthy practices, such as massages, walking barefoot on the earth, and spending time in a sauna. (Who's going to say no to those things, am I right?)

YOUR BODY'S
SELF-CLEANING PATHWAYS

Have you heard anyone say, "I need to do a detox"? Does that make you think of juice cleanses or twenty-one-day fasts? The good news is that we don't need to go to such extremes, thankfully; our bodies are designed with extremely sophisticated self-cleaning systems. *Detox* simply means giving our bodies the time to employ these systems.

Instead of a "detoxification *program*," what you need is a "detoxification *lifestyle*."

When the body is working well, we excrete accumulated toxins through our organs: the liver, kidneys, lungs, skin, lymphatic system, glymphatic system, and colon. We don't need to "do" a detox. We never *stop* detoxing. These are essential processes that keep us alive.

Our bodies aren't just fighting against external toxins coming in from the world around us, which are known as *exogenous toxins,* but we also have to manage something called *endogenous* toxins. These are the by-products of our metabolism and the various natural processes that go on within a healthy and well-functioning body. While our bodies are designed to manage these endogenous toxins, they keep our bodies busy, and when we also have too many exogenous toxins coming in, our bodies can't keep up. The Lucy-and-Ethel analogy from the earlier chapter can apply here, as well.

When the body is working well, many of the toxins we are exposed to have the potential to be dealt with successfully by our bodies' efficient detoxification systems. Unfortunately, the modern environment puts a strain on these systems. Our bodies' ability to manage the increased toxic loads (from the rise of the external toxins I talked about in part 1 of this book) hasn't risen sufficiently to support the exponentially larger demand. Chronic inflammation, which is widespread in today's world, is one of the signs that our bodies can't keep up with the pace.[1]

The good news is that the human body has an amazing capacity for defending itself against invaders, repairing injuries, and healing. That being said, we have to support the body as it does its work. For the body's detoxification processes to occur, we have to consume the nutrients that our bodies need: proteins, phytonutrients, minerals, fats, and carbohydrates. More about that in the "What's Food Got to Do with It?" chapter.

For now, let's take a brief tour of some of our amazing bodies' self-cleaning organs and systems.

THE LIVER

Your liver is a hardworking organ, responsible for more than five hundred functions within the body, and one of its main jobs is to work as your body's filtration system. It's recognized as the major detoxifying organ in the body.[2] It also turns nutrients from food into substances your body can use and breaks down fats.[3]

You may only think of the words *detox* and *the liver* through the lens of *doing a liver detox,* which is a phrase that is tossed around frequently in the health and wellness world. Instead of doing a liver detox, it makes more sense to live a lifestyle that supports your liver's various functions, just as nature intended. This means putting *in* fewer toxins to begin with, as we learned about in part 1 of this book.[4]

Despite our best efforts, however, our livers are always going to be faced with toxins that need to be managed. How does your liver do it? Water-soluble toxins can be sent straight to your kidneys and excreted within your urine. Fat-soluble toxins, however, need to be metabolized within your liver. These fat-soluble toxins require a lot more attention, and your liver springs into action.

The liver detoxification process has three phases. In phase one, your liver uses a group of enzymes known as the cytochrome P450 family, which break down toxins (through oxidation, reduction, and hydrolysis) and converts them to less harmful substances. Phase one results in excess free radicals in your system, which are themselves harmful, and this is where antioxidants from foods come in: a healthy diet provides a great deal of support to phase-one liver detoxification. More on this in the next chapter.

In phase two, the liver makes these less harmful substances (that are still toxins) water-soluble so they can be excreted from your body (through urine or sweat).[5] The phase-two processes are called *conjugation reactions,* and the toxins created during phase one are joined together with other molecules so they are less reactive (and not as dangerous). As with phase one, a healthy diet that includes sufficient nutrients and phytochemicals supports these processes.[6]

Finally, it's on to phase three, which is known as the "liver drainage" phase. The water-soluble toxins are either moved into your blood, filtered through your kidneys and eliminated in your urine, or moved into your bile, released into your digestive tract, and then excreted through your stools.

It's important to understand: if your liver's detoxification system is overtaxed—because toxins are coming in faster than your liver can process them, your liver function is damaged, or you're not taking in sufficient nutrients to support these processes—it can't do everything you're asking it to do. When this type of overload occurs, liver function may become compromised and toxins may accumulate in the body, which can lead to impaired organ function and an increased risk of chronic disease. It can also affect your body's ability to burn fat efficiently and lead to weight gain.

As we already learned, one of the best things we can do to help the liver is purposefully put fewer toxins into our bodies, and we can also help by providing the important nutrients it needs to support its important detoxification work, which are found in foods such as leafy greens, cruciferous vegetables, and others. More about that in the next chapter. No special "detox" protocol required.

How does alcohol factor in?

Over 90 percent of the alcohol you consume must be processed by the liver, and if your liver is busy processing alcohol, other important functions come to a halt.[7] Alcohol always goes to the front of the line and must be processed first before your liver can move on to other things.[8] So, if you are hoping to have efficient detoxification, this is important to understand.

No one is more disappointed about this fact than I am. If you read my first book, *Delay, Don't Deny*, you may remember that I shared with joy that I had one perfect glass of prosecco with dinner every night. Since that time, however, I have realized that genetically I am a slow alcohol metabolizer, which means it takes my body even more time to process alcohol than average. Digging in my heels, I ignored that information for a long time, until I finally realized that if I wanted to feel my best, I would need to have a lot less alcohol in my life and that it shouldn't be a daily indulgence for me.

Because I am clean(ish), I am not going to *never have alcohol again*. But, because I am clean(ish), I want to live a lifestyle that supports my body's detoxification pathways. Consuming alcohol daily doesn't do that, unfortunately. For me, alcohol has become an infrequent treat rather than a nightly indulgence.

THE KIDNEYS

The kidneys are second only to the liver when it comes to importance as a detoxification organ and in the removal of toxins. Every day, they filter our blood about sixty times.

Much of the kidneys' work is to filter out many of the endogenous toxins that are produced within our bodies as a part of our metabolic processes, such as ammonia, urea, uric acid, and creatinine, as well as the toxins produced by phase-two liver detoxification. Besides those internal toxins, the kidneys also filter out a variety of toxins that come into our bodies, such as heavy metals (cadmium, chromium, lead, mercury, platinum, and uranium, which are all damaging to our kidneys) or POPs (such as fluorinated hydrocarbons or glyphosate) that we learned about in part 1. Even medications we take, such as nonsteroidal anti-inflammatory drugs (NSAIDs), may affect the way our kidneys function over time.[9]

In the case of many of these chemicals, if the toxic particles are too large, they don't pass through the filtration system easily. Cadmium, for example, is one heavy metal that may build up in the kidneys over time and cause long-term damage. As we age, and especially if this type of long-term damage has occurred, our bodies end up with decreased kidney function, which allows both endogenous and exogenous toxins to continue to build up over time. One estimate I read said that by the age of ninety, most of us have only one-third to one-half of the kidney function that we had when we were twenty, which means that we have a decreased ability to rid the body of many toxins (including the ones that build up naturally as by-products of the body's metabolic processes).[10]

Have you noticed the rise in dialysis centers popping up in neighborhoods near you? The CDC estimates that as many as 15 percent of adults in the U.S. now have chronic kidney disease.[11] Clearly, we want to prevent the type of damage that leads to kidney disease so our kidneys can do the important work we need them to do.

One of the most important things we can do is to limit the flow of new toxins coming *in*. We can also support our kidneys by taking in important nutrients that help them function more efficiently. Beetroot juice, chocolate, blueberries, turmeric, ginkgo biloba, ginger: all those foods have been shown to either protect or improve kidney function in studies. Does that mean that this is a complete list of exactly what you need to add to your diet to keep your kidneys working well? No. As I will discuss in greater detail in the next chapter, foods have thousands of compounds within them, and we can't isolate which are the "magical" ones. Eating a variety of plant foods, with the complete spectrum of nutrients found within plants, is our best bet.[12]

THE LUNGS

Our lungs are incredibly important, and we rely on them to supply oxygen to our cells. Every cell uses oxygen throughout the day to function. Our brain cells start to die when deprived of oxygen, and this can occur as soon as within five minutes.[13]

While we understand that in the case of drowning or suffocation, death can occur within minutes, poorly functioning lungs can lead to a condition called *chronic hypoxia,* which is when not enough oxygen is coming into the body's tissues on an ongoing basis.[14] Not only does this lead to diminished brain function, but the rest of the body also can't function properly without adequate oxygen.[15]

So, what does this have to do with self-cleaning? Our lungs are an important detoxification organ, designed to filter out toxins from the air we inhale and also to release waste products such as carbon dioxide as we exhale. This starts as soon as the air enters our noses (thank you, nose hairs), and continues as the air comes into our lungs through a series of tubes that branch off and get smaller and smaller . . . Visualize an upside-down tree with its many branches. The tiniest tubes are about the same thickness as a human hair.

As the air comes in, our lungs filter out both carbon dioxide and other airborne toxins. Unfortunately, our lungs become damaged over time when too many contaminants come in. We have all seen the images of smokers' lungs, blackened and damaged. (The relatively new practice of vaping may even be worse, though long-term effects are still not widely known.)[16]

If you've ever changed your HVAC's dirty filter, you can visualize what happens within your lungs when you're breathing in excessive levels of polluted air. And since research shows that the health risks from exposure to indoor air pollution may be greater than those related to outdoor pollution, it's more important than ever to make sure that we are clean(ish) when it comes to our indoor air quality. Breathing in chemical-laden air within our homes is something we can avoid through the use of air purifiers, houseplants, and by choosing safe household and personal care products.[17]

Both regular exercise and targeted breathing exercises can help improve the function of your lungs.[18,19] Proper nutrition can also help our respiratory system function optimally. Scientific evidence tells us that the nutrient-deficient Western diet (full of ultra-processed foods) is linked to overall poor respiratory health, while a diet high in nutrients (including vitamin C, vitamin E, flavonoids—found in a variety of plant foods, vitamin D, minerals, etc.) is protective.[20]

Overall, just as with our other detoxification pathways, the key to better lung health is this: we want to have fewer *toxins* coming in, while we support our bodies' self-cleaning mechanisms by putting more *nutrients* in.

THE SKIN

Our skin is our largest organ, and we each have an average of twenty-one square feet of it, weighing in at about nine pounds—and it renews itself every forty to fifty-six days or so. It's also an important detoxification pathway.[21] In addition, studies suggest that the skin may play a role in the body's total antioxidant defense.[22]

While the skin provides somewhat of a barrier between the body and surrounding environment, our skin is porous, with tiny openings that let things come in and also go out. That's one reason why it is so important to be careful with what you put onto your skin. Studies show that the absorption of chemicals through the skin may represent the most significant exposure pathway for most of us, and many commonly used chemicals enter the bloodstream and eventually may cause health problems. Carefully choosing our personal care and household cleaning products can make a great deal of difference here.[23]

Besides being concerned with what gets in through our skin, we also need to ensure that our skin is able to let things out. We eliminate toxins through our skin through the action of our sweat glands, and when analyzing sweat, scientists found small amounts of drugs and medications, VOCs, and even toxic metals, such as arsenic, cadmium, lead, and mercury.[24,25] One study found that many toxic elements seem to be preferentially excreted through sweat.[26]

A sedentary and climate-controlled modern lifestyle in which we never sweat leads to a decrease in our skin's ability to excrete toxins. There's even some evidence that this may play a role in obesity, and scientists are studying the role of the skin in systemic metabolic disorders.[27] This may be because decreased levels of skin detoxification have been linked to an increased risk for oxidative stress and insulin resistance.[28]

So, to harness your skin's detoxification power, you need to make time to sweat. Exercise is one way to make that happen, of course, but taking a hot bath or spending time in a sauna are also excellent strategies.

UNSUNG HERO: THE LYMPHATIC SYSTEM

Many people don't know much about the lymphatic system, though most of us recognize the experience of having swollen lymph nodes when we are sick. The spleen, tonsils, and thymus are all part of this system.

The lymphatic system is important because it's your body's waste-management system—think of it as the sewer system for your body. Much like the circulatory system, which branches through all parts of your body to distribute blood, the lymph system travels through a complex network of lymphatic vessels, nodes, organs, and tissues. Unlike your circulatory system, which is powered by your heart, your lymphatic system has no pump.

Your lymphatic system works together with your circulatory system and your immune system, sweeping away a wide variety of cellular waste and toxins and transporting this "sewage" to the liver and kidneys to be processed and eliminated. Not only does it remove excess fluids and waste products from your tissues, it also delivers nutrients to your cells. When waste products begin to accumulate and build up faster than they can be eliminated, we see it through water retention, general puffiness, and, in extreme cases, dramatic swelling referred to as *lymphedema*. We are also learning that there's a link between a poorly functioning, sluggish, or overburdened lymphatic system and metabolic syndrome.[29]

I'm about to give you some shocking information: a Western diet high in ultra-processed foods is linked to poor lymphatic system performance.[30] Okay, I was only kidding; I know that by now, this information isn't shocking. Based on what we have learned so far, we should expect that a Western diet is linked to negative health outcomes everywhere we look. On the flip side, a high intake of polyphenols, which are compounds found in plants, is known to have a beneficial effect on lymphatic function.

One of the best ways to keep your lymph system flowing and promote lymphatic circulation is through movement. Hippocrates may be best known for his quote "Let food be thy medicine and medicine be thy food," but he also is quoted as having said, "Walking is the best medicine." Walking is an excellent way to get your lymphatic fluid moving.[31] Personally, I use a vibration platform and also a rebounder as part of my regular exercise routine, and both of those are great at keeping the lymphatic fluid moving. Dry brushing, which is just what it sounds like—you use a stiff-bristled brush to gently brush your skin—is also recommended as a way to stimulate the lymphatic system—and it feels great while you do it.[32]

THE GLYMPHATIC SYSTEM

No, that isn't a typo. We also have something called the *glymphatic system*, which is connected to the lymphatic system. Because it works through the glial cells of the central nervous system, it was first called the *glial-lymphatic* system, but is now simply known as the *glymphatic* system.

The glymphatic system is the brain's waste management system. While we are sleeping, our brains have the ability to flush out toxins (including excess proteins) that build up during the waking hours.[33] Since it works while we are asleep, it's one more reason why we need to make sure that we get sufficient sleep.[34] Sleep as a detoxification strategy?[35] Sign me up!

If the glymphatic system doesn't work properly, toxins can build up in our central nervous system and within the brain itself. This may be a factor in a number of neurodegenerative diseases such as Alzheimer's disease.

Besides sleep, exercise helps the glymphatic system work efficiently, just as it does with the lymphatic system. This is one more reason why our modern sedentary lifestyle leads to negative health outcomes in general.

IT ALL ENDS AT THE COLON

Detoxification includes all our bodies' self-cleaning mechanisms, and we need to keep all these various pathways and systems working so our bodies can remove contaminants and waste products effectively. The digestive system plays a huge role in the removal of waste products, and we all know how awful it feels when that waste gets backed up. "You're full of it" is more than just a figure of speech, am I right?

It's important to keep your bowels moving regularly, as this process is essential for us to expel both waste and toxins from our bodies. While it all ends at the colon, however, it doesn't begin there.

As with our bodies' other self-cleaning systems, the digestive system requires a variety of foods and nutrients to support its various functions, including detoxification. First, we need our foods to be well digested and absorbed, so the essential nutrients found within them can reach the parts of the body where they are needed. Natural enzymes found within the food itself play a key role in this process. These enzymes are found in a variety of foods such as fruits and vegetables, fermented foods, and honey.

The closer a food is to its natural form, the more likely it is to retain the enzymes we rely on for digestion. One example is wheat. When you grind wheat berries (which is the cheerful name for *wheat grains*) into flour, you end up with whole wheat flour that still retains all the components that were within the original wheat grain. This includes the bran, the germ, and the endosperm. Industrial milling, on the other hand, removes the bran and the germ and subjects the endosperm to all sorts of treatments: heat, bleaching, and the "enrichment" process to add back in necessary vitamins. This gives consumers and food manufacturers a shelf-stable white flour that is the foundation for most modern-day baking. But we have lost the protein, the fiber, the flavor, and the natural enzymes that were part of the original package prior to refining. This ultra-processed not-food is a far cry from freshly milled wheat flour.[36]

When food is not digested well, this becomes a problem as the food moves through the intestinal tract. We know that undigested foods and other toxins within your digestive system can cause chronic systemic inflammation as they travel along.[37] This is one reason why we must feed our gut microbiomes well, because they play a key role in the digestive process. The foods we eat determine the composition of our intestinal microbiota, because whichever part of the microbial population we feed is the part that grows stronger.

Efficient digestion relies on our gut-bug communities. Eating a diet rich in foods that support gut health, such as fermented foods, prebiotic and probiotic foods, fibrous fruits and veggies, and so on, ensures that we are feeding the gut microbiome well and also helps your intestines to remove waste effectively. It's probably no surprise to learn that the Western diet feeds the type of gut community that we do *not* want to promote.[38]

The intestinal lining itself has an important role as a barrier against harmful compounds in transit, including microorganisms and toxic chemicals.[39] When this barrier is damaged, these harmful compounds and microbes are able to escape from the intestine, which may trigger a systemic inflammatory response. Many autoimmune diseases are related to this type of damage within our intestinal tract. You may have heard of this referred to as *leaky gut*. What causes leaky gut? That pesky Western diet again.[40]

You may have heard someone say that plant foods and dietary fibers are *damaging* to a healthy gut, but that is actually not true—the key word being *healthy*. Increasing dietary fiber can strengthen your gut lining over time. Let's hear it straight from a 2016 study:[41]

> A study comparing a standard rodent diet (fiber from wheat, corn, and oats comprising 4.3% of the diet by weight) with a diet devoid of any fiber showed that mice fed the fiber-deficient diet had a thinner mucus layer, thus allowing microbes to come in closer proximity to the gut epithelium. Without sufficient amounts of [dietary fiber] in the gut, bacteria may degrade the host mucus layer in order to provide themselves with the substrates necessary to survive, thus breaking down one of the host's physical barriers.

Yes, they were rodents, but these scientists believe these findings can also be applied to humans.

This concept can be really confusing because you've likely read books, blogs, or social media posts that tell you certain types of plant fiber are harmful to your gut lining. In fact, there are many dietary protocols (Paleo, just to name one) that eschew certain plant foods such as grains and legumes, considering them to be damaging to our gut linings and, therefore, our overall health.

Like many people's relationship statuses, however, "it's complicated." If you spent years eating the Western diet, it's likely your gut lining is less healthy than it should be. As that rodent study showed, when there isn't enough dietary fiber, your gut bacteria actually consume your mucus layer instead, leading to a damaged gut barrier. When that happens, too much fiber can indeed cause all sorts of problems, because your gut lining has been damaged. It's a vicious cycle: not enough fiber caused gut damage, but when you add back in more fiber, the damaged gut can't handle it. In that situation, grains and legumes just might be a problem for many people, so that part is true.

Rather than blaming the fruits, vegetables, and grains themselves, however, understand that the root cause of the issues is the gut-lining *damage itself* and not the foods. The gut lining was damaged, and then these foods cause problems. A healthy gut, on the other hand, should be able to tolerate these foods. The good news is that you can heal.

For anyone with known or suspected gut issues, such as leaky gut, small intestinal bacterial overgrowth (SIBO), or irritable bowel syndrome (IBS), addressing gut health by rebuilding a healthy gut microbiome can really help you reduce your body's toxic load in many ways.[42]

Beyond digestion of food and maintaining a healthy gut lining, the digestive system plays a very important role in the detoxification process. Your feces are composed of a variety of things, such as water, protein, undigested fats, polysaccharides, bacterial biomass (both living and dead), and undigested food residues. Slow bowel transit time may result in an accumulation of toxins within the colon.[43] A healthy person should expect to have a bowel movement at least once per day, moving the waste right on out of our bodies on a regular basis.[44] Research shows that eating a diet high in dietary fiber keeps things moving, just as your grandmother probably told you.[45] And, no prunes required . . . though you absolutely can eat prunes if you love them.

ACTION PLAN: SUPPORTING YOUR BODY'S SELF-CLEANING ABILITIES

Use your Clean(ish) Journal (or the worksheets available at ginstephens .com/cleanish) to complete these end-of-chapter prompts and activities.

After reading this chapter, take some time to make a plan for how you can live a detoxification *lifestyle* by supporting your liver, kidneys, lungs, skin, lymphatic and glymphatic systems, and your colon.

Go back and reread each section of this chapter and consider changes you can make today that support these important self-cleaning pathways.

In your Clean(ish) Journal, make a plan for each of your body's self-cleaning pathways by writing a few sentences to complete each one of these.

What I can do:

- to support my liver:

- to support my kidneys:

- to support my lungs:

- to support my skin:

- to support my lymphatic system:

- to support my glymphatic system:

- to support my colon:

Putting it all together:

- What can I do to support my entire body as it self-cleans, fostering an environment where each organ and system is working together to perform all the important detoxification tasks my health depends on?

WHAT'S FOOD GOT TO DO WITH IT?

Wait a minute, why is there another chapter on food? Didn't we spend a great deal of time talking about food in the last part of the book? Isn't food something that belongs solely in the "What Goes In" section of the book?

No, because food is an essential part of the "what comes out" side of the equation, as well.

Let food be thy medicine and medicine be thy food.

—Hippocrates

In the modern world, we have lost much of the traditional food wisdom, going from being intimately connected to our food (growing, harvesting, and preparing our own food) to becoming consumers of industrially produced food products.

Real foods—of both plant and animal origin—have therapeutic effects, protecting us against diseases such as cancer, diabetes, obesity, heart disease, and others. In this chapter, we will learn about all the amazing things foods do for us—besides simply tasting delicious and filling up our bellies. The chemicals we need to run the amazing machines that are our bodies are found within real food. Our bodies can't process toxins without adequate nutrition, so we must support our bodies with a nutritious diet to harness our true self-cleaning power and support our self-cleaning systems.[1]

WHAT ROLE DO FOODS PLAY IN OUR BODIES' SELF-CLEANING PROCESSES?

In the last chapter, I mentioned that our self-cleaning systems rely on support from nutrients found within our foods. Our natural detoxification pathways aren't able to do their work without this nutritional support, in fact.

As an example, we learned that the liver is an important detoxification pathway in the body and we need it to function properly for us to "self-clean" as required. The liver doesn't work alone—it requires support from the foods we eat. These nutrients are literally *required* for our livers to function optimally, and if you aren't taking in these required nutrients, your liver can't do its best work.[2]

Here are some of the nutrients our livers require to perform their important tasks:[3]

Riboflavin (Vitamin B$_2$)	Phospholipids	Thiols
Niacin (Vitamin B$_3$)	Carotenes (Vitamin A)	Bioflavonoids
Pyridoxine (Vitamin B$_6$)	Ascorbic acid (Vitamin C)	Silymarin
Folic acid	Tocopherol (Vitamin E)	Pycnogenol glycine
Vitamin B$_{12}$	Selenium	Taurine
Glutathione	Copper	Glutamine
Branched-chain amino acids	Zinc	Ornithine
Flavonoids	Manganese	Arginine
	Coenzyme Q10	

Many of those nutrients may be familiar to you, but you may not know what all of them are or where to get them. At the end of this chapter, you will understand where to get the nutrients you need, and it isn't as complicated as you may be thinking. Heck, let me go ahead and tell you the secret now:

Eat a variety of real foods.

Notice I didn't say, "Eat a few special foods that will solve all your problems." Thanks to sensational headlines, we have become conditioned to believe that there are magical foods that can provide us with specific benefits that are greater than other "ordinary" foods. Açai berries? Quinoa? Kale? Magical!

While writing this chapter, I did an experiment just to see if I could find some examples of these types of sensational headlines. Which food should I research? Hm. Lots of options.

Most of us would agree that blueberries are probably good for us, right? I've certainly seen them referred to as "superfoods" more than once. So, I took a few minutes to see what recent headlines could tell us about the humble blueberry.

According to the recent news headlines about blueberries:

The One Food to Eat to Avoid Heart Disease, According to RDs,[4] February 9, 2021

> *Really? There is one food that will help you avoid heart disease??? And it's blueberries??? I think it's really cool that we have finally found the missing link in the mystery of how to avoid heart disease! Who knew it was so simple??? Hooray for blueberries!*

How to Live Longer: Blueberries May Reduce Age-Related Diseases to Boost Longevity,[5] February 17, 2021

> *I'm going to live longer by eating blueberries? It sounds like the fountain of youth is blueberries!*

Daily Blueberry Consumption May Help Manage Diabetes, Study Finds,[6] October 20, 2020

It just gets better and better, doesn't it? Blueberries really are magical. Time to buy some blueberries.

From Improving Gut-Health to Managing Diabetes, 6 Reasons Why You Must Eat Blueberries,[7] June 24, 2020

*Wait, I **must** eat blueberries? Is there no other way to improve my gut health or manage diabetes other than blueberries? That seems odd.*

Blueberry-Enriched Diet May Help Women's Muscle Growth, Repair: Study,[8] August 6, 2020

It DOES get better and better! We all want more muscle. Hmmm. Wait a minute. Upon reading the study, it appears the study participants ate almost two cups of blueberries a day. That's a lot of blueberries.

Single Dose Of Blueberry Polyphenols Boosts Cognitive Performance in Middle Aged Adults,[9] August 5, 2020

But! This article tells me I only need a single dose! Wow!

Are blueberries healthy? Surely. Do they have many potential health benefits? Yes. Are they the one superfood that can cure all your ills? No.

Why do blueberries get all the press? According to Dr. Barbara Shukitt-Hale, a nutrition researcher and blueberry expert, "It may be just because blueberries are one of the more well-studied fruits," she said. "I don't know if you studied, say, peaches, if it would be the same."[10] In the article where Dr. Shukitt-Hale was interviewed about blueberries, she went on to make this recommendation: "I think they're one of the healthiest fruits," she said. "But eating a wide range of fruits and vegetables, that's your best bet."

Even one of the world's premiere blueberry experts agrees: while there is no denying that blueberries are part of a healthy diet and lifestyle, our "best bet" comes from eating a *variety* of fruits and vegetables.

Just as we can't point to any one potentially dangerous chemical and say, "This is the one that is the root of all our health problems," because the effects of chemical exposures are cumulative and synergistic, we also can't point to any one *food* and say, "This is the one magical food that will make us all better." We can't even say, "This is the one magical component within food that will solve all our problems." No, the beneficial chemicals in our foods don't work independently, they work synergistically. Even when it comes to blueberries.

"Nutritionism" is when we fixate on individual nutrients and ignore the truth about food: food really is the sum of its parts. A carrot is so much more than just a vehicle for beta-carotene. It has many other powerful compounds within it, such as fiber, vitamin K_1, potassium, and various antioxidants. Let's take some time to understand the powerful role these compounds play in our bodies' self-cleaning processes.

WHY ARE PLANT FOODS SO HEALTHY?

Foods play a role in removing toxins from our bodies. As an example, coriander, citrus fruits, and chlorella all exhibit natural chelating properties, and therefore, they assist our bodies in the removal of toxic metals such as cadmium and lead. Chlorella also appears to help with the removal of POPs.[11]

No, that still doesn't mean that coriander, citrus fruits, and chlorella are the three magical foods that will solve every problem we have.

Plants have many thousands of compounds within them: vitamins, minerals, and medicinal chemicals called *phytonutrients,* as well as lots of fiber, and all of this means that they are powerful tools within our self-cleaning toolboxes.

Let's understand what all these chemicals do for us.

Phytochemicals:

> *Phytochemicals are any biologically active compounds found in plants.*
>
> Scientists estimate there are over five thousand phytochemicals, and we don't even know what they all do. That's one reason why it's difficult to make effective supplements: if we don't know what all these chemicals are doing, we certainly don't know which ones to put into supplements. And we can't do a better job than real food, even when we try.[12]

Polyphenols:

> *Polyphenols are an example of phytochemicals.*
>
> Polyphenols are a large family of naturally occurring compounds found in plants *(that all happen to contain more than one phenolic hydroxyl group, hence the* phenol *in the name, which doesn't mean anything to me, but my chemist husband gets it).*

Antioxidants:

> *Polyphenols can act as antioxidants in the body.*
>
> Antioxidants are substances that can prevent or slow damage to cells caused by free radicals, which are unstable molecules that the body produces as a reaction to environmental and other stressors.

PHYTOCHEMICALS

Have you ever heard "Eat the rainbow"? No, not "Taste the rainbow," the slogan for Skittles. We want to eat the rainbow of real foods from nature. Plant-based foods get their colors from pigments that typically correspond to a phytonutrient category. As an example, orange foods tend to be high in beta-carotene, green foods are high in chlorophyll, and purple foods are high in flavonoids.[13]

What are phytochemicals? They are naturally occurring compounds in plant foods, such as fruits, vegetables, whole grains, beans, nuts, and seeds. Many phytochemicals act as antioxidants, neutralizing free radicals and removing their power to create damage.

POLYPHENOLS FOR THE WIN

Plants are healthy, and (almost) everyone agrees. One of the reasons has to do with the polyphenols found in plants. There are more than eight thousand types of polyphenols that have been identified, but they fall into four main groups:[14,15,16,17,18,19]

Type	Intake Is Protective Against . . .	Where Do We Find Them?
Flavonoids	Inflammation, high blood pressure, cancer, liver disease	Fruits, vegetables, legumes, apples, onions, dark chocolate, red cabbage, tea, cacao, beer, wine
Phenolic acids	Diabetes, cancer, inflammation, ulcers, heart disease, liver disease, neurological conditions	Fruits, vegetables, whole grains, seeds
Stilbenes	Neurological diseases, obesity, cancer, diabetes, atherosclerosis, high blood pressure, cardiovascular diseases	Grapes, red wine, peanuts, legumes, berries, rhubarb, passion fruit, white tea
Lignans	Heart disease, menopausal symptoms, osteoporosis, breast cancer	Seeds (particularly sesame and flax), cashews, grains, olive oil, a wide variety of fruits and vegetables

Polyphenols are typically a part of the plant's defense system and are also involved in the defense against ultraviolet radiation or a variety of pathogens. Many of these compounds evolved as toxins within the plant, designed to repel insects and other predators. That sounds scary. We are eating plant toxins? Yes, but we consume them at what's known as *subtoxic* doses. *Hormesis* is a process in which we receive benefits from low doses of something that would be toxic at higher doses.[20] Think back to the exercise example I used earlier. When we are building muscle, we experience micro-tears in our muscle fibers. As the muscle heals post-workout, the body builds it back stronger than it was before. So, these micro-tears are an important part of the muscle-growth process and not something to be scared of. Exercise is a hormetic stress, meaning the low level of stress caused by exercise has a positive effect on our bodies overall.[21] The same can be said for what happens when we take in these plant chemicals: they have a protective effect at the dose that is found within our foods.

In general, anything that is considered to be a hormetic stress tends to have a positive effect on the aging process. These mild stresses force the body to respond to what is a minor threat, leading to an enhanced ability over time to cope with more severe stresses and resist disease.[22] This is why we can ignore any book that tells us to avoid plant foods because they have scary-sounding chemicals that may be bad for us in large doses. In the doses we consume within our foods, they are not only *not bad* for us, they are *very good* for us.

Both epidemiological studies and meta-analyses of research studies (which is when scientists review all the studies on a subject to draw overall conclusions) suggest that long-term consumption of a diet rich in plant polyphenols offers protection against development of cancers, cardiovascular diseases, diabetes, osteoporosis, and neurodegenerative diseases, among other things.[23]

We get the polyphenols our bodies need from consuming a diet high in plant foods overall: fruits, vegetables, whole grains, nuts, seeds, legumes, spices and seasonings, and also beverages such as coffee, tea, and red wine.

Research on phytochemicals has found several that are either equally as effective or *more effective* for lowering inflammation than typical anti-inflammatory drugs such as ibuprofen. These phytochemicals also regulate a variety of protective mechanisms within the body and regulate cell growth.[24]

WHAT ABOUT ANTIOXIDANTS?

Where do we find antioxidants? Plant polyphenols act as antioxidants in the body and counter the harmful effects of oxidative stress on the body.

There's not any one magical antioxidant that has been found to be useful in isolation. Instead, we find benefits from increasing the intake of antioxidant-rich foods in general. These compounds are designed to protect every part of the plant's cells against oxidative damage, in ways we may not even fully understand, and these benefits also transfer to *us* when we eat them.

Besides being delicious, herbs and spices are especially beneficial. Some spices have been studied for their relationship to health, such as turmeric and ginger, but many others, such as clove, oregano, and thyme, are also known to have high levels of antioxidants. In general, plants that have been used traditionally as herbal or traditional "medicines" tend to be the highest antioxidant-containing foods available.[25]

THE POWER OF ENZYMES

In the last chapter, I briefly mentioned the role of enzymes within our foods. Not only do we take in enzymes within our foods themselves, but we have other types of enzymes that occur within our bodies.

Our metabolic enzymes play a role in all body processes and also help us neutralize toxins, changing them into less toxic forms. Digestive enzymes are mostly made in the pancreas, and they help us break down our foods. Food enzymes come from foods themselves. The enzymes present in raw foods (including raw foods that have been fermented) help start the process of digestion.

Enzymes help speed up chemical reactions in the human body. They bind to molecules and alter them in specific ways. They are essential for respiration, digesting food, muscle and nerve function, among thousands of other roles.[26]

For enzymes to work effectively in the body, we must have adequate vitamins and minerals present. Where do we get "adequate vitamins and minerals"? From eating a wide variety of foods from day to day.

WHY IS FIBER IMPORTANT?

Remember that plants feed us, but they also feed our gut microbiomes. We talked about this in the last chapter. Our gut microbiomes are made up of a community of up to one hundred *trillion* bacteria, along with other microbes such as fungi, parasites, and a few mini viruses. That sounds absolutely horrifying if you have always thought of bacteria, fungi, parasites, and viruses as the enemy of health. Actually, though, we count on the symbiotic relationship we have with the various things that live in our guts.[27]

The microbes that live inside of us are each capable of producing hundreds of chemicals of their own, powered by the foods (and chemicals) that we send down to them through our eating and drinking. These chemicals they produce regulate our immune systems, affect our mood, and even our appetites. According to Dr. Tim Spector:[28]

Thousands of food chemicals interact with thousands of different microbe species to produce over 50,000 chemicals that affect most aspects of our body. When we consume food, it is as much for the benefit of our gut microbes as it is for us.

How important is dietary fiber? We know that it alters the gut, which specifically affects intestinal, liver, and kidney functions, all of which are key players in our bodies' detoxification systems. Low dietary fiber intake is also linked to conditions such as diabetes, cardiovascular disease, nonalcoholic fatty liver disease (NAFLD), and chronic kidney disease (CKD).[29]

CHOOSING FOODS TO SUPPORT DETOXIFICATION

We want to include foods that have the important phytochemicals we need, including polyphenols and antioxidants. We also need to make sure we have plenty of naturally occurring enzymes and also sufficient fiber within our diets. When we include a wide variety of plant foods, we ensure that we are getting all these components within our foods.

Here are some of the foods that support our bodies' self-cleaning processes:[30]

Food	How Does This Food Support Self-Cleaning?
Nuts and seeds	Great sources of fiber
Proteins	Provide a source of amino acids necessary for phase-one and phase-two detoxification
Legumes	Great source of fiber and also a source of amino acids for phase-one and phase-two detoxification
Fruits	Contain a variety of phytonutrients essential for detoxification and are a great source of fiber
Whole grains	Provide both soluble and insoluble fiber, which are beneficial for intestinal health
Vegetables	Contain a variety of phytonutrients essential for detoxification and are a great source of fiber, just like fruits Vegetables also provide antioxidant support and support both phase-one and phase-two detoxification
Herbs and spices	These tend to be the highest antioxidant-containing foods available

Now those are some "superfoods" you can count on!

ORGANIC FOODS HAVE MORE NUTRIENTS

If you don't remember the details, go back to the "Food, Glorious Food" chapter, but I want to remind you of something very important here:

> Organic foods contain more nutrients and phytochemicals (that's good for us) and also fewer toxins (that's *also* good for us). More of what we want and less of what we don't. Even if the amounts are small, remember that small amounts add up over time.

So, when you are choosing foods to be a part of your self-cleaning arsenal, choose organic foods whenever you can. It makes a difference.

REFLECT AND TAKE ACTION: CONSIDER YOUR DIET DIVERSITY AND FOCUS ON NUTRIENTS

Use your Clean(ish) Journal (or the worksheets available at ginstephens .com/cleanish) to complete these end-of-chapter prompts and activities.

Look back at the chart on page 196 that lists the types of foods that support detoxification within the body.

What does your overall intake of these foods look like? Think about the past seven days and write down what you ate, but *only write down those foods that would fit into the NOVA classification scale in groups 1–3*. Record individual foods such as nuts, meats, whole grains, greens, beans, tomatoes, carrots, apples, oatmeal, potatoes, and even recipes such as hummus, guacamole, salads, soups . . . but don't include ultra-processed foods such as potato chips, crackers, hot dogs, pasta, and so on. We rarely eat foods in isolation, so consider the individual ingredients within what you're eating.

Don't overthink this; if you aren't sure what to write down, do your best. I promise I'm not taking a grade.

Here's how I might record my day for today. I had a tomato sandwich on high-quality, whole-grain sprouted bread, and then for dinner, I plan to make a black bean and quinoa bowl with guacamole. The whole-grain bread that I choose is made from sprouted grains and legumes, so it's not what I would consider to be ultra-processed. The mayonnaise I put on my sandwich, however, is ultra-processed, so I didn't record it.

This is how I would record it:

1	Whole-grain sprouted bread, tomato, black beans, quinoa, onion, garlic, red bell pepper, zucchini, avocado

Now, it's your turn.

If you can't remember—and, HELLO, I get it—then you should plan to keep track of the foods that you eat for the next seven days and write them down day by day.

Day	Foods That Support My Body Nutritionally List only foods that fit into groups 1–3 on the NOVA food classification scale
1	
2	
3	
4	

5	
6	
7	

How did you do? Did you eat a wide variety of foods over the week, or did you find that you ate the same few things over and over? Write about it in your Clean(ish) Journal.

When you are planning what you will eat this week, find a new recipe that includes foods you don't normally eat, and add it to your weekly rotation. Focus on foods from plants so you increase your intake of the powerful phytochemicals and fiber found within these foods.

- In your journal, write down at least one new recipe to try.

This week when you are doing your grocery shopping, buy at least one or two items from the produce section that you haven't purchased or eaten in the past year.

- In your journal, write down what new items you plan to purchase.

INTERMITTENT FASTING:
A POWERFUL SELF-CLEANING TOOL

Intermittent fasting is one of the best—if not *the* best—self-cleaning tools that we have in our toolboxes. I'm going to explain why within this chapter, but first I want to give you a little background on what intermittent fasting entails. If you came across this book without first reading one of my earlier books about intermittent fasting (also known as IF), you may not know much about IF other than what you have heard on the news or from friends who have tried it. You may even be someone who tried it yourself and had limited to no success (and if that sounds like you, then you definitely need to read *Fast. Feast. Repeat.*, because I wrote it to help you understand how to develop an IF approach that works for you, and you'll likely understand what may have gone wrong before).

Whether you're completely new to IF or you're someone who dabbled in it before, I'm going to discuss the basics in this chapter, but to really understand how and why to live an intermittent fasting lifestyle, plan to read *Fast. Feast. Repeat.* It's called *The Comprehensive Guide to Delay, Don't Deny Intermittent Fasting* for a reason. This single chapter can't go into the depth that I went into in that book.

By the way, even if you are an experienced intermittent faster, I still recommend that you read *Fast. Feast. Repeat.* if you haven't read it yet. Why? Because of the conflicting information out there, there are several mistakes you may be inadvertently making. *Fast. Feast.*

Repeat. explains what those mistakes are and how to maximize your approach to help you meet your health and wellness goals.

INTERMITTENT FASTING BASICS

If you are new to IF, you may wonder: What exactly is intermittent fasting? Even if you eat three meals a day plus snacks like most people in our modern society, you are somewhat of a faster, whether you realize it or not. We all fast while we sleep, and we wake up every morning in the fasted state. Most intermittent fasters simply extend that fasted state throughout the day rather than eating a traditional breakfast in the morning. Just like everyone else, we break-fast, but it may be when most people are having their dinner. *Breakfast* literally means "break the fast." We all do it, just at different times of the day. For me, break-fast, which I usually eat in the late afternoon or early evening, really is the most important meal of the day!

There's a period of the day when intermittent fasters fast, sticking to clean-fast approved beverages only (plain water, black coffee, plain tea, and unflavored sparkling water), and there's a period of the day when we eat, which is called our *eating window.* IF is a flexible lifestyle that doesn't have to be exactly the same from day-to-day, but the most common eating windows vary between one and eight hours a day.

To illustrate how this looks, let's say someone follows an intermittent fasting lifestyle with a four-hour daily eating window. Since a day has twenty-four hours, twenty hours of each day would be spent fasting (including the time you are asleep), and all your eating for the day would take place during the consecutive four-hour eating window that you choose. We would call that approach 20:4, representing twenty hours of fasting and a four-hour eating window. Most people who use the daily eating window approach end up with anything between 16:8 (sixteen hours of fasting and an eight-hour eating window) and 23:1 (a twenty-three-hour fast and a one-hour eating window). Because it's a flexible lifestyle, your eating window can vary from day to day, based on your schedule and even your varying appetite.

Here's how this might look as a day in my life. Every morning, I wake up and start the day with black coffee. After my coffee, I switch over to water and unflavored sparkling water until I am ready to eat. I usually open my eating window at some point between 2:00 and 5:00 p.m. with a snack of some type. A couple of hours later, I prepare dinner for my husband and me, and we eat together. After dinner, I will often have a dessert of some type, or just a little something sweet to close my window. Overall, my eating window usually lasts for somewhere between two and six hours most days.

The daily-eating-window approach isn't the only way to live an intermittent fasting lifestyle, and there are other options that involve longer fasts of up to thirty-six to forty-two hours. These are based on the concept of alternate daily fasting (ADF), which is a well-researched practice. True ADF would include a fast (or "down day") over a thirty-six-hour period followed by an "up" day with unrestricted eating, and the pattern would continue as: down day (fast), up day (feast), down day (fast), up day (feast).

You can even combine the two approaches into what I call a *hybrid approach,* where you choose a couple of days a week to be fasting days (which are always followed by up days) and then the remaining days are eating window days. A week following the hybrid approach might look like this:

Sunday	Monday	Tuesday	Wednesday	Thursday	Friday	Saturday
19:5 19 hours fasting, 5-hour eating window	Fasting Day	Up Day Eat 3 meals within 12 hours	19:5 19 hours fasting, 5-hour eating window	Fasting Day	Up Day Eat 3 meals within 12 hours	18:6 18 hours fasting, 6-hour eating window

Keep in mind that this chart is not designed to give you the impression that this is the "best" intermittent fasting schedule to follow. This is just one example of how someone might design a hybrid IF approach. IF is extremely flexible, and once you understand the various options, you can design a plan that fits your changing schedule and feels like a lifestyle you can continue forever.

Confused? Don't be. Once you read *Fast. Feast. Repeat.* it will make a lot more sense.

IS INTERMITTENT FASTING EXTREME OR DANGEROUS?

For people who have never heard of intermittent fasting or who don't understand the many health benefits that come along with the IF lifestyle, this type of schedule may seem bizarre or even possibly dangerous. What?!?!?! You go most of the day without eating? Every *day*? You might even fast for thirty-six hours? Don't you have headaches? Don't you collapse from lack of food? How do you have energy to do day-to-day tasks?

Many intermittent fasters have gotten the speeches from well-meaning friends and family members:

"Of course you're losing weight—you're starving yourself!"

"Everyone knows that breakfast is the most important meal of the day! You need energy to start your day."

"You must eat six small meals per day to keep your metabolism from shutting down!"

Not one of those statements is true, even though we have probably all heard them. You aren't starving yourself, you won't collapse without breakfast, and your metabolism will be just fine. Let's go through these one by one:

Are we starving ourselves? Absolutely not. My book is called *Fast. Feast. Repeat.* after all, not *Fast. Eat a Little Tiny Diet Meal. Repeat.* When I eat, I eat well, and that's true for most IFers. I choose foods that make me feel great, and I eat until I am satisfied. Back in my low-calorie days, whenever I wanted to lose a few pounds, I would restrict my calories throughout the day to about 1,200 (because that's what "they" said I should do), and *that* felt like I was starving myself. (In *Fast. Feast. Repeat.*, I go into a lot more detail about why IF is different from a typical low-calorie diet that you have probably tried before and why you are well-fueled during the fast rather than starving.)

In the research on ADF, they found that participants consumed an average of 125 percent of their bodies' energy needs on alternate "feast days." This means they ate *more* food than their body needed on their up days, so they clearly were not starving themselves. So, are we IFers starving ourselves? No, and the research backs that up.[1]

What about breakfast? Do we need breakfast first thing in the morning to fuel our bodies? That's what we have all been told. The surprising answer to that question is no. If you have ever been "hangry," you know the feeling. You need to eat NOW. Many people imagine that is what IF feels like. While it may feel like that over the brief adjustment period, once we are adapted, *hangry* goes away. The key is that we are well-fueled during the fast . . . by our fat stores, which are there for that very purpose. One of the most common things we hear from new IFers is that they can't believe how great they feel during the fast. Most of us are a lot less hungry while fasting than back in our low-calorie, frequent-small-meal days. The difference is astounding. Instead of getting worse over time, like most low-calorie diets, IF gets better and better as we adjust.

Will fasting slow our metabolic rates over time? The answer to that is also no. We have research that illustrates this. In one study, researchers followed participants over a seventy-two-hour fast.[2] They monitored the metabolic rates of the participants, as well as their levels of ketosis (which increases as fat burning goes up). According to the authors, the participants' resting metabolic rates *increased* after the first thirty-six hours of fasting. In addition, the participants saw no metabolic slowing from where they started, even through the seventy-second hour of fasting. (It is interesting to note that the metabolic rate increased from the twelve-hour point to the thirty-six-hour point, but it did slightly decline again as they headed toward the seventy-two-hour point. The overall metabolic rate at seventy-two hours was still slightly higher than that noted at twelve hours, however.)

The authors attribute the increased metabolic rate to the processes of gluconeogenesis and ketogenesis (which is how the body provides fuel when none is coming in). The body uses a lot of energy to carry out these processes, which may be the key to the slight metabolic boost we experience.

The takeaway from that study is this: scientists found that metabolic rate increased slightly between twelve to seventy-two hours of fasting. Metabolic shutdown? Clearly not! On the contrary, metabolic rate went UP from baseline!

In another research study, this one comparing ADF to a low-calorie diet, scientists found that participants' resting metabolic rates (RMR) decreased significantly in the low-calorie group, but not in the ADF group.[3] According to the scientists: "The apparent impact of ADF on preserving RMR during weight loss could have clinical significance in preventing weight regain after weight loss."

Now that we have a basic understanding of what intermittent fasting is, let's answer this question: How does intermittent fasting help us be more clean(ish)?

While most of us begin living an intermittent fasting lifestyle with the goal of losing weight, IF is about so much more than just weight management. Even if you never lost a pound, I am convinced that IF is one of the healthiest things you can do for your body. Instead of damaging your body or your metabolism, IF has the potential to improve your health in many ways. I actually like to call it the health plan with a side effect of weight loss.

It's such a powerful wellness approach that my husband lives an intermittent fasting lifestyle now, and it's strictly for the health benefits. Unlike many of us, he has never needed to lose weight, and he still fits into the same pants he wore at our wedding back in 1991 (annoying, right?). Based on what I have shared with him about the power of IF, he has decided to follow an eight-hour eating window most days, which gives him at least sixteen hours of daily fasting. During the workweek, he eats within an eight-hour eating window each day, although he is somewhat more flexible on the weekend when he wants to be.

So—what's so special about IF that an always-slim man would adopt it as his lifestyle? It's actually pretty exciting, and it is why I will be an intermittent faster for the rest of my life. Time to dive into the science behind IF!

As I already said, it's really one of the best—if not *the best*—self-cleaning tools we have in our toolboxes. Let me explain.

The biggest news in the intermittent fasting world was without a doubt the announcement of the 2016 Nobel Prize in Medicine. As written in the press release, Yoshinori Ohsumi "discovered and elucidated mechanisms underlying *autophagy,* a fundamental process for degrading and recycling cellular components."

That's a mouthful, so I want to take a minute to explain what that means.

Autophagy is one of our bodies' most powerful self-cleaning mechanisms, and it can be thought of as the recycling/upcycling system that takes place at the cellular level. In today's world, much of our modern lifestyle leads to a decrease in the amount of autophagy that goes on from day to day. Decreased autophagy is linked to neurodegenerative, infectious, and metabolic disorders, as well as cancer and aging, among other things.[4,5]

What stimulates autophagy in humans, you may ask? Lots of things do, such as calorie restriction, exercise, and deep, restorative sleep.[6] Also, certain things we take in tend to stimulate autophagy, including compounds such as resveratrol, coffee, and antioxidants in general.

But guess what *else* stimulates autophagy? If you guessed fasting, you are exactly right! Including intermittent fasting in our lives is one way to experience increased autophagy and the deep self-cleaning that goes along with it.

AUTOPHAGY: OUR SELF-CLEANING SUPERPOWER

Let's take a few minutes to understand what autophagy is, and why it is such a powerful self-cleaning mechanism.

Our bodies are designed to keep us going when times are tough, as our ancestors couldn't count on food to be available 24-7. When we have no food coming in, our bodies have to get creative with what's on hand. Think about it this way: if you haven't been to the grocery store in a while, you dig around in your pantry and fridge to find what might be hanging around, and you can make a meal out of that when you need to. Your body is the same way.

If there is no food coming in, your cells look around and see what's hanging around that may not be needed anymore. Rather than break down valuable muscle tissue, they look for old junky cell parts to break down and reuse. When we eat every few hours, however, our bodies never need to do this. Think about it like this: if you had a hot meal delivered to your doorstep every two hours or so, would you ever need to use up the leftovers in your fridge and pantry? It's only when nothing new is coming in that you need to scrounge around in the back corners, and our bodies operate much the same way.[7]

Fasting has been practiced for thousands of years and is part of most major religions. The first scientific report making the connection between reduced food intake and longevity came out in 1935. Now that we understand autophagy more, this makes sense.

Decreased autophagy is linked to the development of age-related diseases. Many of the known longevity-promoting interventions (eating less food overall, fasting, exercise, various antiaging compounds and substances) are shown to increase autophagy. The increase in autophagy seems to be key when understanding why they have a beneficial effect on longevity.[8]

Autophagy is a complex process, and research is still ongoing. Here are a few of the other exciting discoveries being made about autophagy, all taken from a 2019 review article "A Comprehensive Review of Autophagy and Its Various Roles in Infectious, Non-Infectious, and Lifestyle Diseases: Current Knowledge and Prospects for Disease Prevention, Novel Drug Design, and Therapy."[9] You can read that article in its entirety by searching for the title online.

Autophagy:

- suppresses the formation of tumors;

- clears away protein accumulation in the brain that can lead to neurodegenerative disorders such as Alzheimer's, Parkinson's, and Huntington's disease; and

- plays a beneficial role against infectious diseases by both boosting the immune system and degrading pathogens themselves.

In addition to what autophagy *does* do within our bodies, defects in autophagy pathways or autophagy-related genes are linked to a variety of autoimmune and autoinflammatory diseases, such as multiple sclerosis, lupus, rheumatoid arthritis, psoriasis, inflammatory bowel disease, diabetes, and Crohn's disease. This illustrates that when we don't have sufficient autophagy going on in our bodies, our health will likely suffer.

When we live an intermittent fasting lifestyle, we will have periods of the day—every day—where our bodies are focused on the important work of cellular housekeeping. While fasting, I love visualizing my cells hard at work taking out the cellular trash, keeping me healthy at the cellular level. Hooray for autophagy![10]

MORE GOOD NEWS ABOUT INTERMITTENT FASTING

In 2016, those of us in the intermittent fasting community were thrilled when the Nobel Prize in Medicine was awarded for research related to autophagy. We were even more excited in 2019, when Dr. Mark Mattson from Johns Hopkins University released a paper called "Effects of Intermittent Fasting on Health, Aging, and Disease" in *The New England Journal of Medicine*.[11] Rumor has it that *NEJM*, the world's leading medical journal, knew that doctors had been getting a lot of questions about intermittent fasting from their patients, and so they asked Dr. Mattson, as one of the world's leading experts on the health benefits of IF, to write a review article so physicians would have a resource from which to learn, so they could in turn share the information with patients. Is that rumor true? I don't know, but I sure hope it is. I certainly don't doubt that lots of people are discussing IF with their doctors, because the popularity of IF has exploded over recent years.

The article was released on December 26, and all the news outlets and TV shows ran lead stories about his findings. Intermittent fasting was suddenly on everyone's lips—and not as a weight-loss approach but as a way to live a healthy life. The tide turned that day; instead of being a "weight-loss diet," intermittent fasting firmly cemented itself in our minds as "a healthy lifestyle."

In it, Mattson (and his coauthor, Dr. Rafael de Cabo) highlight the importance of autophagy and the metabolic adaptations that occur after our bodies adjust to IF:[12]

Energy restriction for 10 to 14 hours or more results in depletion of liver glycogen stores and hydrolysis of triglycerides to free fatty acids in adipocytes . . . where they produce the ketone bodies acetoacetate and B-hydroxybutyrate . . . Reduced levels of glucose and amino acids during fasting result in reduced activity of the mTOR pathway and up-regulation of autophagy. In addition, energy restriction stimulates mitochondrial biogenesis and mitochondrial uncoupling.

That's a mouthful, but in plain-speak: when we fast, we deplete our liver glycogen stores, burn fat, get into ketosis, and experience increased autophagy. You may have thought that the only way to get into ketosis was to follow the keto diet, but fasting is actually even more ketogenic, and you're burning your own fat for fuel to make those ketones.

They found that intermittent fasting results in "lasting adaptive responses" that allow us to resist cellular damage and a wide range of stresses; it has positive health effects on obesity, insulin resistance, hypertension, and inflammation, and improves memory and may halt the progression of neurological diseases.

Within the *NEJM* article, Drs. Mattson and de Cabo outlined several clinical applications for intermittent fasting:[13]

- **Obesity and Insulin Resistance:** Intermittent fasting improves insulin sensitivity and is associated with weight loss.

- **Cardiovascular Disease:** Intermittent fasting improves blood pressure, resting heart rate, and levels of cholesterol, blood glucose, and insulin, all of which are indicators of cardiovascular health. It also reduces both systemic inflammation and oxidative stress, which are both associated with atherosclerosis.

- **Cancer:** Intermittent fasting is thought to inhibit the growth of cancer cells. IF also makes the cancer cells more susceptible to medical therapies.

- **Neurodegenerative Disorders:** Intermittent fasting may delay the onset and progression of Alzheimer's disease and Parkinson's disease. IF also increases stress resistance within our neurons and enhances processes that can prevent seizures.

- **Asthma, Multiple Sclerosis, and Arthritis:** Intermittent fasting led to improvements in asthma symptoms, reduced autoimmune demyelination related to MS, and lowers the inflammation that causes increased arthritis symptoms.

You know that I am not a doctor, so I hope I explained all those clinical applications correctly. If you want to read the article for yourself, as well as the sources that Drs. Matson and de Cabo used to write it, you can search for it online. It is available for free through the *NEJM* website, as long as you register for a free membership.

As I already mentioned, intermittent fasting really is the health plan with a side effect of weight loss.

NAIL THE CLEAN FAST: WHY AND HOW TO FAST CLEAN

If you decide that you want to live an intermittent fasting lifestyle to give your body time each day to self-clean, the number one nonnegotiable is this: when you fast, fast clean. Even though we are learning how to be clean(ish), when we fast, clean(ish) isn't enough. We want a squeaky-clean fast every time.

What is a clean fast? I have two chapters that explain it in *Fast. Feast. Repeat.*, so you can see it is more in-depth than I can go into here. To understand all the ins and outs, check out those chapters. In the meantime, I will briefly explain the three fasting goals here and tell you how to accomplish them. Once we understand the *goals* of the clean fast, we can easily understand how to make those things happen.

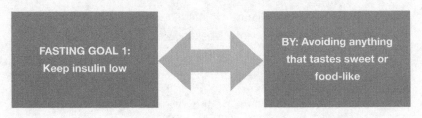

First, we want to keep insulin levels low while fasting so we can tap into fat stores for fuel. You see, insulin is anti-lipolytic, meaning that high levels of insulin prevent maximum fat burning. Fasting itself leads to lowered levels of insulin, whereas eating stimulates insulin release, which your body needs to manage the increased blood glucose levels that occur after we eat.

Besides actually eating, what else might stimulate an insulin release? This can happen anytime your brain thinks you are taking in foods. Sweet tastes are especially problematic because our brains associate sweetness with a source of sugar, and this can lead to a cephalic-phase insulin response that occurs in anticipation of the hit of glucose the body is now expecting from the sweet flavor. Insulin would be needed to manage that sugar load . . . except that sugar load never actually comes if we are consuming artificial sweeteners or artificially flavored, zero-calorie products.

To avoid having an insulin response, during the fast we *avoid* consuming any and all sweeteners (artificial or natural), flavored coffee or water (or anything that adds a food flavor, such as spices, lemon wedges, or apple cider vinegar, just to name a few examples), or herbal teas with a sweet or food-like flavor. Herbal teas with a bitter flavor profile would be okay, as a bitter flavor is not associated with an insulin response. This is also why plain tea and black coffee are okay during a clean fast; they have a bitter flavor profile. In addition to flavors, be cautious with supplements, especially any that are food-like.

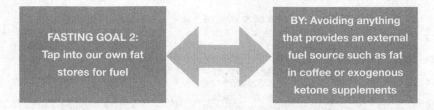

We also want to tap into our fat stores for fuel, and to do that, we avoid taking in anything that might be a source of fuel for our bodies during the fast. Don't add any fat to your morning coffee (or any milks, creamers, or the like) or take exogenous ketone supplements, as those are sources of fuel.

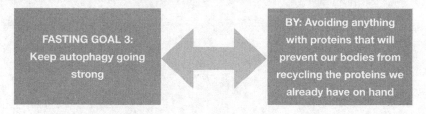

Finally, we want to make sure that we experience increased autophagy. We want our bodies to self-clean during the fast, as that is one of the most important benefits we are hoping for. To do that, we avoid taking in any source of protein during the fast, which would mean eliminating things like pre-workouts, bone broth, and so on. Protein stops autophagy in its tracks. We want our bodies to recycle our old, junky proteins, so we avoid any source of protein completely during the fast.

Now that we understand the three goals of the clean fast, this graphic illustrates it in more detail:

WHAT IS A "CLEAN FAST"?

Yes!	Maybe...	No!
• Water *(unflavored)*	*We call this the "grey area"*	• Food
• Black coffee *(unflavored)*	• Peppermint essential oil for breath freshening only, NOT for water-enhancing *(select food-grade and use sparingly)*	• Flavored water

• Any plain tea brewed from actual dried tea leaves only *(black tea, green tea, etc., unflavored varieties only)*	• Herbal tea with a bitter flavor profile	• Flavored coffee
	• Vitamins and supplements *(There is no easy answer for all vitamins and supplements. Any that are clearly food-like or listed in the "No" column should be taken within your eating window.)*	• Fruity, sweet, or matcha teas
• Mineral water, club soda, sparkling water, or seltzer water *(unflavored)*		• Diet sodas
		• Natural or artificial flavors
• Minerals/electrolytes/salt *(with no additives/flavors)*		• Natural or artificial sweeteners
		• Gum or mints
• Medications, as prescribed by your healthcare professional		• Food-like flavors of any type *(fruit juices, fruit flavors, etc.)*
		• Bone broth, broth, or bouillon
		• Added fats, including coconut oil, MCT oil, butter, etc.
		• Cream, creamers, milk *(of any amount or type)*
		• Supplements such as collagen, pre-workouts, BCAAs, exogenous ketones, etc.

Whenever you aren't sure if something is okay for the clean fast, take a look at the ingredients and compare them against this chart. If it has only ingredients from the "Yes" column, it's fine. If it has ingredients from the "No" column, you know it doesn't work. And if it is something in the gray area, it may or may not work for you.

INTERMITTENT FASTING: IS IT RIGHT FOR YOU?

After reading this chapter, you should now realize that intermittent fasting is not some radical new fad diet that is here today and gone tomorrow. Think about it: fasting is actually an ancient practice that is seen all around the world and in every major religion. The good news is that in intermittent fasting, you are not being asked to go forty days and forty nights without food; with most intermittent fasting plans, you are eating until you are satisfied every day, and the majority of people find that it's a lot more enjoyable than trying to eat tiny, unsatisfying meals spread throughout the day. Once you adjust, it's actually easier than typical diet plans that you've tried before. This is one of those things that most people don't believe until they try it for themselves.

Now you understand that intermittent fasting is a powerful way to allow your body to self-clean and that it is not only a healthy way to live, but it also isn't something to be scared of. There is most likely an intermittent fasting plan that will suit you, whether you are like my never-needed-to-lose-weight husband or someone who does want to lose a few pounds.

One caveat: fasting is not right for you if you are pregnant, breastfeeding, below the age of eighteen (and therefore not yet physically matured), or if you have an eating disorder that would serve as a contraindication to fasting.

As with any major lifestyle change, check with your doctor (or mental health counselor) if you aren't sure if fasting is right for you.

REFLECT AND TAKE ACTION: GIVING YOUR BODY TIME TO CLEAN

Use your Clean(ish) Journal (or the worksheets available at ginstephens .com/cleanish) to complete these end-of-chapter prompts and activities.

- Autophagy is a powerful self-cleaning tool, and intermittent fasting comes along with many health benefits that were described in this chapter. In fact, I like to call IF the health plan with a side effect of weight loss. Which of the health benefits appeal to you?

- If you have never tried intermittent fasting before, how do you feel about trying it now?

- If you did try intermittent fasting in the past but stopped doing it, think about why you stopped. Would you consider trying it again now? Why or why not?

- If you are someone who already incorporates intermittent fasting in your life, consider all the ways that it's a powerful self-cleaning mechanism and reflect upon your *why* for choosing it as a lifestyle. After reading this chapter, is your *why* reinforced?

If you are not currently incorporating intermittent fasting into your life, consider how you could make a few small changes that increase the number of hours you spend in the fasted state each day.

WHAT I AM DOING NOW

I usually eat all my food for the day between the hours of _____ and _____.

That means I currently have an eating window of about _____ hours from start to finish.

(For example, if you currently have breakfast at 8:00 a.m. and finish eating an evening snack by 9:00 p.m. each day, that would be an eating window of thirteen hours from start to finish.)

I could increase the amount of time in the fasted state each day by: *(select all that apply)*

Delaying my breakfast until _____ each day *(list your new time for breakfast)*.

Skipping breakfast and opening my eating window at lunchtime.

Closing my eating window by _____ each day *(list your new time to stop eating)*.

By making these changes, I would have an eating window of about _____ hours from start to finish.

That would mean I spend _____ more hours in the fasted state each day than I do currently.

To learn more about how to customize an intermittent fasting lifestyle that suits you, make sure to read *Fast. Feast. Repeat.: The Comprehensive Guide to Delay, Don't Deny Intermittent Fasting.* You'll learn how to design your intermittent fasting toolbox, how to "tweak it till it's easy," and how to make sure it's a long-term and sustainable lifestyle.

EXTRA CREDIT: MORE TOOLS FOR SELF-CLEANING

At this point in the book, we know that it's important to cut down on toxins that are coming *in* while also working to ensure that our bodies have a handle on what's going *out,* which we do by supporting our bodies' self-cleaning mechanisms through practices such as intermittent fasting and providing sufficient nutrients from the foods we eat. In this short chapter, we are going to take a brief look at a few additional tools you will want to add to your self-cleaning toolbox.

Here's some good news: every one of these tools is something you'll enjoy using. Supporting your body's self-cleaning and enjoying the process? Yes, please!

One thing to keep in mind as you read this chapter: not all things that are toxic to our bodies are chemical in nature. In this chapter, we will also learn about a few things that make our environment (or bodies) more "dirty" in ways you may not consider.

EXERCISE

Let's start with exercise. As I already mentioned, exercise is a powerful tool when it comes to elimination of toxins. When we exercise, we experience increases in circulation, respiration, and sweating.

Exercise is also essential when it comes to keeping your lymphatic system moving. Since your lymph system has no pump of its own, it relies on body movements to pump the fluid and keep it flowing. Walking is a simple and effective way to get things moving.

What are the best exercises to do? The answer to that is: do whatever forms of movement you enjoy. We want to include muscle-building activities and also those that increase your heart rate.

Overall, never forget that exercise boosts the effectiveness of most (if not all) of our bodies' elimination pathways, so find activities you love doing and make sure every day is an active day.

Just as we are not meant to eat the Western ultra-processed diet, we are not meant to be sedentary. There's a new saying: sitting is the new smoking. While I am not sure I would go that far, I do know that to live our healthiest and most vibrant lives, we need to get moving.

SAUNA

Besides exercising, using a sauna is another way to work up a good sweat. I am fortunate enough to have an infrared sauna in my garage, but they are also available in many health clubs and gyms for members to use.

Saunas have been used for hundreds of years, particularly in Scandinavian countries. In general:

> Existing evidence supports the use of saunas as a component of depuration (purification or cleansing) protocols for environmentally induced illness.[1]

What's *depuration*? It's another word for *detoxification*.

There are two types of saunas: radiant-heat saunas and infrared saunas. Of the two, infrared saunas are said to reach deeper into the body and promote a "deeper" level of sweating, leading to increased circulation throughout the body, as well as increased blood flow to the skin, which is the reason behind many of the proposed detoxification benefits. In one case study, a patient with high levels of mercury found that mercury levels normalized with repeated sauna use.

Overall, regular sauna use has shown beneficial effects on blood pressure and cardiovascular function, as well as a lower risk of cardiovascular mortality, sudden cardiac death, stroke, pulmonary diseases, and dementia.[2]

One study in particular found that a moderate to high frequency of sauna use was associated with lowered risks of dementia and Alzheimer's disease.[3] The scientists who conducted that study consider sauna use to be an effective strategy for improving cardiovascular function, which they feel can subsequently prevent or delay the development of neurogenerative diseases such as dementia. Is this related to the detoxification effects of the sauna? While it's not certain what the specific cause/effect is here, we do know that increased levels of environmental toxins are related to neurological diseases, so the relationship seems plausible.[4]

MASSAGE

Most of us have heard that massages are great for detoxification. I have bad news: evidence for this claim is lacking. While that doesn't mean massage is *not* a great detoxification strategy, we simply don't have the scientific evidence to support the concept that your standard massage is leading to detoxification benefits.

There is sufficient evidence that massages are effective for reducing anxiety and lowering blood pressure and heart rate in the short term.[5] Massage therapy has also been shown to reduce pain, anxiety, and muscular tension after surgery.[6] Neither of those are based on detoxification claims, however.

We do have research related to massages and the performance of the lymphatic system, one of our bodies' detoxification pathways, though this research is limited. Evidence supports the use of what is known as *manual lymphatic drainage* for those who experience lymphedema.[7] Manual lymphatic drainage is a specific massage technique that includes very gentle pressure and slow movements that are designed to gently stimulate the lymph vessels and direct the fluid into those vessels. In one meta-analysis, scientists found that most styles of massage therapy made a positive impact on the quality of life of fibromyalgia patients, including manual lymphatic drainage.[8] So, if you have access to a practitioner who performs this specialized type of massage, you may experience benefits from it.

In a very specific example, massage therapy has been shown to help patients who are going through alcohol detoxification.[9] One study found that the group receiving massage treatments had a lower pulse rate, reduced levels of respiration, and also lower scores on the Alcohol Withdrawal Scale during the early stages of their detoxification process. Similar results were found with patients going through a psychoactive drug withdrawal/detoxification program (including alcohol, cocaine, and opiates).[10] While neither of those studies specifically shows that the massage enhanced the detoxification process itself, both illustrate that massage is an excellent companion to those types of detox/withdrawal programs, perhaps due to massage's already known anxiety-reducing benefits.

So, why did I include massage here as a self-cleaning tool, when there isn't strong evidence that your typical spa massage treatment is making a difference? I included massage anyway because it does have a few therapeutic detoxification-related applications that are supported by research. And when I go get a massage from my favorite massage therapist, it may not be stimulating my lymphatic system in any measurable way . . . but it *might*. And, even if it isn't, the anti-anxiety benefits will likely help me sleep better. There *is* evidence that shows that massage therapy is useful in combatting insomnia.[11] So it sounds like a great time for me to talk about . . . sleep!

SLEEP

Quality sleep is essential as a part of our bodies' self-cleaning toolboxes. As we already learned, the glymphatic system is the brain's waste management system, and it works while we are sleeping to flush out toxins (including excess proteins) that build up during the waking hours. If our glymphatic system doesn't work properly, toxins can build up in our central nervous system and within the brain itself.

> *Essentially, sleeping acts as a garbage collector that comes during the night and removes the waste product left by the brain. This allows the brain to function normally the next day when one wakes up from slumber.*[12]

Besides removing the toxic waste by-products that have accumulated throughout the day, while we are asleep, our brains reorganize and recharge themselves. In a typical night, we go through four to six sleep cycles, and each cycle has four stages. Each stage is essential for restoring and rejuvenating the brain. While we sleep, the brain essentially reorganizes itself and creates new pathways that help us learn new information and consolidate memories.[13]

How much sleep do we need? Scientists estimate that on average, we need a minimum of seven hours of sleep each night for optimum cognitive and behavioral function, though this number does vary slightly from person to person. And when we sleep, we need to make sure we sleep well so we experience all the restorative benefits sleep has to offer.

To improve the quality of your sleep, here are some strategies to keep in mind:

- Limit caffeine after noon, as caffeine can keep you from having restful sleep.

- Stick to a consistent sleep routine from day to day. Our bodies thrive when we have a sleep rhythm that matches our personal circadian rhythms. We are not all the same when it comes to sleep timing, however. You may be someone who is naturally early to bed and early to rise, or maybe you're a natural night owl. Designing a sleep routine that matches your body's pre-ferred rhythms makes it more likely that you'll get the right amount of sleep for your body.

- Skip alcohol. While it may help you fall asleep more quickly, it negatively affects the quality of your sleep.

- Darkness matters. The light from an alarm clock, streetlights, or a night-light can keep you from falling into a restful and deep sleep. Your goal is to keep your bedroom as dark as possible. Alternatively, you could wear a sleep mask.

- Consider the temperature. Most of us sleep better when our bedrooms are on the cooler side. Try a variety of temperature settings until you find the one that feels best for you.

- Keep it quiet. A noisy bedroom can keep you from sleeping well. Consider a white-noise machine or fan to block out sounds that would cause you to wake up.

- Reconsider having pets in your bed. We all love our furry family members, but are they keeping you from a restful sleep? For us, the answer was yes, so we close our bedroom door at night and sleep in a pet-free room.

BLUE-LIGHT BLOCKING

You just read about the importance of sleep, but did you know that there is one feature of our modern lifestyle that interferes with sleep, and it's affecting most of us and even our kids? I'm talking about the problem with blue-light exposure. While blue light isn't a toxin in the sense of the word (as it isn't a chemical we take in), it is something that makes our environment "dirty" in a way. Let me explain.

Before I do, I want to let you know that there are three types of people when it comes to the issue of blue light and sleep: One, those who already know that blue-light exposure at night is a problem; and two, those who have never heard of this at all. The third type are people like me, who *know* it is a problem, *know* what the solution is, but still struggle to *apply* the solution. In this section, I am going to be talking to people in group two and three, including myself, because I need to do a better job where this is concerned.

So, what's the problem?

Most of us have electronic devices nearby 24-7, and we stare at their screens from the time we wake up until the time we go to bed. Not only that, but we also have replaced most of our light bulbs with fluorescent or LED bulbs, and we watch LED televisions in the bedroom before we go to sleep. All these screens and bulbs are considered sources of "blue light" because they emit a great deal of blue-wavelength light. (Think back to elementary school, when you learned that white light is a blend of all the colors of the spectrum, with the reds on one end and the blues on the other, and in between, all the colors of the rainbow.)

Research is very clear that when we are exposed to high levels of blue light before bedtime, it contributes to sleep problems. This is because blue-wavelength light suppresses the production of melatonin and causes mental alertness.[14]

Why would light make a difference? Let's think of this from a biological perspective. In the morning, the sun comes up, and we respond well to blue wavelengths throughout the day when the sun is high in the sky—they provide a boost to our attention, our reaction times, and also our moods.[15] We are supposed to be wide awake when the sun is high in the sky, and that's what the blue light tells our bodies. As the sun goes down, however, the sky turns red, and this red light leads to increased melatonin production, prepping us for sleep. Studies show that exposure to red light at night improves the quality of our sleep.[16]

So, what do we do about this? Are we doomed to a life of no lights on after sunset, or do we need to swap out our light bulbs for red bulbs? Do we need to turn off all televisions and put down all devices after sunset? The answer, fortunately, is no.

After the sun goes down, it's time to put on our blue-light-blocking glasses. These glasses have special lenses that block out the blue light wavelengths within our surroundings and give everything a reddish glow. This makes me think of that song from the 1980s: *I wear my sunglasses at night.* Good times.

Here's what you're probably wondering: Does it work? Yes. Studies show that wearing these types of glasses before bed improves sleep.[17] Personally, I own blue-blocking glasses, and as I type this, I vow to do a better job actually putting them *on* at night. My sleep (and my brain) will thank me.

EARTHING

Are you ready to learn about your body's electrical charge and how it affects you in ways you have probably never considered? While the concept may sound foreign to you at first, there is evidence to support the importance of balancing your personal electrical charge, and it's easy to do.

Let's go back to elementary school science for a moment and remember what we learned about static electricity. We have all experienced what happens when a negative charge builds up and then is discharged between two objects—*zap*! Why does this happen? Certain activities—generally involving rubbing or brushing two objects together—transfer electrons and cause a negative charge to build up. This might be something like walking on a rug, rubbing your pet, or taking off a sweater. Electrons move through conductors easily, so when you touch something conductive that has a positive charge, the extra electrons "jump" from you to that object. The *zap* comes from the transfer of those electrons.

I'm sure you know that atoms are the building blocks of all matter, and atoms are made of protons, neutrons, and electrons. This means *you* are made of atoms, as well. You are also very much an electrical being.[18] You've heard of an electrocardiogram, or ECG. Doctors use these machines to observe the electrical pulses within your heart, because the pumping action is regulated by an electrical conduction system that is responsible for coordinating the movements of your heart itself.[19] If the electrical system isn't functioning correctly, it can lead to a heart attack. Our nervous system also requires electricity to do its work.[20] The electrical pulses moving through our nervous system make it possible for us to feel, to move, and even to think. When something interferes with the electrical workings of our bodies, such as injury, illness, or even toxins, we have problems. Epilepsy, Alzheimer's disease, and Parkinson's disease are all related to issues with electrical activity or nerve cell function.[21]

The earth also has an electrical charge. Thanks to lightning strikes, solar radiation, and other atmospheric effects, the earth has built up a supply of free electrons, which results in a natural negative charge on the earth's surface.[22]

We use the earth itself to help us manage electricity in our homes. I'm sure you've heard of *grounding* as it refers to your home electrical system. Your electrical outlets are all grounded, meaning that the third prong of an electrical plug is connected to a path that allows for any excess electrical charge to flow into the ground rather than creating an electrical overload in your home, which could lead to a fire or a dangerous electrical shock were it not grounded properly.[23]

The concept of earthing for our bodies is similar to grounding within your home, except in reverse. Just as the way your home's electrical wiring sends excess electricity into the ground, when we are physically connected to the earth, electrons are able to flow between us and the earth. The negative electrons from the earth flow into our bodies, and this process "cleans up" our personal electrical charge.

What do these electrons do for us? This really is an important self-cleaning mechanism, even though many people haven't heard of it. Electrons act as antioxidants within our bodies and neutralize damaging free radicals, which plays a role in reducing inflammation and promoting the immune response.[24, 25]

Is there scientific evidence that earthing is important? Yes. According to research:[26]

> Earthing could be one of the simplest, and yet most profound, interventions for helping reduce cardiovascular risk and cardiovascular events. Earthing has also produced (1) symptomatic improvements in sleep disturbances and chronic muscle and joint pain; (2) the restoration of normal, day-night, cortisol-secretion profiles; (3) a reduction in the electrical fields that are induced by AC current on the body; (4) a reduction in overall stress levels and tensions; (5) an increase in parasympathetic system function and/or a reduction in sympathetic system function; (6) a speeding of recovery from delayed-onset muscle soreness after exercise; (7) an improvement in heart rate variability; and (8) an improvement in immune system response.

It's also been shown to improve moods, reduce pain, and lower inflammation.

In one review article that I read, the scientists said this about earthing:[27]

> This discovery suggests that the planet we live on is the original painkiller, the original anti-inflammatory: nature's way to counteract inflammation.

Scientists believe that our modern lifestyle keeps us from experiencing the benefits of earthing by keeping us disconnected from the surface of the earth. It's only been in recent times that we have become disconnected: we wear shoes, we stay inside, we sleep in beds—all of this is very different from the way humans traditionally connected to the earth as they lived their lives, both walking and sleeping in direct contact with the surface of the earth. Because of this disconnection, we rarely have the chance to collect the powerful electrons that we need.

The best way to connect with the earth? Walk barefoot on the grass, on the beach, on the ground, or even on concrete. You can also sit on the ground or on a concrete surface that is touching the ground. The key is that you don't want anything between your skin and the earth's surface that isn't conductive, so wearing shoes or walking on asphalt won't provide the same benefits. Is the weather too cold to walk outside barefoot? You can even buy earthing mats and earthing bedding that can be used indoors and/or while you are sleeping.

My favorite way to "clean up" my electrical charge? Walking barefoot on the beach. The sand and salt water make for the ideal earthing experience. This is one example of how something we crave (walking barefoot on the sand) is actually great for our bodies. Our bodies know, even if we don't understand why.

INDOOR AIR QUALITY

The air inside our homes is often more toxic than the air outside. Better construction methods have made our homes airtight, which keeps the indoor air from escaping outside. That is good news for our heating and cooling system efficiency, but bad news for our air quality.

This means that all the toxins that are now present in our indoor air from our cleaning products, personal care items, and from chemicals that may off-gas from our paint, carpets, and other home furnishings are trapped inside. As we discussed in earlier chapters, long-term exposure to these environmental pollutants can lead to health issues such as respiratory diseases, heart disease, or even cancer. For that reason, we should all work to improve the indoor air quality of our homes.[28]

The EPA tells us that "the most effective ways to improve your indoor air are to reduce or remove the sources of pollutants and to ventilate with clean outdoor air."[29] If that doesn't illustrate that indoor air is more of a problem than outdoor air these days, I don't know what will.

Besides bringing in more outdoor air, there are a few ways to "detox" the air within your home. The first methods include the use of high-quality air filtration systems and upgrading the air filter in your HVAC system. You want to look for systems and filters that remove both particles and gases.

It may surprise you to learn that plants may also improve the quality of your indoor air.[30] Bill Wolverton, a NASA scientist, made a discovery in the late 1960s that swamp plants were effectively eliminating Agent Orange that had been inadvertently released into the local waters near Eglin Air Force Base.[31] This led to his later work into using plants to improve indoor air quality. In an early experiment, they created a tightly sealed building called the BioHome, which had high levels of VOCs (which are substances that come from sources such as paint, cleaning products, and home furnishings). NASA first published these findings in 1984:[32]

Air quality tests before and after the placement of plants by mass spectrometer/gas chromatograph analyses revealed that nearly all the VOCs were removed. Moreover, one no longer experienced burning eyes or other classic symptoms of "sick building syndrome" (SBS) when entering the BioHome.

Changing/improving your air filters, selecting high-quality air filtration systems, and adding houseplants to your surroundings: all are easy ways to clean up your house's air, which will lead to a cleaner *you*.

TAKE ACTION: CHOOSE YOUR TOOLS

Use your Clean(ish) Journal (or the worksheets available at ginstephens .com/cleanish) to complete these end-of-chapter prompts and activities.

Which tools will you choose to boost your body's self-cleaning? As you read through this list, check all the ones you want to try, and write a few sentences in your Clean(ish) Journal with your thoughts about each one that you checked.

Exercise

☐ Time to get moving! We want to keep our lymphatic system flowing, as well as increase our circulation and respiration and work up a good sweat.

How can you increase your daily movement in a way that you enjoy?

Sauna

☐ Promote a deeper level of sweating by spending time in a sauna. See if any gyms or health clubs in your area include access to a sauna as a part of their membership plans. List options in your journal.

Massage

☐ Schedule regular massages to reduce anxiety and boost mood.

In your journal, remind yourself why you deserve to include massages as a part of your self-care routine.

Sleep

☐ Our glymphatic system requires restorative sleep to flush toxins from our brains. If you know you are not getting the sleep your body needs, make a plan for ways you can improve the quality of your sleep.

Look back at the list on page 222 for ideas and write down the ones you want to try.

Blue-Light Blocking

☐ Is your house full of "dirty" blue light after dark, coming from bulbs and screens everywhere you turn?

What can you do to decrease your blue-light exposure after sunset?

Earthing

☐ Connecting to the earth helps us "clean up" our personal electrical charge by increasing the flow of electrons, which act as antioxidants within our bodies and neutralize damaging free radicals.

How can you spend more time connecting with the earth?

Indoor Air Quality

☐ Since indoor air is often more toxic than outdoor air these days, it's more important than ever to have a plan for cleaning up our home's air.

What strategies will you choose to clean up the air within your home?

PART 3

HERE WE GO!
BECOMING CLEAN(ISH)

In this section of the book, you'll pull together what you learned in parts 1 and 2 to develop your own personalized and practical action plan for cleaning up where it counts.

Our goals? We want to find products that won't harm us, our kids, our pets, or the environment (or add to our body burdens), choose foods that nourish our bodies (and are also delicious), and support our bodies' self-cleaning pathways, all while living a balanced life where we are empowered by knowledge but not burdened by fear.

- First, you'll consider your own evolution to clean(ish), reflecting upon your past and present and then envisioning what a clean(ish) future looks like for you.

- You'll create your own definition of clean(ish) eating, with a goal of eating (mostly) clean.

- You'll also create a personal definition of clean(ish) living so that you can develop personal care and cleaning routines that are (mainly) clean.

- Do you need to get your family on board? You'll make a plan for that, as well.

- Finally, you'll choose your clean(ish) timeline and address nine focus topics in the order that you choose.

THE PRECAUTIONARY PRINCIPLE

Before we begin to develop our personal definitions of clean(ish) eating and living, let's talk about something called *the Precautionary Principle* and understand how it applies to our lives.[1,2] This chapter is short by design, but I want you to take time to reflect upon this principle before moving forward.

You may remember that I concluded the introduction with this saying:

An ounce of prevention is worth a pound of cure.
—Benjamin Franklin

That, in a nutshell, is what the Precautionary Principle embodies, and it's what guides my own personal definition of clean(ish).

You see, there is still a lot of scientific uncertainty when it comes to dangers from daily toxin exposure, and you may have noticed that I used a lot of words like *may* and *could* or *has been linked to* within previous chapters. That's because much of our scientific evidence is not absolute, and research is ongoing. Also, as I have mentioned before, a lot of the research involves studies of chemicals in isolation, yet we don't live in a way that exposes us to one chemical at a time. Our buckets become full from tiny exposures that add up over time, just as the ocean became salty over time.

Industries use this scientific uncertainty to cast doubt on whether certain chemicals are dangerous, and that leads to delays in taking action. The tobacco industry did this for years, and the companies and scientists who develop and use the chemicals I mentioned in part 1 of this book are doing the same thing now. They attempt to discredit watchdog organizations such as Consumer Reports or the Environmental Working Group, labeling their work as "junk science" and "pseudoscience" and insisting that consumers have nothing to worry about when it comes to the chemicals in our foods or household products.

Besides the resources I used to write this book (and have listed in the references section), I also read a lot of articles produced by industry/pro-industry scientists as I did the research for this book, wanting to understand both sides of every argument, and when these articles criticize the watchdog organizations, it feels a lot like the fox guarding the henhouse to me. Their *one job* is to convince you that the watchdog organizations have got it wrong, that those groups are full of kooks and people who don't understand science, and that people like me are confused and misled by the wacky watchdog organizations. They want us all to believe that our biggest problem is that we probably aren't smart enough to understand that everything is *fine*, and we have nothing to worry about. *Trust us*, they say, *and ignore the wackos spreading fear.*

These are the exact same strategies that were developed by the tobacco industry in the 1950s, and their goal was to cast doubt on the growing evidence showing that smoking was harmful. They also characterized the research against smoking as "junk science," and anyone speaking out against smoking was portrayed as an alarmist. Big tobacco actively worked to discredit both the warnings and those who gave them.

In a 2001 article within the *American Journal of Public Health*, the authors discuss how this happened in the tobacco industry and continues today in other areas:[3]

A major component of the industry attack was the mounting of a campaign to establish a "bar" for "sound science" that could not be fully met by most individual investigations, leaving studies that did not meet the criteria to be dismissed as "junk science." The campaign also included attempts to characterize relative risks of 2 or less as highly questionable and not amenable to investigation by epidemiologic methods.

Such tactics are not unique to the tobacco industry . . . Research on a number of current environmental issues is often labeled "junk science": particulate air pollution, electromagnetic radiation, and environmental estrogens, for example.

We now know with complete certainty that smoking is dangerous for our health and that smoking causes lung damage. There is no more *may* or *could* about it. Smoking causes lung damage. Period. Among other things. No one disputes this now, and we have clear evidence that the tobacco companies were involved in internal cover-ups for decades. That should make all of us angry.[4]

We are at a similar crossroads today, where the number of scientists and concerned citizens speaking up about these types of dangers is increasing, yet industry and *their* scientists are discrediting the message whenever they can. In the meantime, we continue to live within the big chemistry experiment, crossing our fingers that it's all going to be okay in the long run.

This is why I prefer to use the Precautionary Principle as I make my buying decisions.

The Precautionary Principle is grounded in the belief that if we wait until we are completely sure, it may be too late.[5]

When an activity raises threats of harm to human health or the environment, precautionary measures should be taken, even if some cause-and-effect relationships are not fully established scientifically.[6]

As we develop our own personal definitions of what it means to be clean(ish), let's apply the Precautionary Principle to our own lives. Isn't it better to err on the side of caution when we can, making choices that help us limit the number of toxins *coming in* as we also include strategies that support our bodies' natural processes involved in toxins *going out*?

Let's act *before* we get hurt.

REFLECT AND TAKE ACTION:
APPLYING THE PRECAUTIONARY PRINCIPLE

Use your Clean(ish) Journal (or the worksheets available at ginstephens .com/cleanish) to complete these end-of-chapter prompts.

- As you read about how big tobacco misled the public for decades, how did that make you feel?

- Have you ever been confused by contradictions surrounding the safety of the chemicals in our foods and household/personal care products? As a consumer, how do you know who to trust?

- Consider the saying: "An ounce of prevention is worth a pound of cure." How can you apply the Precautionary Principle to your life as you become clean(ish)?

EVOLUTION TO CLEAN(ISH)

I'm sure you are eager to get started (though you really have laid the groundwork already, as you worked through the end-of-chapter Reflect and Take Action sections throughout the book). In this chapter, we will consider your own personal evolution to clean(ish).

My own personal evolution has taken time, and I'm sure yours has (and will), as well. The good news is that every step along the way of this process, you are completely in charge at all times. You can pick and choose from the strategies and suggestions and incorporate what feels right to you.

As I mentioned in the introduction, it's been quite a process for me.

My personal evolution toward clean(ish) follows:

Birth Through High School: While I was definitely a picky eater, food wasn't stressful. I went merrily on my way, eating whatever foods I wanted to eat. If I liked it, I ate it. If I didn't like it, I didn't eat it. Grown-up foods, such as vegetables? No, thank you. Along with vegetables, diets were also for grown-ups. Nobody around me gave a thought to food quality or how many funky chemicals may or may not have been in any of our products that I can recall. I remember going over to babysit for a family who was very unusual for the mid-1980s: their kids brushed with all-natural toothpaste, the snacks they had on hand were weird, and to this day, I remember how disappointing it was to be told, "Help yourself to whatever you want," at their house.

The "hot dogs" in their fridge? I am not sure what they were made of, but I certainly didn't want to eat them.

College: A whole new world of eating opened up to me, thanks to the college cafeteria. Food was available 24-7, and there were a lot of late-night pizzas. Tomato sauce is a vegetable, right? And there was so much beer. I gained the "freshman fifteen," and dieting officially entered my life. My preferred strategy was calorie counting, and I never gave a thought to the quality of what I was eating or what personal care or cleaning products I used, other than: *Can I afford this?*

BK (Before Kids): As a young adult, managing my weight became a bit trickier. Besides counting calories, now the world was counting fat grams. During a good bit of this time period, my diet was almost 100 percent ultra-processed, low-fat not-food. The closest thing I ate to a vegetable was corn or peas from a can . . . they were fat-free! SnackWell's, SpaghettiOs, and other fat-free convenience foods were my go-to items. When I wasn't dieting, I ate whatever I wanted, and it was all pretty much ultra-processed. I continued to choose my personal care and cleaning products based on price, and safety never crossed my mind.

Early Mom Years: Just like every other mom in the 1990s, I read *What to Expect When You're Expecting* and also the follow-up books for the baby and toddler years. I felt their stance on eating vegetables and creating a toxin-free home was a bit out there. Sigh. Still, I bought the fancy baby laundry detergent (grudgingly), and I enthusiastically popped my prenatal vitamins, because they gave me everything I needed, right? I was so confused. Because Cal was born five weeks early, he had difficulty nursing, and the pediatrician's nurse convinced a crying me to feed a crying him some baby formula. He stopped crying, *I* stopped crying, and we never looked back. My boys ate the same ultra-processed diet I grew up on. I ditched the baby detergent and stocked the kids' medicine cabinet with kid-flavored toothpaste and kid-colored-and-scented bath products. Bath time was a chemical extravaganza, in fact, looking back on it.

The Feingold Years: As I explained in the introduction, a caring teacher set us on the path of discovery when it came to how foods and chemicals affected the behavior of my kids. Instead of an ultra-processed diet of standard American grocery store brands, we switched over to still-highly-processed-yet-additive-free foods. I stocked the cleaning cupboard with unscented and natural products and tossed out all the toxic personal care products for the kids—though I held on to the ones I used. I didn't think *I* needed to watch what I put on my body. It was only a problem for the kids—or so I thought.

The Diet-Struggle Years: As the kids "grew out" of needing special foods and products, we went back to our old ways for the most part. An ultra-processed diet reigned supreme for all of us. Drive-through, frozen family-size microwavable meals, other convenience foods . . . that's what we ate most of the time. I went from one diet to another, and my weight yo-yoed mostly within the 150–200 pound range, depending on whether I was in the "I must diet now" or "I will eat whatever I want now" phase. I did realize that I didn't like heavily scented products, so we never brought back scented laundry detergent or air fresheners. I also chose a few "clean" products for the home, though I realize now I was a victim of greenwashing for most of them.

My Weight-Loss Turning Point: When I got home from a family vacation in 2014 and realized I weighed 210 pounds, it was time to do something, once and for all. That was the year I embraced intermittent fasting. Other than the brief period in the spring of 2015 where I ate "clean" to lose the last 20 pounds, I continued to eat whatever I wanted. I did make a mental note of how much better I felt when I avoided ultra-processed foods. And the weight melted off at a rate of about 2 pounds per week when I ate real foods rather than all the not-food I was used to. Hmmm. Something to think about.

The Early IF Years of Maintenance: Once I hit my goal weight in 2015, I went back to eating all foods. I was still eating a highly ultra-processed food diet, but I was able to maintain without struggle. After all the years of dieting, it felt like a miracle. Intermittent fasting allowed me to eat whatever I wanted and maintain my weight loss. Gradually, though, what I wanted to eat was starting to change.

IF after *Feast Without Fear*: In 2017, when I began to research for my second book, *Feast Without Fear,* my whole mindset toward food changed. Thanks to the work being done in the area of personalized nutrition, I realized that we were all different when it came to what foods worked best for our bodies, and a lot of that had to do with our gut microbiomes. I read about the Blue Zones and learned about how important it was to feed our gut inhabitants well. I finally understood the power of real food. By that time, I had been drinking my coffee black for over a year, and I think the bitterness of the black coffee opened up my palate to the world of vegetables. Suddenly, I was not only eating more vegetables . . . I *liked* them. The more vegetables I added to my diet, the better I felt. We signed up for a meal kit delivery company (can we have a moment of silence for Plated, who has since gone out of the meal kit delivery business), and I ordered foods that were exotic-to-me each week. Slowly and over time, I noticed I was eating completely differently from my ultra-processed diet of before. Real food was delicious, and most ultra-processed foods no longer tasted good to me.

The Menopausal Transition: As I went through menopause, I realized that my body was suddenly more sensitive to both alcohol and sugar, so I cut back on them both. I didn't do it for weight loss or "diet-y" reasons: I did it because I wanted to feel great. It shocked me to realize how much better I felt, in fact. I also began to take a closer look at the chemicals in my foods, my personal care products, and my cleaning products. I switched over to a safe beauty line, and the more I learned, the more I wanted to learn.

THE IDEA FOR WRITING THIS BOOK WAS BORN.

Today: I am a completely different person from who I was even a few years ago. I am grateful that two of my pivotal moments occurred while researching for books I was writing.

What I learned while writing *Feast Without Fear* changed my understanding of food forever. I finally comprehended the power of food within our bodies and how health and longevity depend on how well we nourish ourselves. I realized that we don't simply make decisions about what to eat to manage our weight. Choosing what foods we eat is about much more than how it affects our weight.

The second pivotal moment has been while writing this book. I thought I was making good choices for the most part. Nope. What I learned while researching was so powerful that I knew it was time to stop adding to my toxic load through the products I buy. I also learned how very duped I have been by greenwashing, and that led to me switching over almost every product in my kitchen, bathroom, and laundry room—and I finally feel equipped with how to know which products are better than others. I consider myself to be clean(ish) because I'll still eat a Dorito from time to time if someone offers one to me, but I don't usually buy them. Today, I make choices that support my health goals, yet I don't obsess over perfection.

Never forget: **If I can change, *you* can change.**

REFLECT: YOUR OWN EVOLUTION TOWARD CLEAN(ISH)

Use your Clean(ish) Journal (or the worksheets available at ginstephens .com/cleanish) to complete these end-of-chapter prompts and activities.

Consider my own evolution toward clean(ish) that I shared with you in this chapter, and recall all the stages I went through over the years. It's a process! I'm a little bit embarrassed to admit how much of the process has been recent. Knowledge is power.

Now it's time to reflect upon your own personal evolution toward becoming clean(ish).

Write about it in your Clean(ish) Journal. Alternately, go to ginstephens.com/cleanish to download and print the pdf that contains these pages in worksheet format.

Remember that you aren't yet at the end of your clean(ish) journey, and over the next few chapters, you'll be taking more steps. For now, you're simply reflecting on the past and present, knowing that your future will look different.

- Reflect on your past and present. What have you done in the past? And what are you doing now? Consider writing it as a timeline.

- Envision your clean(ish) future. What will your life look like decades from now? How will eating (mostly) clean and living (mainly) clean change future-you?

ONLINE RESOURCES
FOR BECOMING CLEAN(ISH)

In the next two chapters—"Eat (Mostly) Clean" and "Live (Mainly) Clean"—I'll share some strategies you can use as you transition to clean(ish), and then you'll craft your own definitions of clean(ish) eating and clean(ish) living, making sure it all feels doable for you. Then I'll discuss how you can get your family on board, particularly if you live with picky eaters (whether they are your kids or even your partner). Finally, you'll decide on the timeline you prefer to follow.

As you continue your evolution to clean(ish), you'll rely on resources to guide many of your shopping decisions. This chapter contains a list of a few of the resources I have found to be valuable, and I have ranked them in order of personal usefulness to me. At the end of this chapter, there's a place for you to take notes as you explore some of these resources. Keep in mind that this list is far from exhaustive. There are more resources out there than I could compile in one place, and also the internet is never static and therefore always changing.

I also have links to some of my favorite companies and product lines on my website at ginstephens.com/cleanish, and I'll keep them updated over time as I find new favorites. I don't want to spend a lot of time making decisions about what foods to eat or what products to buy, so I shop with companies that have high standards, and then I trust what they sell. Do you remember the Ronco infomercial of the early 1990s, where the tagline for their rotisserie chicken oven was "Set it and forget it"? That's one of the best taglines ever, and it's how I approach my shopping: I "set it and forget it," meaning I take the time to do my research on the front end, and then I don't have to think about it anymore, freeing up my mind for other things. The products I list at ginstephens.com/cleanish are perfect examples of how I *set it and forget it.*

ONLINE RESOURCES

Environmental Working Group
www.ewg.org
> *"Know your environment. Protect your health."*

This is the number one resource in my clean(ish) toolbox, and I think you'll want to add it to yours.

The website is a treasure trove of resources. If you have enjoyed the (very small and only the tip of the iceberg) amount of science I have shared here in this book and want to learn more, you will absolutely want to go to ewg.org right away. They have page after page of science-backed reports that summarize the key issues.

Big industry loves to refer to the EWG as a bunch of pseudoscientists who are presenting us with false information to alarm us unnecessarily, but is that true? To determine if I could trust the information coming out of EWG, I dug in to see just who makes up their scientific team. I discovered that they are staffed by scientists with a variety of PhDs (as well as an assortment of master's and bachelor's degrees) in many fields, and a perusal of the Our Team section tells me their staff has degrees in biomedical sciences, chemistry, environmental science, environmental science and policy, environmental chemistry and technology, environmental health, agricultural economics, dairy science, conservation and resource studies, nutritional sciences and toxicology, molecular biology and immunology, marine biomedicine and environmental science, and more. Their degrees are from major universities, such as Johns Hopkins, Cornell, the Medical University of South Carolina, Virginia Tech, UCLA, and many other top-notch schools. If these highly educated people are what we call "pseudoscientists," then we can't trust any scientists anywhere, am I right?

I have their app EWG Healthy Living and use it daily when I make purchasing decisions. The app is free and has many helpful sections: *EWG Verified* (all products are free from EWG's "chemicals of concern" and meet their highest standards for safety), *Personal Care, Food, Sunscreens,* and *Household Cleaners.* You can search for specific products, browse, scan barcodes, and more. There's also a list of the yearly "Dirty Dozen" and "Clean Fifteen" based on EWG's guide to pesticides in produce.

Consumer Reports
consumerreports.org

"Consumer Reports works to create a fair and just marketplace for all. As a mission-driven, independent, nonprofit member organization, CR empowers and informs consumers, incentivizes corporations to act responsibly, and helps policymakers prioritize the rights and interests of consumers in order to shape a truly consumer-driven marketplace."

Founded in 1936, Consumer Reports does a lot more than tell you which brand of mattress will give you a good night's sleep (though I love reading their product testing and recommendation articles, and I have relied on their testing data since the 1990s to help me buy everything from a washing machine to a new car). Over the years, they have highlighted many key dangers in the marketplace, such as fallout from nuclear testing on the rise in milk products (1950s), the dangers of cigarette smoking (1960s), the importance of cleaning up our water supply (1970s), the pitfalls of the supplement industry (1980s), the safety of seafood (1990s), and the accumulation of PFAS in our water supply (2020). If you go to the Issues That Matter tab, they share ways you can take action, but there is also information there that you can use, such as the food label decoder. The food label decoder lets you fill in the blanks in this statement: "When I am shopping for _____, what labels tell me that _____."

If you subscribe to only one magazine, this is the one I would recommend, as being a subscriber supports their work and also gives you access to subscriber-only content on their website.

Earth 911
earth911.com

"We believe humans can successfully reduce their impact by using less, reusing and recycling more, and constantly making small improvements through their daily decisions at home, while shopping, at work, and at play. More ideas make less waste."

This is a great site for a variety of resources as you become clean(ish). They have thoughtful blog posts about all sorts of topics that will help you focus on making sustainable choices that make a difference. Their focus began with recycling but has expanded to encompass a much broader knowledge base.

The Organic Center
www.organic-center.org

"The Organic Center is your trusted resource for scientific reporting on agriculture and food. We serve up our unbiased scientific findings in distilled bites so you can make more informed decisions, and protect wild places and biodiversity through environmentally friendly farming. Worry Less. Know Better."

This website is a great resource for all of us, especially the Resource Library tab. They have a repository of videos, articles, and even recipes.

One of the most valuable sections is the "Organic Infographics and Fact Sheets" section. You can find helpful tips such as "Seven Simple Swaps to Detox Your Home," "Top 8 Organic Lunchbox Tips," "Five Organic Gardening Tips," and more.

Campaign for Safe Cosmetics

www.safecosmetics.org

"The Campaign for Safe Cosmetics coalition, a project of Breast Cancer Prevention Partners (formerly the Breast Cancer Fund), works to protect the health of consumers, workers and the environment through public education and engagement, corporate accountability and sustainability campaigns and legislative advocacy designed to eliminate dangerous chemicals linked to adverse health impacts from cosmetics and personal care products."

This website has a variety of resources such as reports related to regulations, chemicals of concern, health and science, and also links to safer cosmetics companies. In addition, they have a partner app called Think Dirty, which helps you find safe options.

Gimme the Good Stuff

gimmethegoodstuff.org

"A resource for conscious moms and healthy kids."

My favorite part of this web page is their product guides section. They have done the work of filtering through various product categories and recommending the safest options. As an example, you can go to their safe cookware product guide and read a thorough summary of what constitutes "safe cookware" and find a list of products they recommend. You may remember from reading my other books that I am ~~lazy~~ efficient (recall that my favorite exercise is standing on a vibration plate) and so I love when someone else has done the legwork for me.

Environmental Protection Agency
www.epa.gov

"Our mission is to protect human health and the environment."

The EPA website has a wide variety of resources that can help you make informed decisions. Information is divided into categories such as air, chemicals and toxins, and greener living. The goal is to ensure that we have clean air, land, and water and to help us reduce environmental risks of all kinds.

Fair Trade Certified
www.fairtradecertified.org

"Fair trade is a global movement made up of a diverse network of producers, companies, consumers, advocates, and organizations putting people and planet first."

Fair Trade USA believes that it's important for companies to make sure their employees have safe working conditions and also protect the environment. They provide a Fair Trade Certified seal that indicates that the company has met their social, environmental, and economic standards. On the website you can find links to a wide variety of products, such as foods, coffee, personal care items, cleaning products, and more.

Certified Humane
certifiedhumane.org

"Create a more humane world for farm animals."

The Certified Humane organization developed a set of standards to ensure that meat, poultry, egg, and dairy products come from animals who have been raised in an environment that meets their stringent criteria. These animals are certified to have not received unnecessary antibiotics and also to have been raised in a humane manner. Animals that are both raised and fed well are healthier, and their meat and other products are superior in many important ways.

They have a free app that you can use to help you find products while you are shopping.

Monterey Bay Aquarium Seafood Watch

www.seafoodwatch.org

"We protect the ocean now and for the future, through trusted seafood recommendations and collaboration with businesses, governments, consumers and partners worldwide."

The Seafood Watch program helps consumers choose safe seafood that is harvested in an environmentally sustainable manner. You can download seafood guides that are specifically tailored for any region of the U.S. These guides have lists of best choices, good alternatives, and options you should avoid.

Green and Healthy Homes Initiative

www.greenandhealthyhomes.org

"Creating and advocating for healthy, safe and energy efficient homes for families, children, and older adults in need."

This group was initially founded in 1986 as Parents Against Lead and has evolved over time to provide resources and to ensure that our homes are safe for all. They have resources such as "The 8 Elements of a Green and Healthy Home," "Home Health Hazards," and "Steps to Take to Protect Your Family," as well as a collection of videos and webinars on a wide variety of topics.

ACTION PLAN: EXPLORING RESOURCES

Use your Clean(ish) Journal (or the worksheets available at ginstephens .com/cleanish) to complete these end-of-chapter prompts and activities.

Time to do some digging! Visit a few of the websites and/or

download the apps that I shared with you in this chapter and take notes of what you find there, so you'll know where to go when you need information in a hurry.

With all these great resources, you never have to stand in the store staring with confusion at the products on the shelves (ending with you grabbing whatever looks good, rather than making an informed decision). Instead of grab-and-go, you'll be armed with knowledge to guide your selections.

Create a section in your Clean(ish) Journal where you can take notes about each resource that you find.

You may want to organize your resources in this format:

Name of organization / Website: _____

_____

What I found there: _____

_____

_____

_____

_____

_____

_____

_____

EAT (MOSTLY) CLEAN

As we live a clean(ish) lifestyle, we eat (**mostly**) clean. The *mostly* is what makes this doable long term.

Never forget that clean(ish) eating is centered around prioritizing foods that nourish your body while also *avoiding* a restrictive mindset. That's easier said than done, particularly since we just spent a lot of time learning about the importance of eating high-quality foods and limiting ultra-processed foods that are full of funky chemicals and additives.

The truth is that it can take time to find balance, particularly as you get started. You may be tempted to do a complete cleanout of your kitchen pantry and fridge, and I want to encourage you not to do that. I think that one of the worst things you can do is go into your kitchen and throw away every food that isn't a whole food right now on day one. We have all done that in the past when starting a restrictive diet, am I right? And how did that work out for you? It never did work well for me. Whenever I tell myself, "I can't," and whenever I try to make too much of a change at once, it all crashes and burns around me. Don't let that happen to you. Remember that going clean(ish) is a process and is also not intended to be restrictive.

Keep this in the back of your mind at all times. As we live a clean(ish) lifestyle:

- We don't aim for rigid perfection. Perfection (in any aspect of our life) is an illusion at best, and the desire for perfection usually leads to self-doubt when we can't live up to unobtainable and unrealistic standards.

- We don't label foods as "dirty" or judge ourselves as "bad" when we eat. No matter what.

- We aren't scared of carbs, grains, dairy, fat, lectins, gluten, and so on. We understand that *no* whole foods that have been eaten by humans for thousands of years are "bad foods," no matter which dietary guru tries to convince us otherwise. Over time, we become aware of what foods may not work well for our bodies, we learn to listen to how we feel after we eat, and we avoid foods that make us feel unwell. The power lies within *you,* not from a dietary theory written by someone who is not living in your body.

- We distinguish between *food* and *not-food.* We eat (mostly) *food.* We (mostly) avoid *not-food.*

> Our number one goal for eating clean(ish) is to be *mindful* of what we put into our bodies while not developing a restrictive mindset.

I have great news for you: we have an entire world of delicious and satisfying foods at our fingertips!

I promise you this: if your food isn't delicious and satisfying, you're absolutely doing it wrong. Food is meant to be pleasurable, and I reject the train of thought that food is only fuel and we are meant to simply "eat to live." I'm sure you've seen that before in diet circles—the notion that if we enjoy eating simply for the sake of eating, we are falling into the world of gluttony and we must repent. No. I want you to wipe that notion from your brain. Food has always been a celebration throughout time, and we can reconnect with this view and appreciate the experience of eating delicious foods once again. In the Blue Zones, they don't beat themselves up for enjoying their food. It's time for us to stop doing that, as well.

There are two factors to keep in mind from day to day:

1. We intentionally *put in* foods that provide the nutritional building blocks our bodies require for vibrant health.

2. We make a plan to *avoid* putting in toxins or chemicals that will add to our body burdens.

Notice that providing your body with adequate nutrition is front and center. As we learned in earlier chapters, the foods we eat do matter a great deal. We want to choose foods that feed us well, as well as the inhabitants of our gut microbiomes. We also want to ensure that we are providing nutritional support for our bodies' self-cleaning pathways. We want to avoid adding to our body burdens when we can. And we want to do all of this while finding balance and enjoying our lives. That's why taking time to develop your own definition of clean(ish) eating is so important. You aren't just going to wing it. You're going to be intentional about the choices you make.

So, this is what your overall Clean(ish) ~~Diet~~ Living Plan will look like:

Eat MORE	Eat LESS
Real food of all types, with ingredients you recognize and can pronounce *(or, better yet, no ingredients list required—asparagus doesn't need an ingredients list, for example)*	Not-food, composed of mostly ultra-processed ingredients that you don't recognize or can't pronounce

You'll decide what "eat more" and "eat less" look like to you when you create your own definition of clean(ish) eating. Before you do, let's talk about a few of the strategies that you'll employ as a clean(ish) eater (and shopper).

PRIORITIZING ORGANIC WHERE IT COUNTS

In earlier chapters, we learned that environmental toxins bioaccumulate. That's why I personally prioritize organic dairy products, organic fat sources (butter, cheese, and olive oil), and organic meats.

Besides being less likely to have environmental toxins, organic dairy products have superior fatty-acid ratios, with lower levels of omega-6 and higher levels of omega-3.[1,2] I also choose organic produce whenever I can. Heck, I almost always choose organic *anything* whenever I have a choice. Notice the words *almost always*. More about that in a minute.

Do I always have a choice? No, because sometimes I eat at restaurants, sometimes the item I need or want at the store isn't available in an organic form, and sometimes I am not the person making the purchasing decisions. And sometimes, I have a favorite brand and the organic or "cleaner" option just doesn't taste as good to me. That's where the *almost always* comes in.

One example of that? Duke's Mayonnaise. It has soybean oil that is probably GMO, "natural flavors" that could be anything, and some kind of funky preservative—but I love the way it tastes. I've tried to make the switch to a cleaner mayo, but none of them make me happy. I don't eat mayonnaise every day, but when I do, it needs to be Duke's.

Because I am clean(ish), I know that because I am careful about what I choose *most of the time,* it doesn't fill my bucket to have non-organic options *some of the time.* If I *did* eat mayo every day, I would most likely consider my options more carefully. But when an item is a sometimes choice, it isn't making as large of an impact from day to day. I don't have to feel guilty about choosing the brand of mayonnaise I prefer because I have made room for it by prioritizing quality in the other foods that I eat. Yesterday, I had an egg sandwich, and the ingredients were organic bread, organic scrambled eggs from free-range chickens, cooked in organic butter, and I spread just the right amount of Duke's mayo on the bread. It was delicious. It was clean(ish). It was just right.

One important factor that I don't want to minimize: as you intentionally add in more organic foods, you'll realize that organic foods typically cost more, which can be a limiting factor for many families. Why do organic foods tend to cost more? If you think back to an earlier chapter, you'll remember that the U.S. government subsidizes certain crops: corn production receives the highest subsidies, followed by soybeans, sugar, cotton, and wheat. The largest part of these subsidies goes to big agribusiness, and smaller farmers who grow organic foods are given little to no support. Organic farms are also more labor intensive, which drives up costs even more.

Yes, organic foods are generally more expensive. That being said, there are cost-effective ways to increase the number of organic foods that you can afford. Even big-box discount stores increasingly have their own lines of organic canned or frozen veggies that are a bargain. When you buy store-brand organic foods, they are often cheaper than name-brand nonorganic options, so you can save money by doing comparison shopping. Smaller stores such as ALDI or Lidl tend to have very reasonable prices on higher-quality and organic foods. Farmers' markets are also a great choice during growing season.

How can you make your shopping dollars go further when shopping for organic foods?

- **Buy ingredients:** Rather than buying ready-made or packaged foods, buy ingredients and cook your meals yourself. The money you save by not buying convenience foods can give you enough of a savings to choose organic options.

- **Comparison shop:** My husband is the king of comparison shopping. We have a perfect partnership: he likes to go to the store, and I like to let him. *(I consider it his way of modern-day hunting-gathering while I stay home around the hearth.)* He has a circuit of about six different stores that he frequents, and he knows where our favorite organic sandwich bread is on sale and where's the best place to get a good price on organic butter. Even big-box retailers often have lots of organic options these days, and the cost savings can be significant.

- **Buy in season:** When foods are in season, they are often a bargain. One of my favorite times of the year is berry season, when all the local grocery stores have fresh organic strawberries and blackberries at great prices.

- **Choose the store brand:** Often, an organic store-brand item may be cheaper than a conventional big-brand option. Don't be brand loyal in this case.

- **Buy in bulk:** Many grocery stores (particularly those that are more health-focused) have organic dry goods in large bins. If you shop in that department, you may find big savings over prepackaged items.

- **Choose whole grains:** High-quality organic whole grains (brown rice, quinoa, oats, pastas, etc.) are not expensive and can form the basis of many different meals.

- **Stock up during sales:** When common pantry items are on sale, stock up! Organic canned goods and dried items like beans and pastas, for example, will last a long time on the shelf.

- **Go frozen:** Fruits and vegetables are frozen at the peak of ripeness and retain their nutritional value. These frozen options are often a lot less expensive than buying them fresh.

- **Canned goods are a great value:** As with frozen foods, many canned foods were processed soon after being harvested. Because they are shelf stable, you can stock up and you'll have less food waste versus buying fresh foods that may go bad before you can eat them.

- **Get creative:** There are many ways to save money by being creative with your purchases. As an example, rather than purchasing expensive cooking sprays, buy a spray bottle and fill it with organic olive oil.

- **Grow your own:** Last summer, Chad grew tomatoes in our backyard. With a little of his sweat equity, we had free tomatoes all season. Not only were they free, they were so much better than anything you can get in the grocery store. Here in Georgia, we love a tomato sandwich during the peak of summer. If you've never had a tomato sandwich made from a tomato that was on the vine five minutes ago, you're missing out. Even in a small space like a city apartment, you can grow things like fresh basil in a pot on the windowsill, and you can tell yourself you're living off the land.

WHAT IF YOU STILL CAN'T AFFORD ORGANIC?

Sometimes, you just can't swing it, and that's okay. Don't avoid produce completely just because you can't afford the organic options. Conventional produce is a better option than ultra-processed foods every single day of the week. Wash all produce thoroughly (scrubbing under running water is fine—no need to use fancy produce washes[3]) and choose a variety of options from day to day. Besides feeding your gut microbiome well due to increased diversity in your diet, variety may help limit your exposure to any one kind of pesticide.

The Environmental Working Group puts out a new list every year known as the "Dirty Dozen." These can always be found at www.ewg .org/foodnews/dirty-dozen.php. The "Dirty Dozen" are the *worst* offenders in stores; these are the ones that have the most concerning levels of pesticide contamination.

The EWG "Dirty Dozen" for 2021:

1. Strawberries	7. Cherries
2. Spinach	8. Peaches
3. Kale, collard, and mustard greens	9. Pears
4. Nectarines	10. Bell and hot peppers
5. Apples	11. Celery
6. Grapes	12. Tomatoes

When possible, make sure that you prioritize organic options for those twelve items from the produce department. If you can't buy organic, wash them well.

The Environmental Working Group also has a "Clean Fifteen" list, and these are the conventional items that had the *least* amount of pesticide contamination. If you can't afford to go completely organic, these conventional options are some of your safest bets.

The EWG "Clean Fifteen" for 2021:

1. Avocados	9. Broccoli
2. Sweet corn	10. Cabbage
3. Pineapple	11. Kiwi
4. Onions	12. Cauliflower
5. Papaya	13. Mushrooms
6. Sweet peas (frozen)	14. Honeydew melon
7. Eggplant	15. Cantaloupe
8. Asparagus	

Keep in mind that these lists change from year to year, so always make sure that you are using the most up-to-date lists.

BECOME A DEDICATED LABEL READER AND MAKE SIMPLE SWAPS

When you are making food decisions at the grocery store, read the labels. You may find that you can make a simple swap that will improve the quality of what you're eating, but with no sacrifice in taste or enjoyment. You may even enjoy the high-quality version *more*, especially as your taste buds adjust to real food vs. ultra-processed foods.

Let me give you a couple of examples of what I mean.

I love crackers and chips. Yes, they are ultra-processed, and that is even true for organic options. Foods *can* be both ultra-processed and also made with organic ingredients. That doesn't mean I never choose crackers or chips—I eat them pretty much every day in one form or another. Because I do enjoy these foods, it's key to ensure that I am making the best choice I can with what I buy.

These are the ingredients from a big name-brand wheat cracker, sun-dried tomato and basil flavor.

Whole Grain Wheat Flour, Canola Oil, Sugar, Cornstarch, Malt Syrup (from Corn and Barley), Refiner's Syrup, Salt, Leavening (Calcium Phosphate and Baking Soda), Tomato Powder, Sundried Tomato Powder, Paprika, Garlic Powder, Spices (Includes Basil), Onion Powder, Dried Red and Green Bell Peppers, Yeast Extract, Natural Flavor (Contains Celery), Sulfur Dioxide (Sulfites) to Preserve Freshness. BHT added to packaging material to preserve freshness.

Other than the first ingredient, which sounds wholesome (whole grain wheat flour), it's full of problematic ingredients: highly refined oils, lots of GMO commodity crop ingredients, mystery added flavors, yeast extract (which is generally code for MSG), and a variety of preservatives. This cracker is full of inflammatory and funky ingredients. I would leave this one right there on the shelf of the grocery store and make a different choice.

The good news is that there is a type of cracker I can choose that gives me every bit of the same flavor and salty-crunch experience as the name-brand cracker, but with higher-quality ingredients. Well, it isn't going to give me that same MSG high that the other cracker gives me, but that's actually a *good thing*. The MSG keeps us eating and eating past the point where we would normally stop, which is why we tend to overeat those foods.

These are the ingredients of the crackers I purchase instead, also sun-dried tomato and basil flavor, and labeled as non-GMO:

Nut and seed flour blend (almonds, sunflower seeds, flaxseeds), tapioca starch, cassava flour, organic sunflower oil, sun-dried tomatoes, sea salt, organic onion, organic basil, organic garlic, organic oregano, organic pepper, rosemary extract

Yes, these crackers are still highly processed, but notice how few troublesome ingredients are listed. It does have sunflower oil, which is one of the oils I limit when I can, but because I am clean(ish), I know that some of the products I choose will have these oils from time to time. I'm not willing to give up all crackers and chips for the rest of my life, so I have made the switch to clean(ish) options that serve my body better than the name-brand options, and because I am not living a rigid life of perfection, it works for me. Those crackers are definitely clean(ish).

Here's another example. These are the ingredients and nutrition facts from a brand-name soup from the grocery store:

TOMATO AND LENTIL SOUP

Water, Lentils, Tomato Puree (water, Tomato Paste), Carrots, Modified Food Starch, Diced Tomatoes In Tomato Juice, Contains Less Than 2% Of: Spinach, Salt, Potassium Chloride, Dehydrated Onions, Flavoring, Cheddar Cheese (milk, Cultures, Salt, Enzymes), Parmesan Cheese (milk, Cultures, Salt, Enzymes), Sugar, Concentrated Lemon Juice, Spices, Dehydrated Garlic, Garlic, Yeast Extract, Dehydrated Tomato, Tomato Paste, Olive Oil, Soy Sauce (water, Soybeans, Wheat, Salt), Disodium Inosinate And Disodium Guanylate, Tomatoes, Lactic Acid.

140 calories, 4 g fiber [calcium, iron, and potassium are not reported on the label]

It's full of funky ingredients such as modified food starch, unidentified flavorings, yeast extract (which is usually code for MSG), and a few other questionable ingredients that may be just fine (since we can't determine safety just because the word has a lot of syllables—remember the example of dihydrogen monoxide?) but may *not* be fine. I don't want to have to look up every ingredient while I am standing in the grocery store.

Instead of buying that soup, I could make my own from scratch. Sometimes I do. But sometimes (okay, many times) I need convenience. I've found a brand of foods that's frozen and has only high-quality ingredients as if I had made it myself.

Here are the ingredients in the frozen organic harvest bowl that I enjoy:

LENTIL AND TOMATO BOLOGNESE

organic green lentils, organic cremini mushrooms, organic tomato puree, organic tomatoes (organic tomatoes, calcium chloride), organic carrots, organic kale, leeks, organic extra virgin olive oil, water, organic yellow onion puree, Himalayan sea salt, garlic, organic black garlic puree, organic basil, oregano, organic black pepper, organic red chili

230 calories, 12 g fiber, 93 mg calcium, 5 mg iron, 1219 mg potassium

---

There is not *one* funky or hard-to-identify ingredient within that list other than perhaps the calcium chloride that is in the tomatoes. What is calcium chloride? It's a form of salt that I'm not concerned about. Regular table salt, as you likely know, is sodium chloride.

Let's look beyond the ingredients of the two soups and focus on the nutrition information. If someone is a dieter, they might be inclined to choose the grocery store soup because it has fewer calories per serving. But let's look deeper. Notice that the organic version has twelve grams of fiber in every serving and also nutrients such as calcium, iron, and potassium. The fiber is going to feed our gut microbiomes well, and the nutrients will support our bodies' important behind-the-scenes work.

Because I don't have time to always make foods from scratch, label reading helps me have a clean(ish) option on hand. I can grab that frozen lentil and tomato bolognese, heat it up, and enjoy it with a handful of non-GMO sun-dried tomato and basil crackers on the side. Think back to the two factors I identified on pages 254 and 255:

1. By choosing the organic harvest bowl, I intentionally *put in* foods that provide the nutritional building blocks my body requires for vibrant health.

2. By choosing the non-GMO crackers with no funky ingredients, I made a plan to *avoid* putting in toxins or chemicals that will add to my body burden.

The experience of eating that meal is not *dramatically* different from how it would be to eat the other soup and crackers, but it is *noticeably* different. It's actually *more* delicious because my taste buds have adjusted to the flavors found in real foods and I appreciate the higher-quality options, and the fake flavor of the name-brand soup and crackers is a real turnoff to me now. Don't even get me started on how gross I find most bottled salad dressings to be these days. My taste buds *love* the flavors of real food rather than artificial ingredients, so I'm not only *not* making a sacrifice when I choose higher-quality foods, I enjoy my food more now. That's a real clean(ish) win.

LIFE IN A HURRY: GOOD FOOD, FAST

As I mentioned in the last section, I don't have time to make everything from scratch. I'm busy. You're busy. Life is busy. While I do love to cook, I appreciate shortcuts and the convenience of grab-and-go when necessary. Keep in mind that convenience has a price. Either it costs you your *health* (cheap convenience foods are usually not-food), or it costs more *money* (for higher-quality food that is ready to eat), or it costs you *time* (the time spent in preparation and planning ahead).

What do you do to ensure that what you're grabbing is clean(ish)?

Being prepared really is the key. I'm sure you've heard the saying: "If you fail to plan, you might as well plan to fail." That really is true. If you are not prepared, that's when you dash to the drive-through or find that convenient not-food stashed at the back of your pantry. You end up unsatisfied because your body isn't well nourished, and that often leads to overeating as your body searches for the nutrients it requires. Our bodies always drive us to eat more food when we aren't meeting our nutritional needs, and so never forget that.

To keep this from happening, make sure to have a variety of staple products on hand, which will make it much more likely that the foods you grab are nutritious. My freezer and pantry are always stocked with options. When you find favorites on sale, particularly nonperishables for freezer or pantry, stock up!

You may also be someone who enjoys meal planning on the weekends. Shop once, prep what you need for the week, and also consider planned leftovers to make the most of your time.

What's really saved me has been meal kit delivery companies. I have tried almost all of them over the years, and they played a huge role in my willingness to experiment with new foods because they send exactly the right portions of each ingredient. I currently use two different companies each week, with one delivery on Monday and the other on Thursday. The ones I use right now focus on organic ingredients, and so that's one more way I can be clean(ish) without having to stress about it. While they may seem at first glance to be more expensive than doing your own grocery shopping (and that's more likely to be true if you have a large family to feed), they save us money each week since I am only cooking for two—no more food waste because they send exactly how much we need for each meal. I get to cook a delicious meal from scratch each night, but I didn't have to meal plan or go to the store, and I don't have extra ingredients to throw away later.

You may worry that these companies are not good for the environment because of the packaging and also because you're having everything delivered to your home, but the truth is that a 2019 study found that meal kits actually have a smaller carbon footprint than when you shop at the grocery store.[4] That study was performed in 2019, and I know the companies I use today are doing even more in 2021 than they were doing two years ago, so I feel good about the environmental impact of my choice.

What if you are on the go and don't have time to cook at home every night, even with the time savings of meal kits? That is a real concern because as a society, we are busy, leading us to eat outside the home more than ever. If you have a lifestyle that requires frequent meals on the go, there are a number of strategies that you can keep in mind:

- Review restaurant menus online before you go to see if there are clean(ish) options for you and your family.

- Look for options with more vegetable ingredients. While most restaurants (in my area, at least) don't offer organic ingredients, conventional produce is preferable to ultra-processed food every single time.

- It's okay to not be "perfect" . . . we are clean(ish), after all. However, if you are driving-through the "golden arches" (or another similar fast-food restaurant) several times a week, it's time to consider making a change. Come up with grab-and-go or quick-to-prepare options that you can have on hand for those nights when you need them. We are all busy, but remember that we are building healthy bodies, and that needs to be prioritized.

One thing is common as you become clean(ish): the more you get used to high-quality foods, the more you'll feel it when you choose foods that are in the not-food category, even when on the go. You'll be ready for a delicious home-cooked meal after a few restaurant meals in a row. The first time I craved vegetables instead of fast food, I didn't recognize myself, but it's the norm now.

PRIORITIZE CLEAN(ISH) SWEETENERS

In healthy eating circles, sugar gets a lot of negative attention. It's definitely an ultra-processed food, and much of the sugar out there is derived from GMO crops. There are documentaries, books, and blog posts about how bad sugar is for us, and a call from more and more dietary experts to avoid sugar entirely.

It's not easy to do that, by the way. If you decide you want to minimize sugar, it is almost impossible to buy any packaged foods because most of them have sugar or something that is equivalent to sugar on the ingredients list, and that is true whether you are talking about ketchup, crackers, salad dressings, or really any packaged foods. Sweeteners are everywhere.

You'll need to consider your viewpoint on sugar (in all its forms) when developing your own personal definition of clean(ish). Before you do, keep in mind that there are cleaner options that you can choose from, as not all sweeteners are created equal.

Here are some of the better options:

Blackstrap molasses: A by-product of the sugar-refining process, it contains all the good stuff that was in the original sugarcane (B vitamins, calcium, iron, magnesium, potassium, chromium, and antioxidants).

Coconut palm sugar: The sap from the coconut palm is evaporated down into a crystal form. It has the minerals iron, zinc, calcium, and potassium, as well as a fiber called *inulin,* which may slow the rate of glucose absorption.

Date sugar: These are dehydrated dates that have been ground into granules. All the fiber, vitamins, and minerals that were found in the original dates are still there.

Organic whole cane sugar, or sucanat: This is produced by pressing the juice from raw sugarcane and then removing the water through an evaporation process. This retains many of the vitamins, minerals, and antioxidants from the sugarcane juice.

Raw honey: Raw honey has been taken from the beehive and not heated above 105 degrees, and it retains important enzymes, as well as being high in antioxidants, vitamins, and minerals.

Maple syrup: Pure maple syrup is made from the sap of maple trees, and it contains calcium, zinc, manganese, and a wide variety of anti-oxidants.

CHOOSE YOUR BEVERAGES CAREFULLY

One time I was at a big-box warehouse store and I had a stunning realization while walking through the beverage department: I felt like I was looking smack-dab *directly at* the obesity epidemic, right there on the shelves. In the intermittent fasting chapter, I mentioned insulin and that one of our goals is to keep insulin low during the fast. Hyperinsulinemia—meaning that you have elevated levels of insulin in your blood—is on the rise in the U.S., and this condition has been linked to many chronic health conditions, such as obesity, diabetes, hypertension, renal failure, nonalcoholic fatty liver disease, polycystic ovary syndrome, sleep apnea, certain cancers, atherosclerosis, and cardiovascular disease, not to mention metabolic syndrome as a whole.[5] Having high levels of insulin at all times is not good for our bodies, for so many reasons.

Even if you are not an intermittent faster (and even if you never want to be), insulin matters to your body because hyperinsulinemia is something to avoid, for all of us. You don't want to live a life where you are causing frequent insulin release all day long. This happens when we eat frequently throughout the day (meal, snack, meal, snack, meal, snack . . .), but it also happens when you choose sweet or flavored beverages. When we consume something that tastes sweet or makes our brains think food is coming in, we experience cephalic phase insulin response, and our pancreas releases insulin to manage the glucose that our brains assume will be coming in.

When I looked at the beverages for sale in that warehouse store, almost every one of them was flavored or sweetened in some way. It's harder and harder to find plain water these days, in fact. I've been in convenience stores and coffee shops trying to purchase unflavored sparkling water and all that is on the shelf is bottle after bottle of flavored options.

If you decide to practice an intermittent fasting lifestyle, it's easy to know what to choose during the fast because options are limited: when we fast clean, we stick to plain water, unflavored sparkling water, black coffee, and plain tea.

But what if you aren't an intermittent faster? Does it matter what *you* drink during the day?

I believe the answer is yes.

When I was obese, I remember that I always had a flavored or sweetened beverage at my fingertips from the moment I woke up until time for bed.

I started my morning with a latte, and I sweetened it with zero-calorie stevia. After breakfast, I had at least one more of those lattes midmorning, and after that, I usually switched to zero-calorie (yet still sweet-tasting) diet soda. When I was trying to be "clean," I would choose stevia-sweetened options, but other times, my choices included aspartame or Splenda, or even sugar- or corn-syrup-sweetened sodas. With meals, I always drank soda. In the afternoon, I switched to flavored water or used a water enhancer to give my water more flavor. Plain water? No, thank you. In the evening, I would have flavored herbal teas, usually those with dessert flavors like apple cinnamon or pomegranate, and I added even more stevia.

Does that sound familiar?

And as I finished up my teaching career, I saw that the students in my classes did the same thing. At some point, we started allowing kids to bring water bottles to school and to keep them on their desks during the day. "A hydrated brain is a more-focused brain" became our mantra. What did the kids put in these bottles? Even though we had a "water only" policy, most of the kids added water enhancers (full of flavors and sweeteners).

If your goal is avoiding hyperinsulinemia, it's worth considering what you're drinking during the day. My recommendation? Whether you are an intermittent faster or not, if you aren't having a meal, consider avoiding beverages that are flavored or sweetened. Stick to plain water and unflavored sparkling water, and have black coffee or plain tea. Skip the flavored waters, throw away the water enhancers, shun diet sodas, put down the juices, and stop nursing the sweetened milky coffee beverages and energy drinks all day long.

I have a theory that if every person in the world changed their beverages in this manner—and that is the *only* change they made—we would see a decline in the obesity epidemic and overall health would improve—and hyperinsulinemia would decrease within the population. Can I prove it? No, it's just a theory. But what do you have to lose? Give it a try.

Plain water? Black coffee? Plain tea? Embrace them. See what happens.

WATER, WATER, EVERYWHERE ... BUT WHAT TO DRINK?

Now that I have convinced you to drink more plain water, you will need to find a source for your water. Is bottled water "safer" than tap water?

The short answer: Not necessarily, and it might actually be *less* safe. Or not. It depends.

That may not have been very helpful, so let's dig into the issues with bottled water versus tap water so that we are better equipped to make an educated decision.

Most of us have come to think of bottled water as a higher-quality choice than tap water, and a lot of that is thanks to the marketing practices of the bottled water industry.[6] They spend a lot of money designing logos and product names that let us know that their water is as *pure as a mountain stream.* (By the way . . . have you ever seen the water in a mountain stream? I grew up in the mountains of Virginia, and we had a stream on our property. The water was certainly not "pure" as it flowed, and the water was definitely *not* something I would have consumed directly from the stream. Our neighbors upstream had cows, and the stream also had fish living in it. Use your imagination.)

If you remember from an earlier chapter, Consumer Reports tested a variety of bottled water products in 2020 and found that many of those tested had detectible levels of PFAS chemicals.

It may surprise you to know that tap water is generally held to a higher standard than bottled water.[7] In addition, many popular bottled waters are simply repackaged tap water from their city of origin, with no crystal-clear mountain stream anywhere in sight.

Some bottled water brands even make fancy health claims (based on the water's pH level or added minerals). Some of those claims may actually be true, believe it or not. Alkaline mineral waters have been linked to positive health benefits, and the minerals found in various waters (such as magnesium, sulfur, and calcium, just to name a few) can be used by the body. For that reason, mineral waters can be a great choice.[8,9]

When choosing a bottled water product, packaging is also a consideration for many. Choosing glass bottles over plastic may make a difference in the overall safety of the water inside, as chemicals within plastic bottles may leach into the water inside, and it may be more likely to happen when the bottles are exposed to heat.[10] While there isn't consensus as to whether it's enough to make a difference, if you want to err on the safe side, choose glass.[11,12,13]

REFLECT: CREATING YOUR PERSONAL DEFINITION OF CLEAN(ISH) EATING—WHAT MATTERS MOST?

There are many definitions of "clean eating" out there. In one book that I read, clean eating involved committing to being a vegetarian, and even dairy was off limits. In another, you could have dairy as long as it was low fat. Why isn't full-fat dairy "clean" in that plan? I have no idea. One clean-eating plan had whole grain foods as front and center, while another insisted that you must be gluten-free and avoid grains entirely. In another, meat was to be avoided but fish was okay. Confused yet?

In general, what do these varied definitions of clean eating have in common? Most of them include a focus on natural foods that are free of chemicals, artificial ingredients, and other potentially harmful additives, and an avoidance of ultra-processed foods. But many may stress an unhealthy level of perfection, and some also add in other restrictions based on the author's personal dietary preferences (such as avoiding dairy, gluten, grains, meat, etc.).

Now, it's time to forget about everyone else's idea of what it means to "eat clean" and define *yours*.

First, we can agree on a fairly general definition that fits everyone: clean eating is when you prioritize whole foods and avoid both ultra-processed foods and foods that don't work well for your body. Clean(ish) eating, then, is when you make choices that honor your health and wellness, yet also provide you with flexibility so you can enjoy your life.

As you create your own definition of clean(ish) eating, also remember this: we are supposed to eat for pleasure. Your definition of clean(ish) eating should include choosing foods that you love, and you also want to make sure you have the freedom to live in the real world. You *will* eat foods that are ultra-processed on occasion (or maybe even daily), and you will also eat foods prepared by others that contain ingredients you would avoid when cooking at home.

If I am at a restaurant, I eat the food that sounds good to me, while also considering how I will feel after I eat. As an example,

I know that eating a meal that includes french fries deep-fried in cheap or old cooking oil is likely to give me a stomachache later. I don't want to have a stomachache, so I usually choose a different side dish. There is a local restaurant, however, that features quality burgers and fries, and I've never had a stomachache after eating there. Are their cooking oils the type I prefer to use at home? No. But, because I am clean(ish), I enjoy the heck out of those fries when we eat there, dousing them in malt vinegar and salt. Do I put the vinegar on there because research shows that vinegar reduces the spikes of both insulin and glucose that come after a meal? No. I add it because it's absolutely delicious, and any health benefits are just the cherry on top—or I suppose I should say the *vinegar* on top in this case.

As another example, if I'm at a wedding, I am not going to ask the bride what's in the cake, and I don't even care what's in the cake, to tell you the truth. I am clean(ish), and I will eat cake with zero worries about whether they used organic flour or if the frosting is made with funky oils or sweeteners. I don't even let those thoughts cross my mind, frankly. If I bake a cake at home, I can control what goes in it, and I do. But that doesn't mean I am stuck with only eating cake that I bake for myself for the rest of my life.

FOODS TO EXCLUDE OR LIMIT

Now, I want you to take some time to skim through the previous chapters of the book and decide which of these issues are most important to you. You aren't doing a full reread but simply a skim. You'll record the information within the chart, and I've included the chapters/page numbers in the chart for your convenience.

As you think about each one of these concerns, you're going to identify which are the most problematic to *you* based on what you've learned, and that will help you focus your attention.

I have also left space for you to add a few of your own concerns beyond those I have listed. If you know certain foods don't work well for your body, add them here. For example, perhaps you know a certain food or ingredient (such as gluten or dairy) gives you a stomachache every time you eat it. You'll definitely want to include that as a consideration in your personal definition of clean(ish).

As you think about each concern on the list, your goal is to decide if there are any areas where you want to be completely clean, meaning you'll *always* avoid those ingredients when you know they are present. Or you may decide that clean(ish) is good enough, meaning you'll choose to avoid them some to most of the time, but won't stress about infrequent consumption. Alternately, you may find that you don't find the concerns to be compelling enough to require consideration from day to day.

Before you begin, I want to let you know that I thought about giving you examples from my own personal definition of clean(ish). There are a few ingredients of concern that fall into the "*I will avoid this ingredient completely and at all times*" list for me, a few that are in the "*I am not at all concerned about this ingredient, and I don't plan to avoid it*" group, and most things fall into the "*I will take a clean(ish) approach*" category.

But this isn't about *me*. It's about *you*. So, I decided to leave that part out entirely so you can decide for yourself. You're creating your *personal* definition of clean(ish), not simply following mine.

You can complete this section right here in the book, or you can re-create it within your Clean(ish) Journal if you don't want to write in the book. Alternately, go to ginstephens.com/cleanish to download and print the pdf that contains these pages in worksheet format.

Concern	How I Feel About It	How I Will Apply This to My Life
GMOs "Food, Glorious Food," page 92	☐ I will avoid this completely and at all times. ☐ I will take a clean(ish) approach. I won't consume it frequently, but I won't stress if I encounter it on occasion. ☐ I am not at all concerned about this, and I don't plan to avoid it.	

Nonorganic Meats "Food, Glorious Food," pages 98-101	☐ I will avoid this completely and at all times. ☐ I will take a clean(ish) approach. I won't consume it frequently, but I won't stress if I encounter it on occasion. ☐ I am not at all concerned about this, and I don't plan to avoid it.	
Nonorganic animal products (dairy, eggs, etc.) "Food, Glorious Food," pages 98-104	☐ I will avoid this completely and at all times. ☐ I will take a clean(ish) approach. I won't consume it frequently, but I won't stress if I encounter it on occasion. ☐ I am not at all concerned about this, and I don't plan to avoid it.	
Nonorganic plant foods (fruits, vegetables, grains, etc.) "Food, Glorious Food," pages 101-107	☐ I will avoid this completely and at all times. ☐ I will take a clean(ish) approach. I won't consume it frequently, but I won't stress if I encounter it on occasion. ☐ I am not at all concerned about this, and I don't plan to avoid it.	
Ultra-processed foods in general "Take a Break from Fake," page 117	☐ I will avoid this completely and at all times. ☐ I will take a clean(ish) approach. I won't consume it frequently, but I won't stress if I encounter it on occasion. ☐ I am not at all concerned about this, and I don't plan to avoid it.	
Toxic oils/ highly processed fats "Take a Break from Fake," page 122	☐ I will avoid this completely and at all times. ☐ I will take a clean(ish) approach. I won't consume it frequently, but I won't stress if I encounter it on occasion. ☐ I am not at all concerned about this, and I don't plan to avoid it.	

MSG "Take a Break from Fake," page 123	☐ I will avoid this completely and at all times. ☐ I will take a clean(ish) approach. I won't consume it frequently, but I won't stress if I encounter it on occasion. ☐ I am not at all concerned about this, and I don't plan to avoid it.	
Highly refined grains "Take a Break from Fake," page 124	☐ I will avoid this completely and at all times. ☐ I will take a clean(ish) approach. I won't consume it frequently, but I won't stress if I encounter it on occasion. ☐ I am not at all concerned about this, and I don't plan to avoid it.	
Sugar "Take a Break from Fake," page 124	☐ I will avoid this completely and at all times. ☐ I will take a clean(ish) approach. I won't consume it frequently, but I won't stress if I encounter it on occasion. ☐ I am not at all concerned about this, and I don't plan to avoid it.	
High fructose corn syrup "Take a Break from Fake," page 125	☐ I will avoid this completely and at all times. ☐ I will take a clean(ish) approach. I won't consume it frequently, but I won't stress if I encounter it on occasion. ☐ I am not at all concerned about this, and I don't plan to avoid it.	
Artificial sweeteners "Take a Break from Fake," page 125	☐ I will avoid this completely and at all times. ☐ I will take a clean(ish) approach. I won't consume it frequently, but I won't stress if I encounter it on occasion. ☐ I am not at all concerned about this, and I don't plan to avoid it.	

Other food additives (artificial flavors, colors, preservatives, emulsifiers, etc.) "Take a Break from Fake," page 126	☐ I will avoid this completely and at all times. ☐ I will take a clean(ish) approach. I won't consume it frequently, but I won't stress if I encounter it on occasion. ☐ I am not at all concerned about this, and I don't plan to avoid it.	
Supplements "Take a Break from Fake," page 128	☐ I will avoid this completely and at all times. ☐ I will take a clean(ish) approach. I won't consume it frequently, but I won't stress if I encounter it on occasion. ☐ I am not at all concerned about this, and I don't plan to avoid it.	
My personal ingredient of concern:	☐ I will avoid this completely and at all times. ☐ I will take a clean(ish) approach. I won't consume it frequently, but I won't stress if I encounter it on occasion. ☐ I am not at all concerned about this, and I don't plan to avoid it.	
My personal ingredient of concern:	☐ I will avoid this completely and at all times. ☐ I will take a clean(ish) approach. I won't consume it frequently, but I won't stress if I encounter it on occasion. ☐ I am not at all concerned about this, and I don't plan to avoid it.	
My personal ingredient of concern:	☐ I will avoid this completely and at all times. ☐ I will take a clean(ish) approach. I won't consume it frequently, but I won't stress if I encounter it on occasion. ☐ I am not at all concerned about this, and I don't plan to avoid it.	

| My personal ingredient of concern: | ☐ I will avoid this completely and at all times.

☐ I will take a clean(ish) approach. I won't consume it frequently, but I won't stress if I encounter it on occasion.

☐ I am not at all concerned about this, and I don't plan to avoid it. | |
| My personal ingredient of concern: | ☐ I will avoid this completely and at all times.

☐ I will take a clean(ish) approach. I won't consume it frequently, but I won't stress if I encounter it on occasion.

☐ I am not at all concerned about this, and I don't plan to avoid it. | |

FOODS TO PRIORITIZE

Now that you have identified what foods you may want to avoid, it's time to think about what foods/nutrients you want to intentionally include.

Refer back to "What's a Healthy Diet? And How Do We Know?" from page 134 and "What's Food Got to Do with It?" from page 186.

You'll want to focus on foods that have been part of traditional diets throughout history (including foods that your ancestors ate), foods that are enjoyed in the Blue Zones, foods that feed our gut microbiomes well (plenty of fiber, prebiotics, and probiotics), and foods that have all the vitamins, minerals, and phytochemicals your body needs to function well.

The good news is that they are all the same foods. Overall, your number one goal is to include a wide variety of REAL foods.

Food	What's My Current Intake?	How I Will Apply This to My Life
	☐ I already include this in my diet in amounts that are appropriate for good health.	

Organic foods (in general)	☐ I already include this in my diet, but I know I need to work on including more/greater variety of this food. ☐ I don't include this in my diet now, but I know I need to make an effort to add it in. ☐ I think I may eat *too much* of this food, so I'll work on consuming less of it. ☐ This is a food that I don't eat now, and I also don't think that it belongs in my personal diet.	
Vegetables	☐ I already include this in my diet in amounts that are appropriate for good health. ☐ I already include this in my diet, but I know I need to work on including more/greater variety of this food. ☐ I don't include this in my diet now, but I know I need to make an effort to add it in. ☐ I think I may eat *too much* of this food, so I'll work on consuming less of it. ☐ This is a food that I don't eat now, and I also don't think that it belongs in my personal diet.	
Fruits	☐ I already include this in my diet in amounts that are appropriate for good health. ☐ I already include this in my diet, but I know I need to work on including more/greater variety of this food. ☐ I don't include this in my diet now, but I know I need to make an effort to add it in.	

	☐ I think I may eat *too much* of this food, so I'll work on consuming less of it. ☐ This is a food that I don't eat now, and I also don't think that it belongs in my personal diet.	
Whole grains	☐ I already include this in my diet in amounts that are appropriate for good health. ☐ I already include this in my diet, but I know I need to work on including more/greater variety of this food. ☐ I don't include this in my diet now, but I know I need to make an effort to add it in. ☐ I think I may eat *too much* of this food, so I'll work on consuming less of it. ☐ This is a food that I don't eat now, and I also don't think that it belongs in my personal diet.	
Meat	☐ I already include this in my diet in amounts that are appropriate for good health. ☐ I already include this in my diet, but I know I need to work on including more/greater variety of this food. ☐ I don't include this in my diet now, but I know I need to make an effort to add it in. ☐ I think I may eat *too much* of this food, so I'll work on consuming less of it. ☐ This is a food that I don't eat now, and I also don't think that it belongs in my personal diet.	

Seafood	☐ I already include this in my diet in amounts that are appropriate for good health. ☐ I already include this in my diet, but I know I need to work on including more/greater variety of this food. ☐ I don't include this in my diet now, but I know I need to make an effort to add it in. ☐ I think I may eat *too much* of this food, so I'll work on consuming less of it. ☐ This is a food that I don't eat now, and I also don't think that it belongs in my personal diet.	
Other proteins	☐ I already include this in my diet in amounts that are appropriate for good health. ☐ I already include this in my diet, but I know I need to work on including more/greater variety of this food. ☐ I don't include this in my diet now, but I know I need to make an effort to add it in. ☐ I think I may eat *too much* of this food, so I'll work on consuming less of it. ☐ This is a food that I don't eat now, and I also don't think that it belongs in my personal diet.	
Other animal products (dairy, eggs, etc.)	☐ I already include this in my diet in amounts that are appropriate for good health. ☐ I already include this in my diet, but I know I need to work on including more/greater variety of this food.	

	☐ I don't include this in my diet now, but I know I need to make an effort to add it in.	
	☐ I think I may eat *too much* of this food, so I'll work on consuming less of it.	
	☐ This is a food that I don't eat now, and I also don't think that it belongs in my personal diet.	
Healthy fats/ oils	☐ I already include this in my diet in amounts that are appropriate for good health.	
	☐ I already include this in my diet, but I know I need to work on including more/greater variety of this food.	
	☐ I don't include this in my diet now, but I know I need to make an effort to add it in.	
	☐ I think I may eat *too much* of this food, so I'll work on consuming less of it.	
	☐ This is a food that I don't eat now, and I also don't think that it belongs in my personal diet.	
Herbs/ spices	☐ I already include this in my diet in amounts that are appropriate for good health.	
	☐ I already include this in my diet, but I know I need to work on including more/greater variety of this food.	
	☐ I don't include this in my diet now, but I know I need to make an effort to add it in.	

	☐ I think I may eat *too much* of this food, so I'll work on consuming less of it.	
	☐ This is a food that I don't eat now, and I also don't think that it belongs in my personal diet.	
Clean(ish) sweeteners	☐ I already include this in my diet in amounts that are appropriate for good health.	
	☐ I already include this in my diet, but I know I need to work on including more/greater variety of this food.	
	☐ I don't include this in my diet now, but I know I need to make an effort to add it in.	
	☐ I think I may eat *too much* of this food, so I'll work on consuming less of it.	
	☐ This is a food that I don't eat now, and I also don't think that it belongs in my personal diet.	

WHAT WILL I DRINK?

And, finally, no definition of clean(ish) eating would be complete without considering your beverages. Most of us have a beverage of some sort at our fingertips throughout our day, so you'll want to choose carefully.

Look back at page 268 from earlier in this "Eat (Mostly) Clean" chapter and think about what you're currently drinking throughout the day and with your meals.

Beverage	How I Feel About It	Other Things to Consider About This Beverage

		container, source, organic vs. not organic, ingredients, etc.
Water, unflavored	☐ This is a beverage that I will prioritize throughout my day. ☐ This is a beverage that I will avoid completely and at all times. ☐ I will take a clean(ish) approach. I won't consume this beverage frequently, but I won't stress if I encounter it on occasion.	
Sparkling water or mineral water, unflavored	☐ This is a beverage that I will prioritize throughout my day. ☐ This is a beverage that I will avoid completely and at all times. ☐ I will take a clean(ish) approach. I won't consume this beverage frequently, but I won't stress if I encounter it on occasion.	
Coffee, black	☐ This is a beverage that I will prioritize throughout my day. ☐ This is a beverage that I will avoid completely and at all times. ☐ I will take a clean(ish) approach. I won't consume this beverage frequently, but I won't stress if I encounter it on occasion.	
Tea, plain	☐ This is a beverage that I will prioritize throughout my day. ☐ This is a beverage that I will avoid completely and at all times. ☐ I will take a clean(ish) approach. I won't consume this beverage frequently, but I won't stress if I encounter it on occasion.	
Water or sparkling water, flavored	☐ This is a beverage that I will prioritize throughout my day. ☐ This is a beverage that I will avoid completely and at all times.	

	☐ I will take a clean(ish) approach. I won't consume this beverage frequently, but I won't stress if I encounter it on occasion.	
Coffee or tea, with additives (milk, creamers, sweeteners, etc.)	☐ This is a beverage that I will prioritize throughout my day. ☐ This is a beverage that I will avoid completely and at all times. ☐ I will take a clean(ish) approach. I won't consume this beverage frequently, but I won't stress if I encounter it on occasion.	
Sodas	☐ This is a beverage that I will prioritize throughout my day. ☐ This is a beverage that I will avoid completely and at all times. ☐ I will take a clean(ish) approach. I won't consume this beverage frequently, but I won't stress if I encounter it on occasion.	
Juice-based beverages	☐ This is a beverage that I will prioritize throughout my day. ☐ This is a beverage that I will avoid completely and at all times. ☐ I will take a clean(ish) approach. I won't consume this beverage frequently, but I won't stress if I encounter it on occasion.	
Alcohol	☐ This is a beverage that I will prioritize throughout my day. ☐ This is a beverage that I will avoid completely and at all times. ☐ I will take a clean(ish) approach. I won't consume this beverage frequently, but I won't stress if I encounter it on occasion.	
Other	☐ This is a beverage that I will prioritize throughout my day. ☐ This is a beverage that I will avoid completely and at all times.	

	□ I will take a clean(ish) approach. I won't consume this beverage frequently, but I won't stress if I encounter it on occasion.	

TAKE ACTION: YOUR PERSONAL DEFINITION OF CLEAN(ISH) EATING

Use your Clean(ish) Journal (or the worksheets available at ginstephens .com/cleanish) to create your definition of Clean(ish) Eating.

Now that you've taken the time to consider what to include in your definition of clean(ish) eating, summarize your thoughts.

My personal definition of Clean(ish) Eating:

- There are some foods and/or ingredients that I will avoid *at all times.* These include:

- There are some foods and/or ingredients that I may consume from time to time, but I will limit or avoid them when it is convenient to do so, *or* I'll eat them if avoiding them affects my enjoyment of a recipe, *or* I'll eat them if I don't have another option available. These include:

- There are some foods and/or ingredients that I will actively work to include more of/prioritize in my diet. These include:

When it comes to my beverages, I will choose:

LIVE (MAINLY) CLEAN

I have good news for you—making the transition to living (mainly) clean is easier in many ways than transitioning to clean(ish) eating because the very act of eating is tied up with so many different emotions beyond just nourishing your body. If someone offers you pie, you aren't going to ask them to whip out an ingredients list. (Please don't. If you feel like you can never eat food without reading the ingredients list ever again, I want you to reread the "Paralysis of Analysis" chapter and consider if you may need to work through these tendences with the help of an expert to see if your focus on healthy eating has become problematic.)

There are many day-to-day situations where you aren't fully in control of what you are eating, such as when you're dining at restaurants, if you're eating foods prepared by others, and even when cooking at home—manufacturers use ingredients you wouldn't use, but we still may want to use some of these products in our recipes. As with the examples of my favorite mayonnaise and the crackers and chips that I still choose to eat (even though they may contain oils I wouldn't buy as standalone ingredients to cook with), there are going to be foods that you keep in your life, knowing that some of the ingredients are not ideal. The goal is to lower our *overall* toxic loads, and by eating (mostly) clean, we do that, even though we don't ever reach "perfection."

With the products we buy to clean our homes, apply to our bodies, and furnish our surroundings, however, it's a lot easier to make the swaps to better choices. Almost without exception, natural cleaning products, skin care products, cosmetics, and personal care products work just as well as conventional choices.

Notice how I said "*almost* without exception." That's because you will find examples where you just aren't willing to make the switch to a natural product. As you create your own personal definition for living (mainly) clean, you'll decide what matters most to you, and you always have the freedom to choose products that meet your needs. We are clean(*ish*). Perfection is not required.

I'm going to go ahead and share the number one example from my life where I am thankful for the *-ish*: natural deodorant. Sigh. I have struggled with finding a natural deodorant that works well for me for years. I've finally found one that works 90-plus percent of the time, and so I use it 90-plus percent of the time. However, when it is one hundred degrees in Georgia and I am wearing an outfit with spaghetti straps, there is not one single natural deodorant that does the job I need it to do. Sorry, natural deodorant. It's not you, it's me.

I use natural deodorant 100 percent of the time from September to April, but as soon as it starts heating up, I need additional support when I know I am going to be out in the heat or working up a good sweat. I'm not talking about a sauna sweat here—I don't mind sweating while in the sauna or if I am exercising and then I plan to take a shower. Natural deodorant works just fine in those situations. But if I am going out to lunch with friends and my armpits are going to be exposed to the world and I know I will be sweating, I use regular deodorant that day.

Now, before you say, "But you haven't tried *my* natural deodorant," I need to tell you—yes, I probably have tried it. I tried most of them because I really would like to use natural deodorant 100 percent of the time. The one I use now is fantastic—90-plus percent of the time, as I said. Because I am clean(ish), I know that I have lowered the overall level of my bucket through the other choices I have made, so I am not going to worry about using regular deodorant on the rare occasions when I need additional support.

As you transition to clean(ish) living, your goal is to focus on making swaps that you can live with, just as I have. You'll choose products that make a difference *most of the time,* while also making sure you pick products that work, are convenient, and fit into your budget.

THE BIG PURGE: TO TRASH OR NOT TO TRASH?

As you start sorting through your cleaning and personal care products, you'll want to use the Environmental Working Group app (or any of the other apps or buying guides available) to check what you already have on hand. You may be pleasantly surprised with what you find because some products that don't seem natural or safe when you look at the label are actually great choices. On the flip side, you'll find products you thought were safe (I'm looking at *you,* greenwashing) and realize they are not something that you want to use going forward.

When that happens, you may be tempted to get a huge garbage bag and throw all those things away, immediately.

I want to encourage you *not* to do that. At least, not without careful consideration of each item individually.

Remember that if you decide something is not safe to use in your home or on your body, you may not want to have it seep into our groundwater at the trash dump, either. Read the labels, and if anything has warnings or information about proper disposal methods, check with your local sanitation service.

The EPA also has information about hazardous household waste on their website, and it's important to follow all guidelines for safety.

Also, consider whether you actually do need to dispose of every questionable item you find immediately. If it's on the *not-that-bad-though-it-isn't-that-great* side of the continuum, perhaps you decide to use it up and then buy something else that is safer next time.

That is a legitimate option to consider, especially since becoming clean(ish) is a process. If I found that something was a lot more dangerous than I'd thought, however, I would not keep it around and finish up the bottle. I would safely dispose of it. The choice is always yours.

Before you create your own definition of clean(ish) living, I'll go through some of the categories of items you'll have within your house, discuss issues pertaining to each, and also share some strategies for you to consider.

CLEANING PRODUCTS

When did cleaning products become so complicated and specialized? When I decided to do my own cleaning product purge, I started underneath my kitchen sink. I found FORTY-FIVE different cleaning products in that cabinet alone. That's ridiculous, and I am almost embarrassed to tell you about it. In the pantry, I had twelve individual items, and in the laundry room, there were eighteen various products. That's a total of seventy-five cleaning products just in my kitchen, pantry, and laundry area, and I didn't even go into the bathrooms to see what I had stashed away there, or into the garage, where I know we have even more things that accumulated over the years.

What kind of weirdo has *more than* seventy-five individual cleaning products in her house? Me, that's who.

Under my kitchen sink alone, I had individual products to clean hardwood floors, tile floors, granite, silver, stainless steel, grout, dishes (in the sink), dishes (in the dishwasher), wood tabletops, glass and mirrors, the stovetop, the oven, my hands, stainless steel pots and pans, upholstery, carpet . . . The list goes on. We do not need this many products, y'all. Maybe you don't have the accumulation that I do, or maybe your kitchen is out of control, just as mine was.

Don't even ask me to tell you what happened when I started checking them using the Environmental Working Group's Healthy

Living app, because that let me know just how greenwashed I had been. It would be embarrassing, except that I know I'm not alone.

I did find some very interesting results while checking my products in the app, and I am actually going to tell you what I found, even though I just told you not to ask. Have you ever seen CLR Calcium, Lime, & Rust Remover on the shelf? When you look at the label, it looks like it's probably a dangerous and toxin-filled option. I had it under my kitchen cabinet, so I looked it up. EWG gives it a score of A. That same brand has a mold and mildew stain remover that EWG also gives an A. On the other hand, one "green" brand's "Natural All-Purpose Cleaner, Aloe and Green Tea" that I had under my cabinet gets a C. Another brand's "All-Purpose Cleaner, Free & Clear" option, which seems like such a good choice, being "Free & Clear" and all, gets a D. This once again illustrates that you can't tell if a product is nontoxic by looking at the label.

After contemplating everything I had on hand and eliminating everything I didn't need, I was left with about ten different essentials. Cleaning just got a lot simpler, and it feels amazing to have all that space back.

As you look closely at what you have on hand, you'll realize that you can replace a bunch of your cleaners with *one* nontoxic all-purpose cleaner. You don't need separate options for your countertop, the bathroom, and so on.

Here are a few tips for simplifying your cleaning products and routines:

- Buy concentrated forms of cleaning products. This helps you reduce packaging waste. Most cleaning products that you buy are mostly water, so when you buy the concentrated forms and then add your own water, you also save money in the long run.

- Soap and hot water are enough for many jobs, including handwashing. No need to use hand sanitizers with alcohol or products with triclosan (which is linked to antibiotic resistance).

- Remember that clean has no smell. That being said, essential oils, when used safely, can be a great option, and there are nontoxic cleaning products that use essential oils in a responsible and safe manner.

- Get a vacuum with a HEPA filter. We want to avoid recirculating whatever it is you're sucking up off your floors.

- Choose steam cleaners for your rugs rather than toxic carpet cleaners.

- Nontoxic laundry routines are more important than you may realize . . . the chemicals in your laundry products do not fully wash out and remain in the fabrics, and these clothes touch your skin (almost) 24-7. You don't need fabric softeners or dryer sheets, and you want to avoid heavy lingering scents at all costs.

BECOME A HOME CHEMIST

It can be a lot of fun to make your own household cleaning products. If you do a web search using the phrase "homemade natural cleaning products," you'll get hundreds of recipes that you can experiment with.

Most of them use simple ingredients that you likely already have on hand:

Baking soda

White vinegar

Liquid castile soap

Hydrogen peroxide

Essential oils *(research each to make sure you're using it safely)*

I'll be honest—I do not make my own cleaning products at this stage of my life (with one exception—I deodorize rugs with straight baking soda mixed with a little essential oil). There was a period of time from around 2003 to 2005 where I did make all my own cleaning products, and it was very satisfying to use products that I had formulated myself. Back then, there were a lot fewer options available in stores, and it was also more difficult to research the products that were available to see if they were safe.

Making your own cleaning products can be a lot less expensive than buying premade products, and you can customize everything to fit your needs. If you decide to go this route, have fun with it and start small. You can always add more recipes over time.

LIVING (MAINLY) CLEAN, ROOM BY ROOM

Now that we've tackled cleaning products, let's go from room to room of your house to find simple solutions for some of the most pressing concerns you'll find in each room.

These lists are by no means exhaustive, but they'll get you started.

IN THE KITCHEN

Use nontoxic cookware. If you have PTFE- or Teflon-coated pots and pans in your kitchen, it's time to replace them. At normal cooking temperatures, cookware with this type of nonstick coating releases a variety of gases and chemicals with mild to severe levels of toxicity.[1]

Instead, choose stainless steel, carbon steel, cast iron, or 100 percent ceramic (rather than ceramic-coated, certain brands of which may contain nanoparticles that end up in your foods).

Change out your food storage containers, wraps, and bags. If you're still storing your food in plastic containers, wraps, or bags (or worse yet—microwaving them in plastic), you'll want to swap them out for safer storage options. Mason jars and other glass storage containers are an excellent choice.

Many glass storage containers come with plastic lids, and if you don't want the plastic to come in contact with your foods, you have a couple of options. First, you can cover the food with unbleached parchment paper and place the plastic lid on top of that, or you can choose silicone stretchy lids, which can be washed and reused many times. You can even find a reusable beeswax wrap that is washable and clings to your container.

Silicone food storage bags made from food-grade silicone are another convenient storage solution, and they are both washable and reusable. Silicone has plastic-like properties, but because it contains no petroleum-based chemicals like BPA or phthalates, it is generally considered to be nontoxic. It is also more stable and is less likely to leach into your foods than plastic. One caveat is that when silicone is heated, small amounts of siloxanes may migrate into your foods, so to be on the safe side, avoid heating silicone to high temperatures where there is prolonged contact with your foods.

Replace your cooking utensils. Bamboo, wooden, or stainless steel cooking tools are ideal. Silicone utensils are also a safer option. Avoid standard plastic cooking utensils.

Consider your water filtration options. Earlier, I shared the surprising results found by Consumer Reports when they tested a variety of bottled water brands, and your local tap water may also be contaminated with various things you would rather avoid. I'm sure you've seen news stories about these issues in communities such as Flint, Michigan; Tallulah, Louisiana; or East Chicago, Illinois. One estimate I read suggested that about one-fifth of the United States may have issues with water quality, meaning that as many as sixty-three million Americans may be affected.[2] If you're concerned, it's time to think about water filtration options.

What you choose depends on your budget and space considerations. Pitcher filtration options are the cheapest and take up the least amount of space. You can also find countertop filtration systems, as well as those that mount under your kitchen sink. If you have a larger budget, there are whole-house filtration systems that remove a wide variety of contaminants.

Choose a wooden cutting board instead of plastic. One problem with plastic cutting boards is that you can end up with tiny pieces of plastic within your foods, which is definitely not what you want. But isn't a plastic cutting board more sanitary than wooden options? It turns out that the recent recommendations to use plastic cutting boards to prevent bacterial growth got it wrong—when the plastic surfaces are used over time, the knife cuts actually create crevices that harbor *more* bacteria, whereas bacteria placed on wooden surfaces die out quickly—and any bacteria that end up deeper inside the wooden board don't survive for long.[3] The USDA tells us that bamboo cutting boards are more resistant to bacteria than other woods, making bamboo an excellent choice.[4] Fractionated coconut oil, or MCT oil, is my cutting board conditioner of choice.

Get rid of pests naturally. When you have a pest problem, it's tempting to call an exterminator, but do you really want those toxic chemicals in your home? I sure don't. Instead, research to find nontoxic methods for dealing with your specific pests. As an example, if you have ants, do a web search for "nontoxic ant control" and you'll find solutions such as using dichotomous earth or essential oils like peppermint oil or tea tree oil.

Pests such as ants and cockroaches are attracted to moisture, so make sure that you don't have leaky faucets or dampness under your sink. Rather than using toxic pesticides, there are a variety of different traps that rely on sticky surfaces to target the specific pests you're dealing with. Even better than getting rid of pests—stop them from coming in by locating their entry points and sealing with a nontoxic caulking.

IN THE BATHROOM

Examine your makeup, skin care, and other personal care products carefully. Go through your bathroom and check each product against the Environmental Working Group's Healthy Living app database. One thing you can do is cut back on the number of products that you use on a day-to-day basis. Do I really need to use twenty-six products each day? Okay, yes. Yes, I do. Especially since I have vetted each one of them through the EWG app.

Even products such as nail polish and nail polish remover have safer options that are listed in the EWG database. When you are using options that are not highly rated, however, apply them in a well-ventilated room, or even go outside and give yourself a pedicure in the fresh air.

Address moisture issues. Although mold and mildew are all natural, it certainly isn't nontoxic. High levels of mold and mildew in your home absolutely will add to your toxic load and fill your bucket, so it's essential to make sure you don't have mold or mildew problems. Mold grows best in warm and damp conditions, and proper ventilation can help a great deal. Check under the bathroom vanity cabinets for moist areas, and also keep mold and mildew at bay on shower curtains/ shower doors/the tub surround, on your tile grout, and also in any caulked areas. A mixture of baking soda and vinegar as well as hydrogen peroxide are effective grout/tile cleaners that are safe to use. You can also try non-chlorine bleach alternatives or something like CLR Mold & Mildew Clear, which EWG rates as an A.

Swap out your shower curtain. Vinyl or PVC shower curtains contain endocrine-disrupting chemicals such as phthalates, and as these types of shower curtains off-gas, you breathe in the fumes every time you shower. Instead, replace them with cloth options that you can wash regularly, which will also help decrease mold.

Change your bath mat. If your current bath mat has a plastic backing, opt for something else. Either a bamboo or organic cotton bath mat would be a great option.

IN THE LAUNDRY ROOM

Choose nontoxic laundry detergents. Never forget that you have clothing touching your skin for the majority of the day, unless you live in a nudist colony. And even if you do, you spend your nights sleeping between sheets, with your face touching your pillowcase. Since you are in close contact with laundered fabric almost constantly, it's essential to keep your laundry toxin-free.

Avoid toxic fabric softeners. Conventional fabric softeners are some of the worst products available, though there are a few nontoxic natural versions that meet the EWG standards. Even many of the ones that are marketed as safer options (thank you, greenwashing) tend to score a D or an F in the EWG's Healthy Living app. Vinegar is a natural fabric softener, and if you use a quarter to a half cup, your clothes shouldn't come out smelling like salad dressing.

Skip dryer sheets entirely. You may have grown up with freshly scented laundry that owed its "fresh" smell to the dryer sheets your mom used, but remember that "clean" has no smell. When I checked the EWG Healthy Living app, there isn't a single dryer sheet option that is rated as an A, though there are a few that score a B. Instead of dryer sheets, try wool dryer balls. Here's a bit of a safety warning: do NOT add essential oil to your wool dryer balls, even though you may read this recommendation on any number of blogs—this can increase the risk of a dryer fire.

IN YOUR LIVING AREAS

Choose your furniture wisely. Many of the building products used in furniture construction such as MDF (medium-density fiberboard) off-gas toxins like formaldehyde. As furniture pieces age, however, they emit fewer and fewer of these gases over time. For that reason, consider purchasing vintage pieces of furniture rather than new ones. Not only are they less likely to off-gas toxins, but the construction is generally superior to modern pieces. Most of the dressers, side tables, and wooden furniture in our home came from high-end vintage or consignment stores, and not only is it likely to be a less-toxic choice, but we also saved money versus buying all new furniture. Plus, it's better quality furniture than many of today's pieces, and we won't have the same furniture as our neighbors.

One caveat: you may not want to choose vintage furniture for your upholstered pieces. That's because upholstered furniture from the mid-1980s to around 2015 often contains flame-retardant foams that you'll want to avoid. In one study, they found that up to 85 percent of the couches they tested (produced from 1984 to 2010) contained harmful flame-retardant chemicals in the foam.[5] So, when purchasing upholstered pieces, choose newer pieces (or those that were produced pre-1984). To make sure you're choosing safe and nontoxic options, you'll want to do some research to find brands that avoid toxic chemicals. Look for either the Greenguard Gold certification or the Oeko-Tex Standard 100 certification.

Don't forget about nature's air purifiers—houseplants. Not only do they absorb many dangerous toxins (even VOCs), they also boost oxygen levels.[6,7] They even have positive psychological effects, increasing task performance, promoting overall health and well-being, and lowering levels of stress.[8]

Get a vacuum with a HEPA filter. Did you know that household dust can be loaded with heavy metals, such as lead, VOCs, allergens, and a variety of toxic chemicals? And when you vacuum, some of these particles can become airborne through emission from your vacuum cleaner? That's where HEPA filters come in. When your vacuum cleaner is equipped with a HEPA (high-efficiency particulate air) filter, it reduces the number of contaminants that are released into the air of your home, collecting up to 100 percent of the particles within your vacuum's filtration system.[9]

Choose your floor coverings carefully. Just as furniture can off-gas dangerous chemicals, so can your floor coverings. When you are getting new flooring, look for the Green Label Plus logo, a certification from the Carpet and Rug Institute. This designation ensures that you are choosing the lowest-emitting carpet, adhesive, and cushion products available and avoiding options that emit high levels of VOCs (such as benzene, formaldehyde, ethylbenzene, acetone, styrene, and toluene).[10] The EPA tells us that VOCs cause minor problems like eye, nose, and throat irritation, frequent headaches, and nausea. Even worse than that? They are linked to more severe health issues, such as liver, kidney, and central nervous system damage. Some VOCs have been shown to cause cancer in animals and are suspected or known to cause cancer in humans.[11]

Choose low-VOC paints. VOCs are not just found in your carpets or floor coverings—they are also found in traditional paints. The good news is that most major paint manufacturers now have no-VOC options available. Whenever you take on a new painting project in your home, choose no-VOC paint.

IN THE BEDROOM

Prioritize nontoxic bedding. We spend about one-third of our lives in bed, so we want to ensure that our sleeping time is spent on self-cleaning (thank you, glymphatic system) rather than contributing to an increased toxic load coming from our bedding. As I mentioned in the laundry room section, we are in close contact with the bedding all night long, so it's essential to avoid harsh and/or heavily fragranced detergents, dryer sheets, or fabric softeners.

It may be time for a new mattress. If your mattress was manufactured prior to 2015, chances are it contains harmful flame-retardant chemicals. If this is the case, consider choosing something else. There are several certifications that make a difference when mattress shopping.

GOTS (Global Organic Textile Standard) requires that a minimum of 95 percent of the materials must be certified organic, and the other 5 percent of the materials can't include certain prohibited substances, such as chemical flame retardants or polyurethane.

If you aren't looking for an organic mattress, the Oeko-Tex Standard 100 designation is something to look for. It sets limits for emissions of harmful chemicals such as VOCs and formaldehyde, and also bans the use of chemical flame retardants and dyes.

The CertiPUR-US designation is used for mattresses with polyurethane foam and prohibits certain substances that may be found in many polyurethane mattresses.

Greenguard certification is provided by UL, which was previously known as Underwriters Laboratories, and I am sure you are used to seeing the UL designation on many products you've purchased over the years. If a mattress has a Greenguard certification, it's required to meet specific emissions limits for VOCs. They have an even more stringent certification process for products to be certified as Greenguard Gold.

IN THE YARD

Garden organically! Are you looking for an alternative to synthetic fertilizers, pesticides, and herbicides? Organic gardening practices are your answer. When your soil is chemical-free and healthy, your plants (including your grass) will also be healthy and more robust.

You can start by testing your soil, and your local university extension office can tell you how to go about doing that. That should let you know if your soil has any deficiencies, and they can also help you remedy any deficiencies you find using natural and safe products. Choose organic fertilizers, and you can also improve soil quality by composting. It's not as scary (or as smelly) as it sounds, and it will not only boost soil quality but will also reduce the amount of trash you throw away each week.

The plants you select matter. If you want to use fewer chemicals in your yard, choosing plants that thrive where you plant them is essential. Native plants are your best options, and this is another time when your local university extension office can help you. In my state, they do both on-site and phone consultations with the home gardener, and their experts can help you with any questions you might have. Don't let fear of the unknown stop you. Your local extension office is there to help you become the gardener you dream of becoming.

As for your lawn, make sure to choose varieties of grass that grow well in your yard's specific conditions, and as your lawn gets healthier, you won't need to water it as much or spend as much time weeding.

Fight mosquitoes naturally. In our area, mosquitoes are a real problem, and we've seen a rise in the number of companies that will come to your house and blanket your whole yard with pesticides to kill the mosquitoes. It's certainly an attractive concept, to be able to use your yard all season long with nary a mosquito bite. Whether they are safe for us (or our pets) is another question. The companies that offer these services in our area caution you to keep your pets out of the yard for a few hours after application, which doesn't sound very safe to me.

In addition to concerns about the safety to us, our kids, and our pets, these pesticide applications don't only kill mosquitoes. These chemicals also affect bees,[12] caterpillars, fireflies, earthworms, and many of the other species that live in your yard.

Instead, make your yard less mosquito-friendly by addressing standing water. Choose plants that naturally repel mosquitoes, such as lavender, marigolds, lemon balm, and geraniums, as well as herbs like rosemary, mint, or basil. Use nontoxic insect repellents when you are outside.

REFLECT: CREATING YOUR PERSONAL DEFINITION OF CLEAN(ISH) LIVING—WHAT MATTERS MOST?

Up to now, you've been learning about many of the issues and challenges that face us in today's modern world, but soon you'll be ready to begin the implementation phase of becoming clean(ish). That's coming up in the chapter called "Slow and Steady Clean(ish) Change: Your Nine Focus Topics."

Three of the nine focus topics are covered by the clean(ish) eating definition that you already created, but six of them fall into the clean(ish) living category. Your next task is to create your personal definitions of clean(ish) living as they relate to those six focus topics.

You can complete this section right here in the book, or you can re-create it within your Clean(ish) Journal if you don't want to write in the book. Alternately, go to ginstephens.com/cleanish to download and print the pdf that contains these pages in worksheet format.

HOUSEHOLD CLEANING PRODUCTS

Go back to the "Household Cleaning Products: What's in Your Bucket?" chapter. Decide how concerned you are about each category of product, and within each category, consider which specific products are the most important to you.

Concern	How I Feel	Which Specific Products Am I Most Concerned About?
Bathroom cleaning products	☐ I am extremely concerned. It is important for me to choose products that are considered to be very safe (i.e., rated as Verified or A/B on the EWG Healthy Living app). ☐ I am moderately concerned, so I'll choose products that are very safe when I can, but it's okay if some of my favorites are rated as a moderate hazard. ☐ This is one area where I am not willing to make changes, so I plan to stick with my current options, no matter the scores.	
Kitchen cleaning products	☐ I am extremely concerned. It is important for me to choose products that are considered to be very safe (i.e., rated as Verified or A/B on the EWG Healthy Living app). ☐ I am moderately concerned, so I'll choose products that are very safe when I can, but it's okay if some of my favorites are rated as a moderate hazard. ☐ This is one area where I am not willing to make changes, so I plan to stick with my current options, no matter the scores.	
Laundry products	☐ I am extremely concerned. It is important for me to choose products that are considered to be very safe (i.e., rated as Verified or A/B on the EWG Healthy Living app). ☐ I am moderately concerned, so I'll choose products that are very safe when I can, but it's okay if some of my favorites are rated as a moderate hazard. ☐ This is one area where I am not willing to make changes, so I plan to stick with my current options, no matter the scores.	

Other cleaning products used in my home or garage	☐ I am extremely concerned. It is important for me to choose products that are considered to be very safe (i.e., rated as Verified or A/B on the EWG Healthy Living app). ☐ I am moderately concerned, so I'll choose products that are very safe when I can, but it's okay if some of my favorites are rated as a moderate hazard. ☐ This is one area where I am not willing to make changes, so I plan to stick with my current options, no matter the scores.	

PERSONAL CARE PRODUCTS

Revisit the "Personal Care Products: Adding to your Bucket" chapter. Decide how concerned you are about each category of product, and within each category, consider which specific products are the most important to you.

Concern	How I Feel	Which Specific Products Am I Most Concerned About?
Hair care products	☐ I am extremely concerned. It is important for me to choose products that are considered to be very safe (i.e., rated as Verified or 1–2 on the EWG Healthy Living app). ☐ I am moderately concerned, so I'll choose products that are very safe when I can, but it's okay if some of my favorites are rated as a moderate hazard. ☐ This is one area where I am not willing to make changes, so I plan to stick with my current options, no matter the scores.	
Makeup/ cosmetics	☐ I am extremely concerned. It is important for me to choose products that are considered to be very safe (i.e., rated as Verified or 1–2 on the EWG Healthy Living app).	

	☐ I am moderately concerned, so I'll choose products that are very safe when I can, but it's okay if some of my favorites are rated as a moderate hazard.	
	☐ This is one area where I am not willing to make changes, so I plan to stick with my current options, no matter the scores.	
Skin care products	☐ I am extremely concerned. It is important for me to choose products that are considered to be very safe (i.e., rated as Verified or 1–2 on the EWG Healthy Living app).	
	☐ I am moderately concerned, so I'll choose products that are very safe when I can, but it's okay if some of my favorites are rated as a moderate hazard.	
	☐ This is one area where I am not willing to make changes, so I plan to stick with my current options, no matter the scores.	
Other products used on skin (deodorant, shaving cream, etc.)	☐ I am extremely concerned. It is important for me to choose products that are considered to be very safe (i.e., rated as Verified or 1–2 on the EWG Healthy Living app).	
	☐ I am moderately concerned, so I'll choose products that are very safe when I can, but it's okay if some of my favorites are rated as a moderate hazard.	
	☐ This is one area where I am not willing to make changes, so I plan to stick with my current options, no matter the scores.	
Dental hygiene products	☐ I am extremely concerned. It is important for me to choose products that are considered to be very safe (i.e., rated as Verified or 1–2 on the EWG Healthy Living app).	
	☐ I am moderately concerned, so I'll choose products that are very safe when I can, but it's okay if some of my favorites are rated as a moderate hazard.	
	☐ This is one area where I am not willing to make changes, so I plan to stick with my current options, no matter the scores.	

Feminine hygiene products	☐ I am extremely concerned. It is important for me to choose products that are considered to be very safe (i.e., rated as Verified or 1–2 on the EWG Healthy Living app).	
	☐ I am moderately concerned, so I'll choose products that are very safe when I can, but it's okay if some of my favorites are rated as a moderate hazard.	
	☐ This is one area where I am not willing to make changes, so I plan to stick with my current options, no matter the scores.	

FOOD CONTACT CHEMICALS

Recall the topics from the "Better Living Through Chemistry" chapter, as well as the room-by-room topics listed in the "Live (Mainly) Clean" chapter. Choose which are the most important to you.

Concern	How I Feel	Which Specific Products Am I Most Concerned About?
Toxins in cookware	☐ I am extremely concerned. I plan to make changes to the current items I use to find safer options.	
	☐ I am moderately concerned, so I'll make safer choices when I purchase new items in this category.	
	☐ This is one area where I am not willing to make changes, so I plan to stick with my current options.	
Food storage containers, wraps, and bags	☐ I am extremely concerned. I plan to make changes to the current items I use to find safer options.	
	☐ I am moderately concerned, so I'll make safer choices when I purchase new items in this category.	
	☐ This is one area where I am not willing to make changes, so I plan to stick with my current options.	

Cooking utensils and cutting boards	☐ I am extremely concerned. I plan to make changes to the current items I use to find safer options. ☐ I am moderately concerned, so I'll make safer choices when I purchase new items in this category. ☐ This is one area where I am not willing to make changes, so I plan to stick with my current options.	
Beverage containers/ bottles	☐ I am extremely concerned. I plan to make changes to the current items I use to find safer options. ☐ I am moderately concerned, so I'll make safer choices when I purchase new items in this category. ☐ This is one area where I am not willing to make changes, so I plan to stick with my current options.	

CLEAN UP YOUR HOME AND YARD

Think back to the topics from the "Better Living Through Chemistry" chapter, as well as the room-by-room topics listed in the "Live (Mainly) Clean" chapter. Choose which are the most important to you.

Concern	How I Feel	Which Specific Products Am I Most Concerned About?
Pest control (indoors)	☐ I am extremely concerned. I plan to make changes to the current items I use to find safer options. ☐ I am moderately concerned, so I'll make safer choices when I purchase new items in this category. ☐ This is one area where I am not willing to make changes, so I plan to stick with my current options.	
Pest control (outdoors)	☐ I am extremely concerned. I plan to make changes to the current items I use to find safer options. ☐ I am moderately concerned, so I'll make safer choices when I purchase new items in this category.	

	☐ This is one area where I am not willing to make changes, so I plan to stick with my current options.	
Plastics (shower curtain, bath mat)	☐ I am extremely concerned. I plan to make changes to the current items I use to find safer options. ☐ I am moderately concerned, so I'll make safer choices when I purchase new items in this category. ☐ This is one area where I am not willing to make changes, so I plan to stick with my current options.	
Water quality (from my faucets and bottled waters)	☐ I am extremely concerned. I plan to make changes to the current items I use to find safer options. ☐ I am moderately concerned, so I'll make safer choices when I purchase new items in this category. ☐ This is one area where I am not willing to make changes, so I plan to stick with my current options.	
Home fur-nishings (furniture, floor coverings, paint)	☐ I am extremely concerned. I plan to make changes to the current items I use to find safer options. ☐ I am moderately concerned, so I'll make safer choices when I purchase new items in this category. ☐ This is one area where I am not willing to make changes, so I plan to stick with my current options.	
Mattress and bed-ding	☐ I am extremely concerned. I plan to make changes to the current items I use to find safer options. ☐ I am moderately concerned, so I'll make safer choices when I purchase new items in this category. ☐ This is one area where I am not willing to make changes, so I plan to stick with my current options.	
Gardening practices (fertilizers, herbicides)	☐ I am extremely concerned. I plan to make changes to the current items I use to find safer options. ☐ I am moderately concerned, so I'll make safer choices when I purchase new items in this category. ☐ This is one area where I am not willing to make changes, so I plan to stick with my current options.	

INTERMITTENT FASTING FOR SELF-CLEANING

Go back to your reflections about autophagy and intermittent fasting. Also read what you wrote when you considered how you could apply intermittent fasting to your life.

Now, choose one of these options:

☐ I am already living an intermittent fasting lifestyle, and I love knowing that my body spends extra time self-cleaning each day.

☐ I am interested in incorporating intermittent fasting into my life, and I plan to read *Fast. Feast. Repeat.* when I'm ready to get started. I'll start with the twenty-eight-day FAST Start and go from there.

☐ Intermittent fasting doesn't seem like something that is for me right now. *(Sorry, Gin!)* Maybe one day.

OTHER TOOLS FOR SELF-CLEANING

Go back to the "Extra Credit: More Tools for Self-Cleaning" chapter and revisit these tools. Consider which you plan to include as a part of your personal self-cleaning toolbox.

Tool	How I Feel	My Plans
Exercise	☐ I am all in! This is a tool I plan to use. ☐ This is not a tool that interests me at this time.	
Sauna	☐ I am all in! This is a tool I plan to use. ☐ This is not a tool that interests me at this time.	
Massage	☐ I am all in! This is a tool I plan to use. ☐ This is not a tool that interests me at this time.	

Commit-ting to quality sleep	☐ I am all in! This is a tool I plan to use. ☐ This is not a tool that interests me at this time.	
Blue-light blocking	☐ I am all in! This is a tool I plan to use. ☐ This is not a tool that interests me at this time.	
Earthing	☐ I am all in! This is a tool I plan to use. ☐ This is not a tool that interests me at this time.	
Cleaning up my indoor air quality	☐ I am all in! This is a tool I plan to use. ☐ This is not a tool that interests me at this time.	

TAKE ACTION: YOUR PERSONAL DEFINITION OF CLEAN(ISH) LIVING

Use your Clean(ish) Journal (or the worksheets available at ginstephens .com/cleanish) to create your definition of clean(ish) living.

Now that you've taken the time to consider what to include in your definition of clean(ish) living, summarize your thoughts.

My personal definition of clean(ish) living:

- There are some products that I am ***most concerned about,*** and I plan to prioritize choosing safe products (for each category, list the products from that category that you're most concerned about):

  - Household cleaning products:
  - Personal care products:
  - Food contact products:
  - Products throughout my home and yard:

- There are some products that I am *not as concerned about,* so I'll choose safer products when it is convenient to do so, *or* if it doesn't affect the per-formance of the product (such as the way Gin uses safer deodorant *most* of the year), *or* I'll use them if I don't have another option available. This includes:

- ◉ Household cleaning products:
- ◉ Personal care products:
- ◉ Food contact products:
- ◉ Products throughout my home and yard:

- There are some self-cleaning tools (from "Extra Credit: More Tools for Self-Cleaning" and "Intermittent Fasting: A Powerful Self-Cleaning Tool") that I use in my current routine *or* plan to add to my routine. These include:

GETTING YOUR FAMILY ON BOARD

Now that you've developed your personal definitions of clean(ish) eating and clean(ish) living, it's time to think about others who may live with you in your home. Notice that I titled this chapter "Getting Your Family on Board," but you may not live with family members, and instead you have roommates. Some of this advice won't apply to every possible living situation, but you can still pick and choose from any concepts that may apply to your current living arrangement, whatever it may be.

The takeaway message is the same for anyone who doesn't live alone: sometimes, it can be difficult to make changes in what foods you have on hand or the products that you choose because of your partner and kids, or any roommates you may live with.

Back in the day, Chad happily ate my "delicious" Dorito casserole without complaining (*yes, a Dorito casserole is a thing, and yes, I used to prepare it for my family; it involved canned biscuit dough and Doritos and layers of other ingredients in between*), and now he eats an organic chickpea and veggie bowl without complaining. But maybe you don't have a Chad, and if you try to make the leap from Dorito casserole to chickpea bowl, you'll have a fight on your hands.

Maybe your partner is on board, but your kids aren't. What do you do when you have raised picky eaters? And why did I say that you *raised* picky eaters? Because, just like I did with my kids, that's likely what happened at your house.

Here's what we know: for all eternity, kids ate whatever foods were available. Everyone in the family's having roasted scorpion tail for dinner? Little Junior would happily eat the roasted scorpion tail. Eye of newt on the menu? Junior's eating eye of newt. There was no such thing as a picky eater, or if there was, that behavior certainly wasn't indulged by parents who had no other available options to serve Mr. or Miss Picky Eater. Even today, kids in other parts of the world (and I am writing this from the perspective of a mom in the U.S., so forgive me if you are one of my international readers) are much less picky than American kids. Nowadays, we tend to be a society that indulges our kids' finicky food preferences, and you can tell by reading any restaurant kids' menu.

When we have a picky eater in the family, it's easier to microwave a few chicken nuggets just to get the kid to eat something, and many of us think we are doing the right thing by choosing organic free-range chicken nuggets. We smile, knowing we have made a clean(ish) choice, and if our kids only eat chicken nuggets, at least we are feeding them something organic.

Sigh. I did that.

Recall from the discussions in earlier chapters: we need nutrients from a variety of healthy foods to build a healthy body. And fortified *not-foods* and/or vitamin supplements are not the same thing as getting our nutrients from real food. A healthy body is not built from (organic free-range) chicken nuggets alone. So, it's up to us to make changes that will nourish our kids' bodies. I still cringe when I remember buying a chocolate-flavored beverage product— totally NOT food—and I chose it over actual milk because the label showed a bunch of added vitamins. I had no idea what I was doing because I didn't at the time understand the power of real food. Remember that I was raised by a mom who served me SpaghettiOs with a Flintstones vitamin chaser. So, when the time came, I made the same types of choices. It's too late for a do-over for me, but it's not too late for you if you still have kids at home . . . no matter how old they are.

The truth is: kids are very much creatures of habit, just as we are. And if we expose them to nothing but *not-food*, that's what they will expect and prefer. Remember: those *not-foods* are literally designed in a research lab to hook us through their flavor profiles. On the flip side, if we offer our kids high-quality, nutritious foods, they will eventually eat what you're offering. In a 2004 study, researchers found that parents typically gave up after only three to five times presenting a new food to their kids. Overall, studies show that toddlers need between five and ten exposures to a food before they will eat it, while kids ages three to four may need *fifteen* exposures to the food before they will eat it. So, don't give up too soon.[1]

Research shows that "children's intake of fruits, vegetables, and milk increased after observing adults consuming the foods."[2] What did *not* work was pressuring kids to eat certain things, rewarding them for what they eat, or excessive restriction of highly palatable foods. So, we are more likely to positively influence our kids by modeling positive eating behaviors. According to these Canadian researchers (delightful Canadian spellings and all), "In combination with what is known about the effect of parental modeling on children's eating behaviours there is consistent evidence that the responsive 'do as I do' approach has a stronger positive effect on children's consumption patterns than the unresponsive 'do as I say' approach to parenting."[3]

So, let's talk about some practical strategies for how to implement this into your household.

If your kids are young, no need to go into details. Make swaps they will enjoy, and they likely won't even notice much of a difference. Offer a wide variety of foods and keep at it, even when they reject them the first two, three, or fifteen times. Model eating a wide variety of foods, and they will learn from you that these foods are delicious, and eventually, they will develop into well-rounded eaters.

If your kids are older, this is going to be more of a challenge, and they are absolutely going to notice that you're making changes . . . and they are likely to have strong opinions about it.

I worked with kids for twenty-eight years as an elementary

teacher, and one thing I know about kids today is that they tend to have a heart for ecological friendly choices that help our planet in the long run. I would begin there. Explain that your family is doing something very exciting and new, and tell them why. Remain upbeat and positive, and stress the benefits to the planet and to our bodies. Teach them how to read labels.

As you teach them about food and labels, remember that words matter. Don't use words like *dirty food* or *bad food*. We don't want our kids to be judgmental or act like the food police. We *do* want them to have buy-in, and we do want them to become educated consumers.

Take them to the grocery store with you and involve them in the buying process. Kids love it when you give them a choice. Here's an example of that. Let's say that your kids are big fans of a certain brand of yogurt that you now realize is full of funky ingredients and so you no longer want to buy it.

The wrong way:

"Look at how awful this yogurt is. It's a really bad choice. We will never get this again."

Kids start crying and begging for their favorite yogurt.

A better way:

"Here's the yogurt we normally get. What do you notice about the ingredients?"

Then, after a conversation about the ingredients, say:

"Let's look at the other yogurt choices and read the labels. Which ones look good to you? Which would you like for us to try?"

In the first example, you as the parent are making a unilateral decision without explaining why. You're also reinforcing the "good"/"bad" message about foods. That can be internalized as "being good" when making some choices and "being bad" when making others. One of our goals is to strip away labels that are linked to negative moral judgments about food so our kids grow up without that baggage. Food isn't "bad." It isn't "dirty." Never forget that. It's either "food" or "not food." We want kids to be able to distinguish between "food" and "not food" themselves.

By teaching your kids to read labels, you're setting them up for long-term success. When you raise your kids with the clean(ish) approach to choosing foods, they can calmly make their own food decisions when you aren't there (and one day, you will *not* be there beside them as they choose what products to put in their own shopping carts . . .). Also, when you include your children as decisions makers, help them understand the decision-making *process,* and give them a *choice,* they feel in control and empowered because they have been included in the process. They won't be mad about eating a brand of yogurt that they were allowed to choose.

Okay, truth time. My kids weren't always that easy to reason with. Maybe your kids STILL pitch a fit in the grocery store that first time, even though you phrased the choice calmly and asked for their input. (*Yep. Mine would totally have done that. Bless 'em, I raised some strong-willed boys. Now that they are adults, it works out well because they have the tenacity to be successful, but it was not always a picnic at the time.*) What do you do right there in the moment if that happens and your kids are in full-meltdown mode in the dairy section? Do you cave in and get the yogurt you always got, and decide to try again next time?

No, please don't. Instead, take a deep (calming) breath, and say something like, "Okay. We will try again next time. We won't get any yogurt today, but the next time we shop, you can look at the choices again, and you can help me choose then." And then walk away from the yogurt. Your kids can go without it until the next time you shop because you'll have plenty of other healthy options at home for them to choose from when they are hungry. And eventually, they will choose a yogurt that you are all willing to put into the cart.

Another way to get your kids excited to eat different foods is to involve them in the process of preparing it. In a study called "Children Eat More Food When They Prepare it Themselves," researchers found, well, you know what they found by reading the title, don't you?[4]

If you love to grow things, you can also involve your kids from seed to table. In a study from 2020, researchers found that kids developed a more positive attitude toward fruits and vegetables in general after participating in a gardening program that had nutrition education and cooking experiences. This is not the only study to show similar results, so taking time to grow a backyard (or even a flowerpot or kitchen window) garden can have a positive impact on your kids' eating behaviors.[5]

Now imagine if you have them *grow* the food themselves and then they *prepare* it themselves? That sounds like magic to me. Try it and see what happens!

CROWDING OUT

Have you ever heard the phrase *crowding out* in terms of your eating choices? I think it's a great way to approach how you make your food decisions as you develop your personal definition of clean(ish), but it also works very well when managing reluctant family members.

When you practice crowding out personally, you intentionally choose to prioritize nutritious foods, and you place them at the center of your daily eating experiences. Your body gets the nutrients you need, and you feel full and satisfied.

Then you have the freedom and flexibility to select other foods—even ultra-processed foods—to round out your meal or your day.

Because you prioritized nutrition, you'll be less likely to overeat the ultra-processed foods, and you'll finally be able to hear your body's "that's enough" signals.

As an example of how this looks in application, I may plan a meal that includes a big, beautiful salad, full of a variety of different veggies—because I know that diet diversity is the key to feeding my gut well. On the side, I have a handful of tortilla chips because the salty crunch of those chips makes me feel satisfied in a way that the salad alone wouldn't do. I crowded out the chips by focusing on nutritious foods that filled me up, but I didn't eliminate the chips entirely. And because I'm full and satisfied, I won't keep eating after the meal in search of whatever I was missing. For me, that handful of chips was the key to enjoying and feeling satisfied by the salad, while the salad was the key to feeling satisfied by just a handful of chips. A whole bag of chips alone wouldn't have satisfied my body the way the salad and a few chips did. A giant bowl of salad alone might have physically filled me up, but it wouldn't have satisfied me fully.

You can apply this same strategy to family meals. Crowd out the foods you want to de-emphasize with a variety of nutritious (and delicious!) foods that you want your family to eat.

WHAT IF YOUR FAMILY (OR YOUR PARTNER) IS STILL STRUGGLING TO ADAPT?

No matter what happens, don't force your partner to make changes they are not ready for, and never judge them if they aren't ready for change. The same for your kids. The younger they are, the easier it will be, but don't give up on older kids or teens. Remain positive and do your best. Don't blame yourself (*though it is easy to do, am I right?*) if they were raised by you to be picky eaters. In the words of one of my heroes Maya Angelou, "Do the best you can until you know better. Then when you know better, do better."

Overall, you may need to make changes slowly. Add in and crowd out. Offer quality. Don't be upset if they push back. Calmly do the shopping, and make clean(ish) substitutions they can live with.

And one day, maybe your picky son who only ate beige foods when he was a little guy will marry a beautiful girl he met in college, move to San Francisco, and become a vegetarian. That, my friends, is a true story. Cal-who-only-ate-beige-things is now a vegetarian who eats absolutely anything that beautiful girl wants him to eat. And they lived happily ever after. The end.

I hope that you are feeling inspired to make changes within your home and that you feel empowered to introduce these changes in a way that will be met with positive reactions by your family.

As you make these changes over time, I don't think you can go wrong when you follow, model, and reinforce these guidelines with your family:

- Food is not a reward or a punishment. Food is something we use to nourish our bodies.

- Food is to be enjoyed. We don't feel guilty for eating foods we love.

- We make a practice of prioritizing *food* over *not-food*, but that doesn't mean that we are overly dogmatic about every choice. Remember: we are clean(ish). We choose *mostly* food and allow some *not-food* in our lives, but without drama or judgment.

- The whole family can get involved in choosing, growing, and preparing food whenever possible. Developing routines around food and mealtime promotes positive habits.

- We understand the power of nutrition and how food is the building block of a healthy and strong body. *Food*, not *not-food*, is what nourishes us.

- When sitting down to a meal as a family, there is one meal that is prepared for all family members. We don't make special foods to cater to picky eaters.

(Remember that kids won't allow themselves to starve, and as long as you keep offering healthy foods, they will eventually eat. The only exception would be if you have someone in the family with food allergies, which is a different issue.)

REFLECT: KNOW YOUR FAMILY

Use your Clean(ish) Journal (or the worksheets available at ginstephens .com/cleanish) to complete these end-of-chapter prompts and activities.

- Think about your family or housemates and identify which members may struggle with the clean(ish) changes you want to make. Write about the challenges you anticipate.

If you have kids in your home, consider the strategies that I mentioned in this chapter and choose ideas from the list below that you would like to try. Check all the ones that apply, and make a plan in your Clean(ish) Journal for how to implement each.

☐ Model eating a wide variety of foods, including plenty of vegetables and fruits. Let your family see that you enjoy eating them rather than acting like it's a chore. If you aren't enjoying your veggies, they won't either. And if you *aren't* enjoying them, it's time to find new recipes—I promise that veggies can be delicious when you know what to do with them.

Plan:

☐ Repeatedly expose your kids to unfamiliar foods. As research shows us, it can take an average of *fifteen* exposures before a picky toddler is willing to try a new food. And remember—"average" refers to a number in the middle. Your kid may be above average and need seventeen exposures.

Plan:

☐ Explain to your kids about the importance of nutrients and why our bodies need a wide variety of nutrients to be strong and healthy. When you are shopping or meal planning with your kids, take a few minutes to look up some of the ingredients you'll be using so your kids will understand how they are healthy for our bodies. For example, a web search for the key words "carrots nutrition" brings up all sorts of websites that tout the health benefits of carrots. You can also search for terms like "carrots fun facts" and learn all sorts of things you didn't know, which a lot of kids enjoy. Here's one example: the deeper the orange, the greater the beta-carotene content of the carrot. Kids would have a lot of fun hunting down the "orangest" carrots for sale at your grocery store, and they would be more likely to eat them after doing so.

Plan:

☐ Teach your kids to read food labels. When you are at the grocery store, compare labels and choose foods together. Give your kids the opportunity to verbalize why one option is a better choice than another—when they can explain it to you, you know they understand it.

Plan:

☐ Involve your family in meal planning, food prep, or even in the growing of your food, when possible. When kids have ownership in the process, they are more likely to eat those foods. You're also making memories by doing it together.

Plan:

TAKE ACTION: DOES YOUR CHILD NEED MORE?

I want to take a moment to circle back to the story I told in the introduction. You'll recall that my son Will had a variety of food and chemical sensitivities that manifested as behavioral problems, and swapping out the foods he ate and the products we used around the house was life-changing for our family. If you suspect that this may be true for one or more members of your family, it is even more important to make changes to the foods (as well as the cleaning and personal care products) that you have in your home.

I recommend that you start at feingold.org and explore the resources there. If you go to their shopping tab at www.fgshop .org, you'll find books you can purchase, food lists, and more. The book *Why Can't My Child Behave?* by Jane Hersey really helped me understand what was going on with Will, and you can access a free pdf of the first seventy-nine pages to get you started on their website.

If you go to the resources tab of their website and select *More,* you can find lots of free yet valuable information, including a pdf of *Scientific Support for the Feingold Diet* (with references to scientific studies as recent as 2020), a letter you can share with teachers, and more.

From one parent to another, I wish you nothing but success when it comes to helping your difficult child find success. Yes, it's hard to admit when we have a "difficult" child because we feel like we're failing as parents. I promise that you aren't failing. Our sensitive kids are the proverbial canaries in the coal mine, and the blame falls on the funky chemicals and additives, not on our kids (or us as parents). When we understand that, we can parent our kids in more effective ways. If your child had a stomach virus, you wouldn't punish him for vomiting, because that is a physical reaction that is out of his control. Understanding that chemical sensitivities are also physical reactions makes a huge difference in how we respond to that out-of-control child of ours.

CHOOSE YOUR CLEAN(ISH) TIMELINE

Now that you have taken time to consider what eating (mostly) clean and living (mainly) clean will look like for you, it's time to choose your implementation timeline.

The process of becoming clean(ish) includes three steps:

Step 1: Awareness—*Good news! You've already mastered this step by reading this far and doing the work at the end of each chapter. You understand why it's important to make changes in the products you use and the foods you eat, and you've taken time to determine which changes are most important to you. You are now ready to apply what you've learned.*

Step 2: Change—*This is where you are now. You'll choose the timeline you prefer to follow and make clean(ish) adjustments to your life as your budget—and your time—allow.*

Step 3: Live and Adapt—*This step encompasses the rest of your life. You'll live a clean(ish) lifestyle, continuing to learn along the way—and the more you learn, the more you'll refine your personal definition of what it means to be clean(ish). You'll never actually be "done," because change is inevitable. The clean(ish) life is about embracing this inevitable change while remaining empowered to make the choices that are right for you at any given time. As time goes on, you'll learn new information, new* *problems will be identified, and new solutions will be developed. Because of this, you will be inspired to make additional changes based on what feels right to your body (especially when it comes to what foods you'll eat), what new science emerges (since we are always learning new things), and what new products are developed (that solve issues we may not have even identified yet).*

In the next chapter, I'm going to share nine areas where you will focus your attention as you move through **Step 2: Change.** Maybe you'll want to choose one topic per month, or perhaps you prefer to jump right in and tackle a new focus each week. This means you'll spend anywhere from the next nine weeks to the next nine months moving through the process—or you may fall somewhere in between.

Do you remember those Choose Your Own Adventure books? That's what this experience is going to be like for you. Even though I have outlined nine different focus areas, they don't need to be done in order. You'll choose which one to start with and how long you want to spend working on it. Maybe you don't even want to complete all nine of them. That's also okay. If you only feel inspired to tackle three, or five, or seven of the focus topics, remember that every change you make is a step in a positive direction.

Confession: I was going to include an option that I called Life Swap, where you could throw away everything that doesn't meet your personal definitions of clean(ish) and start completely fresh. The longer I thought about it, however, the more I realized that would be a terrible idea.

As you make changes in your life, the goal is to be intentional and methodical so that you make changes that *stick.* We all know that dramatically rushing into things doesn't usually lead to lasting change. Every time I have tried that in the past, it never worked out well for me.

So, rather than life-swapping the whole process, you're going to take it slow and give yourself as much time as you need, whether that is nine weeks or nine months or somewhere in between.

REFLECT: YOUR IDEAL TIME FRAME

You can complete this section right here in the book, or you can re-create it within your Clean(ish) Journal if you don't want to write in the book. Alternately, go to ginstephens.com/cleanish to download and print the pdf that contains these pages in worksheet format.

Think about yourself for a moment. Which of these descriptions sound most like you?

Check as many as apply.

☐ I prefer to make a plan and stick with it. I work best when I have every-thing all mapped out.

☐ I like to figure out things as I go. If I plan ahead of time *too much,* I often get frustrated with myself and quit entirely. I need to be able to adjust my plans on an as-needed basis.

☐ If I give myself too much time to complete projects, I procrastinate and am less likely to take any action at all.

☐ I need time to work through any process, and I don't work well when I feel rushed.

☐ My time is variable. Sometimes, I have more time to devote than at other times, so it's important for me to remain flexible with any timeline I imple-ment.

Now, depending upon which items you checked, decide how you want to approach your clean(ish) timeline.

- If you chose *"I prefer to make a plan and stick with it. I work best when I have everything all mapped out,"* then consider planning out your clean(ish) timeline ahead of time. Go ahead and fill in the timeline on the next pages with your nine focus topics, in the order that you want to ad-dress them.

- If you chose "*I like to figure out things as I go. If I plan ahead of time too much, I often get frustrated with myself and quit entirely. I need to be able to adjust my plans on an as-needed basis,*" then it's probably best for you to only choose your first focus topic for now. After you complete the first focus, you'll choose your second focus, and so on.

- If you chose "*If I give myself too much time to complete projects, I procrastinate and am less likely to take any action at all,*" then you will want to choose shorter time frames. Nine months may be too long for you, as you may lose interest along the way. Consider choosing one focus per week.

- If you chose "*I need time to work through any process, and I don't work well when I feel rushed,*" then the monthly focus may be right for you.

- If you chose "*My time is variable. Sometimes, I have more time to devote than at other times, so it's important for me to remain flexible with any timeline I implement,*" then you'll want to choose one topic at a time, work on it as long as it takes, and then choose the next topic. Both the topics and the time it takes to complete them will vary as needed.

TAKE ACTION: YOUR INDIVIDUAL TIMELINE

Now that you've considered what approach may work best for you, use the chart on the next pages to organize your timeline. This chart is also available at ginstephens.com/cleanish in the pdf that contains these pages in worksheet format.

- In the **Time Frame** column, record the month or dates for each topic you'll address.

  ◦ *If you want to focus on one topic per month and you are beginning the process in July, you'll write "July" for month 1, "August" for month 2, and so on.*

◎ *If you want to take a week for each topic, you can list the weekly dates as your time frame.*

◎ *Alternately, if you decided that you will take a more open-ended approach, you will fully tackle one topic at a time, spending the amount of time that is right for you for each one. Maybe it takes a week for the first focus topic, but the next one takes you three weeks. You can fill in the dates after the fact, to reflect the amount of time it took you to work through the topic. That's perfectly fine. Make the timeline work for you in a way that feels appropriate and doable.*

- In the **Focus** column, you'll choose one of the nine focus topics from page 328 and list one in each box.

  ◎ For example, in the focus column for time frame 1, you may choose to begin with *Choose Safe Household Cleaning Products,* or perhaps you want to start with topic *Limit Ultra-Processed Foods* or *Extend Your Daily Fast.* What you choose and the order in which you select your topics is completely up to you.

  ◎ You may want to fill in all nine focus boxes now, or you may tackle one at a time and choose the one you want to complete next after you finish the first one, and so on.

- In the **Notes** column, you can make any notes that are helpful for you as you get your timeline organized.

Keep in mind that you do *not* need to plan out your entire timeline all at once if you don't want to. Remember: you are in charge at all times, and I am providing you with suggestions—but they are only suggestions. Make this process work for you, your personality, your budget, and the time you have available.

The nine focus topics are explained in detail in the next chapter, but here is a preview:

Focus: Extend Your Daily Fast

Focus: Choose Safe Household Cleaning Products

Focus: Select Safe Personal Care Products

Focus: Avoid Food Contact Chemicals

Focus: Prioritize Quality Foods

Focus: Limit Ultra-Processed Foods

Focus: Add in Nutrients

Focus: Incorporate Tools for Self-Cleaning

Focus: Clean Up Your Home and Yard

Time Frame	Focus	Notes
1_____		
2_____		
3_____		
4_____		
5_____		
6_____		
7_____		

8_____		
9_____		

Now that you've made an implementation plan, let's get started with the focus topics.

SLOW AND STEADY CLEAN(ISH) CHANGE: YOUR NINE FOCUS TOPICS

Finally! Even though you have spent a great deal of time reflecting on the concepts throughout the book as you read each chapter, now it's your opportunity to make plans to put it all into practice.

Here's one thing to keep in mind as you go through these nine focus topics: swapping out products can get expensive. For that reason, you may want to set aside a budget for making safer swaps. How much you budget depends on how much you can afford to spend—maybe it's $20 a week, or perhaps it's $300 per month. You may even find that you can make the transition without increasing your current budget, particularly if you choose to use the products you currently have on hand until they are used up and then replace them on an as-needed basis. If you've been using the same counter spray for twenty years, for example, finishing the bottle you already have in your kitchen probably isn't a big deal in the long run.

But if you're like me, once you decide to make a change, you want to make the swaps *immediately*. I get it. Let your budget and your personality drive your decisions here. We are clean(ish), so it's always okay to make changes on your own terms.

Remember this—no stress—you have plenty of time to do this right. There is no need to feel rushed because there isn't going to be a test—only life.

I also have to admit something that probably won't surprise you: I'm still such a teacher at heart. I can't help it, y'all. I teach—that's what I do. And I also assign homework—but I promise never to give you busy work. So, expect that I'll be assigning you some tasks for each focus topic.

When you get to each new focus topic, I am going to have you review the information about each one (rereading applicable sections of the book) and I also want you to look back at the work you have already done at the end of each chapter (all the Reflect and Take Action activities) and at what you wrote down in your definitions of clean(ish) eating and clean(ish) living.

You'll follow this outline for each of the focus topics:

1. **Reread: Go back through selected parts of the book**
2. **Revisit: Read and consider what you wrote in the Reflect/ Take Action activities**
3. **Review: Look back at your personal definition of clean(ish) eating or living**
4. **Resolve: Set your personal course of action for implementing the focus**

Why? Because you consumed a *lot* of information as you read the book. There was so much information, in fact, that I'm certain that not all of it is fresh in your mind.

We learn best when we review information more than once, and if you want to make changes that stick, you need to thoroughly understand why you're making those changes in the first place. Revisiting the chapters and the activities you already completed will therefore be foundational when it comes to applying the information to your life going forward.

Equally as important, I want you to remember *your why*.

So, here's your first homework assignment, and I want you to do it now, before you do another thing. Go back to page 24 where you first identified your *why*, and reread what you wrote. Go ahead. I'll wait.

Okay, on to the nine focus topics. Remember: you do *not* have to do the focus topics in order. Even though I wrote them in a certain order, there is no reason to do them in the sequence that I chose. You certainly *may* do them in order, but it's not an expectation.

> Note: For each of the nine focus topics, you may choose to complete them right here in the book, or you can re-create the pages within your Clean(ish) Journal if you don't want to write in the book. Alternately, go to ginstephens .com/cleanish to download and print the pdf that contains these pages in worksheet format.

FOCUS

EXTEND YOUR DAILY FAST

I'm sure you aren't surprised that I put this one first because I'm such a huge proponent of intermittent fasting. I believe it is one of the most powerful things you can do to promote health and longevity, if not *the* most powerful thing. But, as I said already, these focus topics are **not** written in any type of sequential order that you must follow.

So, you can choose to start here with the intermittent fasting focus, or you can leave this one until last. Or maybe you *really* don't want to do any kind of intermittent fasting—ever—in which case, that is also fine.

If and when you do decide to practice intermittent fasting, I encourage you to commit to a month for this particular focus, and that's because there's a very important period of time called the twenty-eight-day FAST Start. You'll understand why that first twenty-eight days is so important when you read *Fast. Feast. Repeat.*

Implementing this focus:

1. REREAD: Go back through selected parts of the book
Reread "Intermittent Fasting: A Powerful Self-Cleaning Tool."

2. REVISIT: Read and consider what you wrote in the Reflect/Take Action activities
Go back to *Reflect and Take Action: Giving Your Body Time to Clean* (page 215) and read what you wrote there.

3. REVIEW: Look back at your personal definition of clean(ish) living
Reread what you wrote about intermittent fasting within your personal definition of clean(ish) living on page 310.

4. RESOLVE: Set your personal course of action for implementing the focus
You'll want to choose tasks to complete as you work through this focus area. I have given you a list of a few suggestions, but I have also

given you space to create your own personalized implementation steps, as well.

Here are some of the tasks you can choose as you complete this focus:

- Read *Fast. Feast. Repeat.* and commit to following the twenty-eight-day FAST Start.

- If your goal is strictly self-cleaning and not weight loss, then you'll choose an intermittent fasting approach that allows you to maintain your current weight. If your goal is self-cleaning *and* weight loss, then you'll choose an approach that is more likely to lead to weight loss.

- Find an intermittent fasting community for support along the way. Go to ginstephens.com to see how to connect with Gin's communities.

- Listen to the *Intermittent Fasting Stories* podcast for inspirational stories from IFers from around the world, or listen to *The Intermittent Fasting Podcast* to hear Gin and cohost Melanie Avalon discuss topics related to IF and answer listener questions about a wide variety of topics.

What other things do you want to do as a part of completing this focus? Add your own personalized implementation steps or tasks here:

_____

_____

_____

_____

_____

CHOOSE SAFE HOUSEHOLD CLEANING PRODUCTS

This focus topic is pretty straightforward: you're going to take all the time that you need to examine the household cleaning products that you currently use and make a plan for making the transition to clean(ish) cleaning (try to say that ten times fast). If you have as many cleaning products stashed away as I did, this may take a lot of time. Remember to go through your kitchen, laundry room, bathrooms, garage, and outside storage areas in search of various cleaning products—I found them *everywhere*. The longer you've been in your current home, the more you'll likely have stashed away.

Implementing this focus:

1. REREAD: Go back through selected parts of the book
Reread "Household Cleaning Products: What's in Your Bucket?" and applicable sections of the "Live (Mainly) Clean" chapter.

2. REVISIT: Read and consider what you wrote in the Reflect/Take Action activities
Go back to "Reflect and Take Action: What's in Your Cabinets?" (page 70) and read what you wrote there.

3. REVIEW: Look back at your personal definition of clean(ish) living
Reread what you wrote about household cleaning products within your personal definition of clean(ish) living on page 310.

4. RESOLVE: Set your personal course of action for implementing the focus
You'll want to choose tasks to complete as you work through this focus area. I have given you a list of a few suggestions, but I have also given you space to create your own personalized implementation steps, as well.

Here are some of the tasks you can choose as you complete this focus:

- Gather all your cleaning products. Ignore any greenwashing on the label and take the extra step to use third-party verification through one of the excellent apps or resources that lets you know whether a product is a safer choice or not, such as the EWG Healthy Living website and app and several sources from the "Online Resources" chapter: Consumer Reports, Gimme the Good Stuff, and the Environmental Protection Agency.

- Put all the products that don't meet your definition of clean(ish) living aside.

  - Decide if you need to dispose of any of them now or if you will use them up before replacing. If you're getting rid of them, call the appropriate local authorities/sanitation department and ask them how to dispose of the items safely if you are unsure.

  - Replace the products you remove (or use up) with safer choices.

- Less is more: a general all-purpose cleaner can replace many specialty cleaners.

- Consider concentrated formulations that you purchase and then add to your own spray bottle, along with water. You'll save packaging waste and usually save money at the same time.

- Plan for success. The fewer decisions you'll have to make going forward, the easier it will be to stick to the changes you're making now. Identify your core products, the companies you can trust, and the best places to obtain these products as they run out. Even better: make sure you never run out by having a backup on hand. This will ensure that you're never stuck making snap decisions that might lead to you grabbing something that is convenient (but not up to your clean(ish) standards).

What other things do you want to do as a part of completing this focus? Add your own personalized implementation steps or tasks here:

SELECT SAFE PERSONAL CARE PRODUCTS

This focus topic is also fairly straightforward, though it isn't going to always be easy; you're going to take all the time that you need to examine the personal care products that you (and your family) currently use and make a plan for making the transition to clean(ish) living. When it comes to personal care products, you're going to be surprised how much emotion may be tied into some of your choices, and change won't always be easy. (*I love the way toxin-filled deodorant works, darn it. Sigh.*) Never forget that every time you make a switch to a safer option, you have the potential to lower the number of toxins in your bucket.

Implementing this focus:

1. REREAD: Go back through selected parts of the book
Reread "Personal Care Products: Adding to Your Bucket" and applicable sections of the "Live (Mainly) Clean" chapter.

2. REVISIT: Read and consider what you wrote in the Reflect/Take Action activities
Go back to "Reflect and Take Action: What Are You Using?" (page 81) and read what you wrote there.

3. REVIEW: Look back at your personal definition of clean(ish) living
Reread what you wrote about selecting safe personal care products within your personal definition of clean(ish) living on page 310.

4. RESOLVE: Set your personal course of action for implementing the focus
You'll want to choose tasks to complete as you work through this focus area. I have given you a list of a few suggestions, but I have also given you space to create your own personalized implementation steps, as well.

Here are some of the tasks you can choose as you complete this focus:

- Gather all your personal care products. Ignore any greenwashing on the label and take the extra step to use third-party verification through one of the excellent apps or resources that lets you know whether a product is a safer choice or not, such as the EWG Healthy Living website and app. Also, refer to sources from the "Online Resources" chapter: Consumer Reports, the Campaign for Safe Cosmetics, and Gimme the Good Stuff.

- Put all the products that don't meet your definition of clean(ish) living aside.

  - Decide if you need to dispose of any of them now or if you will use them up before replacing. If you're getting rid of them now, call the appropriate local authorities/sanitation department and ask them how to dispose of the items safely if you are unsure.

  - Replace the products you remove (or use up) with safer choices.

- Less is more: Do you really need all the products that you currently use? Pare down the number of items you use to just the essentials. You'll save both time and money in the long run.

- Plan for success. The fewer decisions you'll have to make going forward, the easier it will be to stick to the changes you're making now. Identify your core products, the companies you can trust, and the best places to obtain these products as they run out. Even better: make sure you never run out by having a backup on hand. This will ensure that you're never stuck making snap decisions that might lead to you grabbing something that is convenient (but not up to your clean(ish) standards).

What other things do you want to do as a part of completing this focus? Add your own personalized implementation steps or tasks here:

AVOID FOOD CONTACT CHEMICALS

Some of the swaps you'll make as a part of this focus will be simple and easy, while others will be more complicated and expensive (*I'm looking at you, expensive-yet-toxin-coated pots and pans*). It's okay to take this focus slowly and swap out a few things now and others as you can afford it.

Implementing this focus:

1. REREAD: Go back through selected parts of the book

Reread "Better Living Through Chemistry," and particularly focus on the "Food Contact Chemicals" section (pages 52). Also refer back to the applicable sections from the "Live (Mainly) Clean" chapter, particularly the "kitchen" section.

2. REVISIT: Read and consider what you wrote in the Reflect/Take Action activities

Go back to "Reflect: How Full Is Your Bucket?" (page 58) and read what you wrote there.

3. REVIEW: Look back at your personal definition of clean(ish) living

Reread what you wrote about avoiding food contact chemicals within your personal definition of clean(ish) living on page 310.

4. RESOLVE: Set your personal course of action for implementing the focus

You'll want to choose tasks to complete as you work through this focus area. I have given you a list of a few suggestions, but I have also given you space to create your own personalized implementation steps, as well.

Here are some of the tasks you can choose as you complete this focus:

- Make an effort to remove plastics and items with nonstick coatings from your kitchen and replace those items with nontoxic options that won't leach into your foods wherever you can afford to do so.

- If you can't replace all your pots and pans/cookware now, get a few basic pieces and use those. You don't need to buy complete cookware sets—instead, choose a few pieces that will meet most of your needs. You can find great deals on individual pieces of high-quality cookware at stores like TJ Maxx and HomeGoods or other stores that focus on closeout products.

- Prioritize making purchases from companies who focus on eliminating toxins from their products.

- Ignore any greenwashing on labels, and take the extra step to use third-party verification through one of the excellent apps or resources that lets you know whether a product is a safer choice or not. Several of the websites listed in the "Online Resources" chapter will be useful here: Consumer Reports, Gimme the Good Stuff, and Green and Healthy Homes Initiative.

What other things do you want to do as a part of completing this focus? Add your own personalized implementation steps or tasks here:

_____

_____

_____

_____

_____

_____

_____

PRIORITIZE QUALITY FOODS

When completing this focus, you're going to emphasize choosing high-quality foods that are non-GMO and organic, including meats and animal products that come from animals raised as nature intended. This is a separate topic from whether your foods are ultra-processed or not; remember that foods can be both ultra-processed and made with organic ingredients. For now, you're only examining any foods in your kitchen that are *not* ultra-processed. (If you can't remember how to tell the difference, reread the section about the NOVA Food Classification Scale from pages 119.) There's a separate focus for limiting ultra-processed foods, and that is the next one coming up.

However, since *you* are in charge of how this process works, if you want to combine this focus and the next one into one big food-focus, you can. It's totally up to you.

Implementing this focus:

1. REREAD: Go back through selected parts of the book
Reread *"Food, Glorious Food"* and sections from the "Eat (Mostly) Clean" chapter that apply to this topic.

2. REVISIT: Read and consider what you wrote in the Reflect / Take Action activities
Go back to "Reflect and Take Action: What's in Your Kitchen?" (page 107) and read what you wrote there.

3. REVIEW: Look back at your personal definition of clean(ish) eating
Reread what you wrote within your personal definition of clean(ish) eating (on page 286) that relates to topics within these chapters/sections (organic foods, non-GMOs, sustainably raised foods, etc.).

4. RESOLVE: Set your personal course of action for implementing the focus

You'll want to choose tasks to complete as you work through this focus area. I have given you a list of a few suggestions, but I have also given you space to create your own personalized implementation steps, as well.

Here are some of the tasks you can choose as you complete this focus:

- Go through your fridge, freezer, and pantry and take a look at the basic foods you have on hand that would not be considered to be ultra-processed foods: butter, milk, cheese, meats, fruits, vegetables, grains, and so on.

- Set aside any foods that don't meet your definition of clean(ish) eating. Decide if you would rather eat them or get rid of them now. It's totally up to you, but for perishable items like these, it's likely a better choice to go ahead and use them up rather than throwing them away.

- Replace these foods with better choices the next time you shop.

- Understand which food labels really mean something and look for them when shopping.

- Prioritize organic/non-GMO/sustainably raised or grown foods when you can.

- Ignore greenwashing on the label, and take the extra step to use third-party verification through one of the excellent apps or resources that lets you know whether a product is a safer choice or not, such as the EWG Healthy Living website and app. Also, refer to sources from the "Online Resources" chapter: the Organic Center, Fair Trade Certified, Certified Humane, and the Monterey Bay Aquarium Seafood Watch.

- Consider changing your grocery store. We get into the habit of shopping where it is most convenient for us (or where the price is the lowest), but that may not be the best source for what you're looking for now. Some stores offer more options than others, so take a tour of stores you may not have visited recently to see who has the selection you need.

What other things do you want to do as a part of completing this focus? Add your own personalized implementation steps or tasks here:

_____

_____

_____

_____

_____

_____

_____

_____

_____

_____

_____

_____

_____

_____

_____

_____

FOCUS

LIMIT ULTRA-PROCESSED FOODS

To avoid being overfed and undernourished, it's important to consider our intake of ultra-processed foods. Now it's time to make some decisions about which ultra-processed foods need to go and which can stay—and this might not always be easy. You'll rely heavily on your personal definition of clean(ish) eating and look at the ingredient labels of your favorite products to see if they have any ingredients you identified as concerning to you.

Implementing this focus:

1. REREAD: Go back through selected parts of the book

Reread "Take a Break from Fake: Problems with Ultra-Processed Foods" and sections from the "Eat (Mostly) Clean" chapter that apply to this topic.

2. REVISIT: Read and consider what you wrote in the Reflect/Take Action activities

Go back to "Reflect and Take Action: Finding Food" (page 132) and read what you wrote there.

3. REVIEW: Look back at your personal definition of clean(ish) eating

Reread what you wrote within your personal definition of clean(ish) eating (on page 286) that relates to topics within these chapters/sections (reducing your consumption of ultra-processed foods and problematic ingredients).

4. RESOLVE: Set your personal course of action for implementing the focus

You'll want to choose tasks to complete as you work through this focus area. I have given you a list of a few suggestions, but I have also given you space to create your own personalized implementation steps, as well.

Here are some of the tasks you can choose as you complete this focus:

- Go through your fridge and pantry and read labels. Look for ingredients that you included in your *"foods and ingredients I will avoid at all times"* list from your definition of clean(ish) eating. Set any of these products aside in a separate pile.

- Ignore greenwashing on the label, and take the extra step to use third-party verification through one of the excellent apps or resources that lets you know whether a product is a safer choice or not, such as the EWG Healthy Living website and app.

- Use the NOVA Food Classification System to help you identify which foods are ultra-processed. Make a separate pile for *"ultra-processed but still clean(ish) enough for me"* items.

- Consider all the products that you put aside that don't meet your definition of clean(ish) eating. Decide if you would rather use them up or get rid of them now.

  - One thing that you might struggle with: throwing food away. It feels like "wasting it." Keep this in mind: you "wasted" it the day you bought it. Eating food you no longer want to eat isn't going to help. Your body is not a trash can.

  - For anything that is in unopened boxes, cans, and bags, consider donating to a local food pantry. In an ideal world, every person would have access to organic and fresh foods. We are not there yet. Families with food insecurity would rather have the foods you donate now than go without a meal.

  - Replace the products you remove (or use up) with safer choices. The EWG app allows you to search by product name and also makes suggestions of "better rated products" for food items, and that can help you make sensible swaps. While not all the foods in your fridge or pantry will be rated in the app, it is still a great place to start.

- Plan to do more cooking at home. When you control the ingredients, you can make sure they are *food* rather than *not-food*.

- Think of ultra-processed foods as condiments rather than the main attraction. Your goal is to de-emphasize their role in your life as much as possible, while still enjoying your meals and eating experiences.

- Make swaps to less-processed versions with fewer problematic ingredients whenever you can. It may be as simple as changing from one brand to another.

- Prioritize making purchases from companies who focus on eliminating problematic food additives from their products.

- Shop the perimeter of the grocery store and get most of your food in a state close to how it appears in nature.

- Find an online marketplace that specializes in natural and/or organic foods. They are likely to have a wider variety of nonperishable options than your local stores, and prices are often better.

What other things do you want to do as a part of completing this focus? Add your own personalized implementation steps or tasks here:

_____

_____

_____

FOCUS

ADD IN NUTRIENTS

We don't just remove foods that have ingredients we want to avoid—we also make sure that we choose foods that have all the nutrients our bodies need to support vibrant health—not to mention self-cleaning. Hippocrates told us to "let food be thy medicine and medicine be thy food." And as Michael Pollan said a lot more recently, "Eat food. Mostly plants. Not too much." Your goal is to eat a variety of real foods so that you'll maximize the number of phytochemicals you take in. Remember that there are so many phytochemicals in plants that scientists haven't even identified what all of them are or what they all do, so the best way to ensure that you're getting what your body needs is to go for variety.

Implementing this focus:

1. REREAD: Go back through selected parts of the book

Reread "What's a Healthy Diet? And How Do We Know?" and "What's Food Got to Do with It?"

2. REVISIT: Read and consider what you wrote in the Reflect/Take Action activities

Go back to "Reflect and Take Action: Examine the Diet of Your Ancestors" (page 153) and "Reflect and Take Action: Consider Your Diet Diversity and Focus on Nutrients" (page 197) and read what you wrote there.

3. REVIEW: Look back at your personal definition of clean(ish) eating

Reread what you wrote within your personal definition of clean(ish) eating (on page 286) that relates to topics within these chapters/sections (choosing what foods to add in).

4. RESOLVE: Set your personal course of action for implementing the focus

You'll want to choose tasks to complete as you work through this focus area. I have given you a list of a few suggestions, but I have also given you space to create your own personalized implementation steps, as well.

Here are some of the tasks you can choose as you complete this focus:

- Get out of your current food rut—most of us get trapped in one, even though we may not realize it. We're busy, so we gravitate toward the same few meals each week. Our bodies need diversity, so we have to take time to plan for it.

- Buy a few new recipe books that are plant-forward. This is not to suggest that you become a vegetarian—but most of us don't have a problem getting sufficient animal products in our diets. It's the vegetables that need some help.

- Overall, make sure to prioritize plants from day to day to up your intake of phytochemicals and boost your body's self-cleaning abilities. You'll also feed your gut microbiome well.

- Buy organic produce when you can, but don't let whether it's organic or not stop you from buying fresh veggies—a nonorganic zucchini is a better choice when it comes to nutrients than an organic chocolate chip cookie. Still, it's helpful to use the EWG "Dirty Dozen" list (as well as the "Clean Fifteen" list) to guide your choices. If a food is on the "Dirty Dozen" list, choose organic.

- Include foods that your ancestors ate. Look for traditional recipes that are either unfamiliar to you or ones you haven't made before and experiment.

- Make a plan to incorporate at least one or two new plant foods (these can be vegetables, fruits, herbs/spices, etc.) each week.

What other things do you want to do as a part of completing this focus? Add your own personalized implementation steps or tasks here:

INCORPORATE TOOLS FOR SELF-CLEANING

It's time to have some fun! All the tools for self-cleaning are also amazing self-care strategies. You'll be taking care of yourself both physically and emotionally, and that's a real win-win. As you work on this focus, make a plan for incorporating these strategies into your regular routine—not just one time as you complete this focus. As an example, after I get a massage, I always make an appointment for the next one before I leave. That means it's already scheduled and I don't even have to think about it.

Implementing this focus:

1. REREAD: Go back through selected parts of the book
Reread *Extra Credit: More Tools for Self-Cleaning*.

2. Revisit: Read and consider what you wrote in the Reflect/ Take Action activities
Go back to Take Action: Choose Your Tools (page 230) and read what you wrote there.

3. REVIEW: Look back at your personal definition of clean(ish) living
Reread what you wrote about incorporating self-cleaning tools within your personal definition of clean(ish) living on page 310.

4. RESOLVE: Set your personal course of action for implementing the focus
You'll want to choose tasks to complete as you work through this focus area. I have given you a list of a few suggestions, but I have also given you space to create your own personalized implementation steps, as well.

Here are some of the tasks you can choose as you complete this focus:

- If you're not already active, make a plan to add exercise to each day.

- Find a sauna in your local community and schedule regular visits. You can kill two birds with one stone by finding a gym with a sauna—work out and use the sauna on the same visit.

- Make an appointment for a massage. While a massage may or may not help your body's detoxification processes, it'll likely reduce your overall levels of anxiety, and who doesn't need a little anxiety reduction?

- Make your bedroom a sanctuary for sleep. Your glymphatic system will thank you.

- Limit your blue-light exposure after the sun goes down by turning off screens, turning down lights, and/or wearing blue-light blocking glasses.

- Take some time to walk on the earth to balance your body's electrical charge and reduce inflammation.

- Take steps to improve your indoor air quality.

What other things do you want to do as a part of completing this focus? Add your own personalized implementation steps or tasks here:

_____

_____

_____

_____

_____

FOCUS

CLEAN UP YOUR HOME AND YARD

Now it's time to focus on your yard, as well as the various other household items that don't fit into the other categories. This is a big topic, but many of the considerations don't apply to day-to-day activities the same way that our foods and cleaning or personal care products do.

In the chapter on how to live (mainly) clean, I mentioned a variety of concepts that applied to the various rooms of your home, and some of them were big-ticket items (such as getting new furniture) or once-in-a-while projects (such as repainting). While you included these in your definition of clean(ish) living, we all know that it isn't practical for you to rip up all your carpet, throw away all your mattresses, get all new furniture, or repaint your entire house as a part of becoming clean(ish).

Because things like buying furniture, getting a new mattress, replacing your floor coverings, or painting the walls are expensive and infrequent, these situations may not come up during your nine-week to nine-month timeline—but they will all come up in the future as you're living your life. When you face any of these big purchases or home improvements, you'll want to make clean(ish) choices, so always keep that idea in the back of your mind.

Implementing this focus:

1. REREAD: Go back through selected parts of the book
Reread "Better Living Through Chemistry," as well as applicable sections from the "Live (Mainly) Clean" chapter.

**2. REVISIT: Read and consider what you wrote in the
Reflect/Take Action activities**
Go back to "Reflect: How Full Is Your Bucket?" (page 58) and read what you wrote there.

**3. REVIEW: Look back at your personal definition of
clean(ish) living**

Reread what you wrote about cleaning up throughout your home and yard within your personal definition of clean(ish) living on page 310.

4. RESOLVE: Set your personal course of action for implementing the focus

You'll want to choose tasks to complete as you work through this focus area. I have given you a list of a few suggestions, but I have also given you space to create your own personalized implementation steps, as well.

Here are some of the tasks you can choose as you complete this focus:

- Gather all your yard and garden products, and also your pest control products (both indoor and outdoor). Ignore any greenwashing on labels, and take the extra step to use third-party verification through one of the excellent apps or resources that let you know whether a product is a safer choice or not such as sources from the "Online Resources" chapter: Consumer Reports, Earth 911, the Organic Center, the Environmental Protection Agency, Fair Trade Certified, and the Green and Healthy Homes Initiative.

- Put all the products that don't meet your definition of clean(ish) living aside.

  - Decide if you need to dispose of any of them now or if you will use them up before replacing. If you're getting rid of them, call the appropriate local authorities/sanitation department and ask them how to dispose of the items safely if you are unsure.

  - Replace the products you remove (or use up) with safer choices.

- Prioritize making purchases from companies who focus on eliminating toxins from their products.

- Think of your yard as a habitat for native plant, animal, and insect species.

- Make choices that will thrive in your climate without the use of toxic chemical fertilizers, herbicides, or pesticides.

- Connect with your local extension/conservation service (or whatever it's called in your location) and use their services. They can help you plan based on your local area.

- Consider a water filtration system (either simple or more complex) for your home.

- Replace your shower curtain liner with a nontoxic option.

- As you buy new home furnishings or do home improvement projects, use resources from the "Online Resources" chapter to help you make cleaner choices: Consumer Reports, Earth 911, the Organic Center, the Environmental Protection Agency, Fair Trade Certified, and the Green and Healthy Homes Initiative.

What other things do you want to do as a part of completing this focus? Add your own personalized implementation steps or tasks here:

_____

_____

_____

_____

_____

_____

CLEAN(ISH): FOR LIFE

Over the course of working your way through this book, I'm sure you have had many moments where you discovered something that surprised you—or even shocked you—either as you read the chapters or as you looked more closely at the contents of your fridge, cabinets, closets, or pantry. I know I have had many of those moments myself along the way.

Upon completion, I'm left with an even greater motivation to be mindful of what I am putting into (or *onto*) my body, and to examine what I am surrounding myself with as I go about my daily life. I hope you feel the same way. By making intentional choices, we really can slow the drip-drip-drip into our toxic-load buckets. Through our choices, we can also support our bodies as they do the important work of self-cleaning.

While I shared a lot with you here in these pages, there are so many more topics that I could have written about. Your *evolution to clean(ish)* won't stop today, and it also shouldn't be limited to the topics I chose to include in this book. For that reason, I want you to feel empowered to dig deeper into any topic that is of interest to you personally, especially if it's a topic that wasn't addressed within these pages.

Never forget that living a clean(ish) life is very much a process that continues to evolve over time. Some days we are more **clean** and some days we are more *-ish,* but every time we make a positive choice, we can be assured that we are doing something that makes a difference.

Clean(ish) is *not* something you start and stop. It isn't a plan or a program. You don't fall off the clean(ish) wagon.

Going forward, every time you make decisions about what to buy or what to eat, you'll filter them through your very own clean(ish) lens, making the best choice for you for that moment in time.

Being clean(ish) is very much a mindset shift and a way of living your life. Perfection is not required.

As a society, we can be certain that we will continue to learn new things because scientific advancement—both the *good* and the *bad*—never stops. And, as we learn, we will continue to refine and adjust what we are doing accordingly.

From time to time, come back to these chapters to remind yourself of why it's important to make changes that you can stick with long term. Revisit your personal definitions of what it means to be clean(ish) every now and then as well, adding to (or taking away) as necessary.

Here's to your good health!

Gin

AFTERWORD

DO YOU NEED MORE?
DIGGING DEEPER
(WITHOUT LOSING YOUR MIND)

A NOTE ABOUT INDIVIDUAL CHALLENGES

While our bodies have amazing self-cleaning pathways and a variety of self-cleaning mechanisms that never stop working for us, you may be someone who needs more than a few simple dietary changes or product swaps to see the vibrant health you are looking for.

If you have gut issues (such as IBS, SIBO, leaky gut, etc.) that affect your ability to tolerate a variety of foods, or if you suffer from other types of health issues that may be related to your overall toxic load (such as high levels of heavy metals) or an inability to detox efficiently (such as a MTHRF gene mutation), you may need support from a medical professional who understands how to heal your gut, lower your toxic load, manage your condition, and so on.

It's important to understand that I am not qualified to give you a plan for managing any of these potentially serious health conditions, and I'm not even going to try. There are other people to turn to for that.

If you suspect that you have any of these health issues or you already have a confirmed diagnosis, then your best bet is to work with a medical practitioner who understands what you are going through and who can provide the specialized support that you need.

The good news is that our bodies have a remarkable propensity for healing when given the right kind of support. Your first step—becoming clean(ish) when it comes to what you put in—is a step in the right direction. Your second step—finding a medical professional to work with you—may just be the final piece of the puzzle that you'll need to feel better and live a long and healthy life.

ACTION PLAN: FINDING A HEATH CARE PRACTITIONER WHO CAN HELP

If you have struggled to find a physician or health care professional that understands your unique needs, or if you are looking for a practitioner who follows a more holistic approach (*treating symptoms while also looking for underlying causes of these symptoms*) versus a conventional Western medicine approach (*may focus on symptoms and medications to treat the symptoms without addressing the underlying cause*), here are some resources that can help you in your search.

American Osteopathic Association
osteopathic.org

What is a DO? Doctors of Osteopathic Medicine, or DOs, are fully licensed physicians who practice in all areas of medicine. Emphasizing a whole-person approach to treatment and care, DOs are trained to listen and partner with their patients to help them get healthy and stay well.

While primary care remains a strong focus for the osteopathic profession, DOs practice in all medical specialties. During medical school, they receive special training in the musculoskeletal system, your body's interconnected system of nerves, muscles, and bones. By combining this knowledge with the latest advances in medical technology, they offer patients the most comprehensive care available in medicine.

There are more than 121,000 DOs practicing their distinct philosophy of medicine throughout the U.S. today. With approximately 25 percent of medical students enrolled in colleges of osteopathic medicine, the profession is one of the fastest-growing segments of health care.

Osteopathic physicians focus on prevention, tuning into how a patient's lifestyle and environment can impact their well-being. DOs strive to help you be truly healthy in mind, body, and spirit—not just free of symptoms.

You may not be aware that both doctors of osteopathic medicine (DOs) and doctors of medicine (MDs) are considered to be accredited doctors, and both are fully licensed to practice medical care in the United States. DO and MD programs both require rigorous study in the field of medicine. In the U.S., the same licensing boards that license MDs give licenses to DOs, and they must meet the same standards for practicing medicine.

On the American Osteopathic Association website, they have a search tool that will help you find a DO in your area. They also have resources that will help you understand how a DO may be different from a traditional MD.

The Institute for Functional Medicine

www.ifm.org/find-a-practitioner/

> *The Functional Medicine model is an individualized, patient-centered, science-based approach that empowers patients and practitioners to work together to address the underlying causes of disease and promote optimal wellness. It requires a detailed understanding of each patient's genetic, biochemical, and lifestyle factors and leverages that data to direct personalized treatment plans that lead to improved patient outcomes.*
>
> *By addressing root cause, rather than symptoms, practitioners become oriented to identifying the complexity of disease. They may find one condition has many different causes and, likewise, one cause may result in many different conditions. As a result, Functional Medicine treatment targets the specific manifestations of disease in each individual.*

On their website, you can search for functional medicine practitioners near you.

American Association of Naturopathic Physicians

naturopathic.org

> *Founded in 1985, the American Association of Naturopathic Physicians (AANP) is the national professional society representing licensed naturopathic doctors, naturopathic medicine students, and other healthcare professionals allied with the naturopathic profession.*
>
> *The AANP's physician members are graduates of naturopathic medical schools accredited by the Council on Naturopathic Medical Education. CNME is recognized by the US Department of Education as the national accrediting agency for programs leading to the Doctorate of Naturopathic Medicine (ND or NMD) or Doctor of Naturopathy (ND) degree.*
>
> *Together, we work to advance the unique and distinct philosophy of naturopathic medicine, to expand access to naturopathic doctors, and to help its members build successful practices.*

On their website, they have a "Find a Doctor" tab that connects you to naturopathic physicians near you.

Alliance for Natural Health
anh-usa.org

> *The Alliance for Natural Health USA (ANH-USA) is the largest organization in the US and abroad working to protect your right to utilize safe, effective, and inexpensive healing therapies based on high-tech testing, diet, supplements, and lifestyle changes. We believe a system that is single-mindedly focused on "treating" sick people with expensive drugs, rather than maintaining healthy people, is neither practical nor economically sustainable.*
>
> ANH-USA is part of an international organization dedicated to promoting natural and sustainable health—and, in particular, consumer freedom of choice in healthcare—through good science and good law. We utilize grassroots advocacy, effective lobbying, litigation, strategic coalitions, and public education campaigns to fight for your right to stay healthy, naturally.

On their website, you can find a link to DocNet, which is a tool to help you search for health care practitioners who are more holistic in their practice.

RECOMMENDED READING

I'm always going to be a teacher at heart, so consider these books to be your homework assignment. I have them listed in the order that I want you to consider reading them. Most of these books are about food, though there is one about environmental medicine and how chemicals may affect your child's behavior. It's one I read back in the day when I was searching for a way to help my own son deal with his food and chemical sensitivities. Why are there no other books on the list about living (mostly) clean? That's because most of the resources I find to be valuable are online sources, and I already included them as resources in part 3 of this book.

Here's something to understand as you read these books: while I love and recommend all of them, I don't agree with every word or idea you'll find in their pages, and you may not, either. It's rare for any of us to find an author or book in the field of nutrition that agrees with our thoughts 100 percent. That doesn't mean that everything they have to say should be discarded.

Here's an example of what I mean. *Fiber Fueled* was written by a physician who follows a plant-based eating approach, and he recommends that you avoid animal foods in your diet. *Nourishing Traditions,* on the flip side, encourages you to include both plant and animal foods, sticking to the animal foods that were prized parts of traditional diets from around the world.

Rather than letting differences within these books confuse you, take away what you will from each, and appreciate the common thread: eat real food and avoid ultra-processed foods. Every one of these books about food celebrates *real food* as the centerpiece of a healthy life.

Yes, my own book is first on the list, and I am not sorry. If you haven't yet read *Fast. Feast. Repeat.*, I want you to start there, and by the time you are done, I bet you'll be an intermittent faster (if you aren't already). While you don't have to be an IFer to live clean(ish), I think it's one of the most powerful approaches you can implement into your life.

Fast. Feast. Repeat. by Gin Stephens
In this book, you'll learn how to create in intermittent fasting approach that works for you. I'll explain the health benefits of intermittent fasting,

teach you everything you need to know about the clean fast, and then fill your IF toolbox with strategies that ensure success. There's also a thorough FAQ section that includes any question you can think to ask.

Spoon-Fed by Dr. Tim Spector

Tim Spector is a professor of genetic epidemiology at King's College London and one of my favorite health researchers. In *Spoon-Fed*, Dr. Spector examines top myths about health, such as "nutritional guidelines and diet plans apply to everyone," "calories accurately measure how fattening a food is," and "gluten is dangerous."

Fiber Fueled by Dr. Will Bulsiewicz

Dr. Will Bulsiewicz is a board-certified gastroenterologist and gut health expert. In his book, he will teach you how to optimize your gut microbiome by choosing foods that encourage the gut-bug species that you want to thrive. If you've struggled with gut health, this book can help you heal. If you've spent time removing food after food from your diet, thinking that avoidance is the key to better gut health, he can teach you how to safely reintroduce foods rather than eliminate more and more "problematic" foods.

The Blue Zones Solution by Dan Buettner

Author Dan Buettner shares what he has learned by studying the diets, eating habits, and lifestyle practices of the communities known as *Blue Zones*—Okinawa, Japan; Sardinia, Italy; Costa Rica's Nicoya Peninsula; Ikaria, Greece; and Loma Linda, California. It's not just what you eat—it's also how you live.

Nourishing Traditions by Sally Fallon

This classic first came out in 2001, but it's a classic for a reason. In it, Sally Fallon and Mary Enig share principles related to the work of Dr. Weston Price: eat real foods, modeled after traditional diets from around the world. Not only do they explain why certain foods are important nutritionally, you'll find a collection of recipes, because this book is at its heart a cookbook.

In Defense of Food: An Eater's Manifesto by Michael Pollan

Michael Pollan's *In Defense of Food* is also a classic, and it was released in 2008. This book takes you deeper into the world of ultra-processed foods versus whole foods—though the term *ultra-processed foods* wasn't yet being used when he wrote this book. His famous "eater's manifesto"—

Eat food. Not too much. Mostly plants.—is the TL;DR version, but if you want to learn more about how he came up with this manifesto, you'll find it all within these pages.

Is This Your Child? by Dr. Doris Rapp

Dr. Doris Rapp, MD, spent her career as a board-certified environmental medical specialist and a pediatric allergist. In her 1991 book, which is marketed as a solution "for children who are complaining, cranky, slow learners, aggressive, hyperactive, unwell, or depressed," she expands on the traditional concept of "allergy." Most of us consider hay fever, asthma, hives, or eczema to be outward signs of allergies, but Dr. Rapp understood that our brains can also be affected by allergies or food and chemical sensitivities. A powerful sentence from the book: *"Substances called chemical mediators are released during allergic reactions and travel all over the body, not just to 'accepted' areas such as the lungs or nose."* You can find a practitioner who follows a similar approach by visiting the American Academy of Environmental Medicine (www.aaemonline.org).

NOTES

INTRODUCTION

1. "Adult Obesity Facts," Centers for Disease Control and Prevention. https://www
   .cdc.gov/obesity/data/adult.html
2. "Obesity pandemic: causes, consequences, and solution—but do we have
   the will?," Fertility and Sterility. https://www.fertstert.org/article/S0015
   -0282(17)30223-6/fulltext
3. "Food and Agriculture Data," Food and Agriculture Organization of the United
   Nations. http://www.fao.org/faostat/en/#home
4. "Nutrition Is a Better Way," The Feingold Association of the United States.
   https://www.feingold.org
5. "Sensitivity to food additives, vaso-active amines and salicylates: a review of
   the evidence," Isabel Skypala, M. Williams, L. Reeves, R. Meyer, and C. Venter,
   Clinic and Translational Allergy.https://www.ncbi.nlm.nih.gov/pmc/articles
   /PMC4604636/
6. https://www.ncbi.nlm.nih.gov/pmc/articles/PMC6389720/
7. https://www.ncbi.nlm.nih.gov/pmc/articles/PMC6835893/
8. https://www.google.com/url?sa=t&rct=j&q=&esrc=s&source=web&cd
   =&ved=2ahUKEwiM2IP2_9XuAhWQGs0KHc0OD0oQFjAJegQIAxAC&u
   rl=https%3A%2F%2Fenveurope.springeropen.com%2Ftrack%2Fpdf%2F10
   .1186%2Fs12302-014-0034-1.pdf&usg=AOvVaw1veUfPQ9OOd5nsLiEkXdJk

PART 1: WHAT GOES IN: YOU ARE WHAT YOU EAT (AND WHAT YOUR ABSORB)

1. https://d124kohvtzl951.cloudfront.net/wp-content/uploads/2018/09/26092837/BCPP
   _Right-To-Know-Report_Secret-Toxic-Fragrance-Ingredients_9_26_2018.pdf

BETTER LIVING THROUGH CHEMISTRY

1. http://www.fao.org/news/story/en/item/80096/icode/
2. https://www.ids.ac.uk/download.php?file=files/dmfile/wp105.pdf

3. https://www.thelancet.com/journals/lancet/article/PIIS0140-6736(15)00480-8 /fulltext?rss%3Dyes

4. https://sustainablefoodtrust.org/articles/21st-century-famine-a-long-time-in-the -making/

5. https://thewaterproject.org/why-water/health

6. https://www.epa.gov/pfas/basic-information-pfas

7. https://www.consumerreports.org/bottled-water/whats-really-in-your-bottled-water/

8. https://www.sciencedirect.com/science/article/abs/pii/S014765131400253X

9. https://www.nrdc.org/issues/toxic-chemicals

10. https://www.epa.gov/mercury/health-effects-exposures-mercury

11. https://pubmed.ncbi.nlm.nih.gov/16551676/

12. https://www.cdc.gov/biomonitoring/Arsenic_FactSheet.html

13. https://www.cdc.gov/exposurereport/pdf/FourthReport_ExecutiveSummary.pdf

14. https://pubmed.ncbi.nlm.nih.gov/19552505/

15. https://www.epa.gov/toxics-release-inventory-tri-program/persistent -bioaccumulative-toxic-pbt-chemicals-covered-tri.

16. https://www.who.int/news-room/q-a-detail/food-safety-persistent-organic -pollutants-(pops)

17. https://www.epa.gov/international-cooperation/persistent-organic-pollutants -global-issue-global-response

18. https://www.scientificamerican.com/article/food-additives-mimic-hormones/

19. https://pubmed.ncbi.nlm.nih.gov/19502515/

20. https://www.ncbi.nlm.nih.gov/pmc/articles/PMC3365860/

21. https://www.ncbi.nlm.nih.gov/pmc/articles/PMC2713042/

22. Ibid.

23. "Environmental Obesogens: Mechanisms and Controversies," Heindel, Jerrold J and Bruce Blumberg, *Annual Review of Pharmacology and Toxicology*. https://pubmed.ncbi.nlm.nih.gov/30044726/

24. "Persistent Organic Pollutant Leads to Insulin Resistance Syndrome," Ruzzin, Jerome et al. https://www.ncbi.nlm.nih.gov/pmc/articles/PMC2854721 /pdf/ehp-118-465.pdf

25. "Minireview: The Case for Obesogens," Grun, Felix and Bruce Blumberg, *Molecular and Cellular Endocrinology*. https://www.ncbi.nlm.nih.gov/pmc /articles/PMC2718750/

26. Ibid.

27. Ibid.

28. "White adipose tissue: storage and effector site for environmental pollutants," Mullerova, D. and J. Kopecky. *Physiological Reviews*. https://pubmed.ncbi.nlm .nih.gov/16925464/

29. "Adipose Tissue as a Site of Toxic Accumulation," Jackson, Erin, Robin Shoemaker, Nika Larian, and Lisa Cassis, *Comprehensive Physiology*. https://www .ncbi.nlm.nih.gov/pmc/articles/PMC6101675/

30. "Biochemistry of adipose tissue: an endocrine organ," Coelho, Marisa, Teresa

Oliveira, and Ruben Fernandes, *Archives of Medical Science*. https://www.ncbi
.nlm.nih.gov/pmc/articles/PMC3648822/

31. "The role of leptin and ghrelin in the regulation of food intake and body weight
in humans: a review," Klok, M. D., S. Jakobsdottir, and M. L. Drent, *Obesity
Reviews*. https://pubmed.ncbi.nlm.nih.gov/17212793/

32. "Adiponectin: More Than Just Another Fat Cell Hormone?" Chandran, Manju,
Susan A. Phillips, Theodore Ciaraldi, and Robert R. Henry, *Diabetes Journals*.
https://care.diabetesjournals.org/content/26/8/2442

33. "Toxicology Function of Adipose Tissue: Focus on Persistent Organic
Pollutants," La Merrill, Michele, et al. https://www.ncbi.nlm.nih.gov/pmc/articles
/PMC3569688/pdf/ehp.1205485.pdf

34. "Fate and Complex Pathogenic Effects of Dioxins and Polychlorinated
Byphenyls in Obese Subjects before and after Drastic Weight Loss," Kim, Min-Ji,
et al. https://www.ncbi.nlm.nih.gov/pmc/articles/PMC3060002/pdf/ehp-119
-377.pdf

35. "Impacts of food contact chemicals on human health: a consensus statement,"
Muncke, Jane, et al, *Environmental Health*. https://pubmed.ncbi.nlm.nih.gov
/32122363/

36. "The placenta as a barrier for toxic and essential elements in paired maternal
and cord blood samples of South African delivering women," Rudge, Cibele V.,
et al, *Journal of Environmental Monitoring*. https://pubs.rsc.org/en/content
/articlelanding/2009/EM/b903805a#!divAbstract

37. "Cumulative Chemical Exposures During Pregnancy and Early
Development," Mitro, Susanna D., Tyiesha Johnson, and Ami R. Zota,
Current Environmental Health Reports. https://www.ncbi.nlm.nih.gov/pmc
/articles/PMC4626367/

38. "Body Burden: The Pollution in Newborns," Environmental Working Group.
https://www.ewg.org/research/body-burden-pollution-newborns

HOUSEHOLD CLEANING PRODUCTS:
WHAT'S IN YOUR BUCKET?

1. "Safer Choice: Fragrance Free," United States Environmental Protection Agency.
https://www.epa.gov/sites/production/files/2016-10/documents/saferchoice
-factsheet-fragrancefree_0.pdf

2. "Household Hazards Hunts," United States Environmental Protection Agency.
https://www.epa.gov/sites/production/files/2014-06/documents/lesson2
_handout.pdf

3. "Household Hazardous Waste (HHW)," United States Environmental Protection
Agency. https://www.epa.gov/hw/household-hazardous-waste-hhw

4. "Fact Sheet: Analysis of Dioxin in Sediments of San Francisco Bay," United

States Environmental Protection Agency. https://archive.epa.gov/region09/water
/archive/dioxin/sediment.pdf

5. "Pharmaceuticals, Hormones, and Other Organic Wastewater Contaminants in
U.S. Streams," United States Geological Survey. https://toxics.usgs.gov/pubs/FS
-027-02/

PERSONAL CARE PRODUCTS:
ADDING TO YOUR BUCKET

1. "Why Skin Deep?" Environmental Working Group. https://www.ewg.org
/skindeep/contents/why-skin-deep/

2. "FDA Authority Over Cosmetics: How Cosmetics Are Not FDA-Approved,
but Are FDA-Regulated," U.S. Food & Drug Administration. https://www.fda
.gov/cosmetics/cosmetics-laws-regulations/fda-authority-over-cosmetics-how
-cosmetics-are-not-fda-approved-are-fda-regulated

3. "What Are Parabens, and Why Don't They Belong in Cosmetics?" Tasha Stoiber,
Environmental Working Group. https://www.ewg.org/californiacosmetics
/parabens

4. "State of the evidence 2017: an update on the connection between breast cancer
and the environment," Gray, Janet M., Sharima Rasanayagam, Connie Engel, and
Jeanne Rizzo, *Environmental Health*. https://www.ncbi.nlm.nih.gov/pmc/articles
/PMC5581466/

5. "Parabens as Urinary Biomarkers of Exposure in Humans," ye, Xiaoyun Ye,
Amber M. Bishop, John A. Reidy, Larry L. Needham, and Antonia M. Calafat,
Environmental Health Perspectives. https://www.ncbi.nlm.nih.gov/pmc/articles
/PMC1764178/

6. "Commission Implementing Decision," *Official Journal of the European
Union*. https://eur-lex.europa.eu/legal-content/EN/TXT/HTML/?uri
=CELEX:32013D0674&from=EN

7. "Cosmetics," European Commission. https://ec.europa.eu/growth/sectors
/cosmetics_en

8. "Fragranced consumer products: effects on asthmatics," Steinemann, Anne,
Air Quality, Atmosphere & Health. https://www.ncbi.nlm.nih.gov/pmc/articles
/PMC5773620/

9. "Contact Allergy: A Review of Current Problems from a Clinical Perspective,"
Uter, Wolfgang, Thomas Werfel, Ian R. White, and Jeanne D. Johansen,
International Journal of Environmental Research and Public Health. https://www
.ncbi.nlm.nih.gov/pmc/articles/PMC6025382/

10. https://d124kohvtzl951.cloudfront.net/wp-content/uploads/2018/09/26092837
/BCPP_Right-To-Know-Report_Secret-Toxic-Fragrance-Ingredients_9_26_2018
.pdf

11. "Why the toxic tampon issue isn't going away," Rune Leith, Environmental Paper

Network. https://environmentalpaper.org/wp-content/uploads/2018/03/RL
_7mars_2018-1.pdf

12. "'Hypoallergenic' Cosmetics," U.S. Food & Drug Administration. https://www
.fda.gov/cosmetics/cosmetics-labeling-claims/hypoallergenic-cosmetics

13. "'Cruelty Free/Not Tested on Animals," U.S. Food & Drug Administration. https://
www.fda.gov/cosmetics/cosmetics-labeling-claims/cruelty-freenot-tested-animals

FOOD, GLORIOUS FOOD

1. "Farm Subsidy Primer," Environmental Working Group. https://farm.ewg.org
/subsidyprimer.php

2. "Examining America's Farm Subsidy Problem," Scott Lincicome, CATO Institute.
https://www.cato.org/commentary/examining-americas-farm-subsidy-problem

3. "Apples to Twinkies: Comparing Federal Subsidies of Fresh Produce and Junk
Food," U.S. Public Interest Research Group. https://www.foodsafetynews.com
/files/2011/09/Apples-to-Twinkies-USPIRG-1.pdf

4. "2020 Top 100 Food & Beverage Companies," *Food Engineering Magazine*.
https://www.foodengineeringmag.com/2020-top-100-food-beverage-companies

5. "9 Ways You May Not Realize Cotton Is in Your Food," Rodale Institute. https:
//rodaleinstitute.org/blog/9-ways-you-may-not-realize-cotton-is-in-your-food/

6. "Where do all these soybeans go?," Kendra Wills, Michigan State University.
https://www.canr.msu.edu/news/where_do_all_these_soybeans_go

7. "GMO Crops, Animal Food, and Beyond," U.S. Food & Drug Administration.
https://www.fda.gov/food/agricultural-biotechnology/gmo-crops-animal-food
-and-beyond

8. "About Genetically Engineered Foods," Center for Food Safety. https://www
.centerforfoodsafety.org/issues/311/ge-foods/about-ge-foods

9. "No scientific consensus on GMO safety," Hilbeck, Angelika, et al, *Environmental
Sciences Europe*. https://enveurope.springeropen.com/articles/10.1186/s12302
-014-0034-1

10. "Glyphosate: the cancer-causing Roundup chemical found in children's cereal,"
Environmental Working Group. https://www.ewg.org/key-issues/toxics
/glyphosate

11. "EWG Tests of Hummus Find High Levels of Glyphosate Weedkiller," Alexis M.
Temkin and Olga Naidenko, Environmental Working Group. https://www.ewg
.org/research/glyphosate-hummus/

12. "Glyphosate Contamination in Food Goes Far Beyond Oat Products,"
Environmental Working Group. https://www.ewg.org/news-and-analysis/2019
/02/glyphosate-contamination-food-goes-far-beyond-oat-products

13. "FDA Glyphosate Testing Conspicuously Skips Oats, Wheat Products,"
Environmental Working Group. https://www.ewg.org/release/fda-glyphosate
-testing-conspicuously-skips-oats-wheat-products

14. "Chemical Pesticides and Human Health: The Urgent Need for a New Concept in Agriculture," Nicolopoulou-Stamati, Polyxeni, Sotirios Maipas, Chrysanthi Kotampasi, Panagiotis Stamatis, and Luc Hens, *Frontiers in Public Health*. https://www.ncbi.nlm.nih.gov/pmc/articles/PMC4947579/

15. "Glyphosate-based herbicides and cancer risk: a post-IARC decision review of potential mechanisms, policy and avenues of research," Davoren, Michael J and Robert H Schiestl, *Carcinogenesis*. https://www.ncbi.nlm.nih.gov/pmc/articles /PMC7530464/

16. "Glyphosate: Its Effects on Humans," Andrew William Campbell, *Alternative Therapies in Health and Medicine*. https://www.researchgate.net/publication /261800913_Glyphosate_Its_Effects_on_Humans

17. "Bio-organic fertilizer with reduced rates of chemical fertilization improves soil fertility and enhances tomato yield and quality," Lin Ye, Xia Zhao, Encai Bao, Jianshe Li, Zhirong Zou, and Kai Cao, *Scientific Reports*. https://www.ncbi.nlm .nih.gov/pmc/articles/PMC6957517/

18. "Increased organic fertilizer application and reduced chemical fertilizer application affect the soil properties and bacterial communities of grape rhizosphere soil," Linnan Wu, Yu Jiang, Fengyun Zhao, Xiufeng He, Huaifeng Liu, and Kun Yu, *Scientific Reports*. https://www.nature.com/articles/s41598-020-66648-9

19. "Effects of organic fertilizer on soil nutrient status, enzyme activity, and bacterial community diversity in *Leymus chinensis* steppe in Inner Mongolia, China," Lirong Shang, Liqiang Wan, Xiaoxin Zhou, Shuo Li, and Xianglin Li, *PLOS One*. https://journals.plos.org/plosone/article?id=10.1371/journal.pone.0240559

20. "Antibiotic Use in Agriculture and its Consequential Resistance in Environmental Sources: Potential Public Health Implications," Manyi-Loh, Christy, Sampson Mamphweli, Edson Meyer, and Anthony Okoh, *Molecules*. https://www.ncbi.nlm.nih.gov/pmc/articles/PMC6017557/

21. "Exposure to exogenous estrogens in food: possible impact on human development and health," Andersson, A. M. and N. E. Skakkebaek, *European Journal of Endocrinology*. https://pubmed.ncbi.nlm.nih.gov/10366402/

22. "Food Additives and Child Health," Trasande, Leonardo, Rachel M. Shaffer, and Sheela Sathyanarayana, *Pediatrics*. https://www.ncbi.nlm.nih.gov/pmc/articles /PMC6298598/

23. "Clinical effects of sulphite additives," H. Vally, N. L. A. Misso, and V. Madan, *Clinical & Experimental Allergy*. https://pubmed.ncbi.nlm.nih.gov/19775253/

24. "Food Dyes: A Rainbow of Risks," Center for Science in the Public Interest. https://cspinet.org/sites/default/files/attachment/food-dyes-rainbow-of-risks.pdf

25. "Sensory influences on food intake control: moving beyond palatability," K. McCrickerd and C. G. Forde, *Etiology and Pathophysiology*. https://onlinelibrary .wiley.com/doi/full/10.1111/obr.12340

26. "Reshaping the gut microbiota: Impact of low calorie sweeteners and the link to insulin resistance?," Nettleton, Jodi E., Raylene A. Reimer, and Jane Shearer, *Physiology & Behavior*. https://pubmed.ncbi.nlm.nih.gov/27090230/

27. "Plausible Biological Interactions of Low- and Non-Calorie Sweeteners with the Intestinal Microbiota: An Update of Recent Studies," Plaza-Diaz, Julio, Belén

Pastor-Villaescusa, Ascensión Rueda-Robles, Francisco Abadia-Molina, and Francisco Javier Ruiz-Ojeda, *Nutrients*. https://www.ncbi.nlm.nih.gov/pmc/articles/PMC7231174/

28. "The Impact of Artificial Sweeteners on Body Weight Control and Glucose Homeostasis," Pang, Michelle D., Gijs H. Goossens, and Ellen E. Blaak, *Frontiers in Nutrition*. https://www.ncbi.nlm.nih.gov/pmc/articles/PMC7817779/

29. "Neurophysical symptoms and aspartame: What is the connection?," Choudhary, Arbind Kumar and Yeong Yeh Lee, *Nutritional Neuroscience*. https://pubmed.ncbi.nlm.nih.gov/28198207/

30. "Feedgrains Sector at a Glance," U.S. Department of Agriculture. https://www.ers.usda.gov/topics/crops/corn-and-other-feedgrains/feedgrains-sector-at-a-glance/

31. "Sector at a Glance," U.S. Department of Agriculture. https://www.ers.usda.gov/topics/animal-products/cattle-beef/sector-at-a-glance/

32. "Diet, Escherichia coli O157:H7, and cattle: a review after 10 years," Callaway, Todd R., M. A. Carr, T. S. Edrington, Robin C. Anderson, and David J. Nisbet, *Current Issues in Molecular Biology*. https://pubmed.ncbi.nlm.nih.gov/19351974/

33. "Meet Real Free-Range Eggs," Cheryl Long and Tabitha Alterman, *Mother Earth News*. https://www.motherearthnews.com/real-food/free-range-eggs-zmaz07onzgoe

34. "Free Dietary Choice and Free-Range Rearing Improve the Product Quality, Gait Score, and Microbial Richness of Chickens," Siyu Chen, et al, *Animals*. https://www.ncbi.nlm.nih.gov/pmc/articles/PMC6025111/

35. "Effect of Free-range Rearing on Meat Composition, Physical Properties and Sensory Evaluation in Taiwan Game Hens," Lin, Cheng-Yung, Hsiao-Yun Kuo, and Tien-Chun Wan, *Asian-Australasian Journal of Animal Sciences*. https://www.ncbi.nlm.nih.gov/pmc/articles/PMC4093180/

36. "A review of fatty acid profiles and antioxidant content in grass-fed and grain-fed beef," Daley, Cynthia A., Amber Abbott, Patrick S. Doyle, Glenn A. Nader, and Stephanie Larson, *Nutritional Journal*. https://www.ncbi.nlm.nih.gov/pmc/articles/PMC2846864/

37. "Lipid oxidation in meat: mechanisms and protective factors—a review," Amaral, Ana Beatriz, Marcondes Viana da Silva, and Suzana Caetano da Silva Lannes, *Journal of Food Science and Technology*. http://www.scielo.br/scielo.php?script=sci_arttext&pid=S0101-20612018000500001

38. "2019 Summary Report on Antimicrobials Sold or Distributed for Use in Food-Producing Animals," U.S. Food & Drug Administration. https://www.fda.gov/media/144427/download

39. "Antibiotic Residues in Chicken Meat: Global Prevalence, Threats, and Decontamination Strategies: A Review," Muaz, Khurram, Muhammad Riaz, Saeed Akhtar, Sungkwon Park, and Amir Ismail, *Journal of Food Protection*. https://pubmed.ncbi.nlm.nih.gov/29537307/

40. "Detection of tetracycline and streptomycin in beef tissues using Charm II, isolation of relevant resistant bacteria and control their resistance by gamma radiation," Araby, Eman, Hanady G. Nada, Salwa A. Abou El-Nour, and Ali Hammad, *BMC Microbiology*. https://pubmed.ncbi.nlm.nih.gov/32600267/

41. "Antibiotic Use in Agriculture and Its Consequential Resistance in Environmental Sources: Potential Public Health Implications," Manyi-Loh, Christy, Sampson Mamphweli, Edson Meyer, and Anthony Okoh, *Molecules*. https://www.ncbi.nlm.nih.gov/pmc/articles/PMC6017557/

42. "Stop using antibiotics in healthy animals to prevent the spread of antibiotic resistance," World Health Organization. https://www.who.int/news/item/07-11-2017-stop-using-antibiotics-in-healthy-animals-to-prevent-the-spread-of-antibiotic-resistance

43. "Organic 101: Can GMOs Be Used in Organic Products?," U.S. Department of Agriculture. https://www.usda.gov/media/blog/2013/05/17/organic-101-can-gmos-be-used-organic-products

44. "Accumulation of cadmium and uranium in arable soils in Switzerland," Bigalke, Moritz, Andrea Ulrich, Agnes Rehmus, and Armin Keller. *Environmental Pollution*. https://pubmed.ncbi.nlm.nih.gov/27908488/

45. "Uranium and heavy metals in Phosphate Fertilizers," Ashraf E. M. Khater, *Uranium, Mining and Hydrogeology*. https://link.springer.com/chapter/10.1007/978-3-540-87746-2_26

46. "Organic foods contain higher levels of certain nutrients, lower levels of pesticides, and may provide health benefits for the consumer," Walter J. Crinnion. *Alternative Medicine Review*. https://pubmed.ncbi.nlm.nih.gov/20359265/

47. "A Systematic Review of Organic Versus Conventional Food Consumption: Is There a Measurable Benefit on Human Health?," Vanessa Vigar, et al, *Nutrients*. https://www.ncbi.nlm.nih.gov/pmc/articles/PMC7019963/

48. "Some Differences in Nutritional Biomarkers are Detected Between Consumers and Nonconsumers of Organic Foods: Findings from the BioNutriNet Project," Julia Baudry, et al, *Current Developments in Nutrition*. https://www.ncbi.nlm.nih.gov/pmc/articles/PMC6397420/

49. "Still No Free Lunch: Nutrient levels in U.S. food supply eroded by pursuit of high yields," Brian Halweil, The Organic Center. https://ucanr.edu/datastoreFiles/608-809.pdf

50. https://www.ams.usda.gov/sites/default/files/media/Labeling%20Organic%20Products%20Fact%20Sheet.pdf

51. "Non-GMO Project Standard," The Non-GMO Project. https://www.nongmoproject.org/wp-content/uploads/Non-GMO-Project-Standard-Version-16.pdf

52. "Organic 101: What the USDA Organic Label Means," U.S. Department of Agriculture. https://www.usda.gov/media/blog/2012/03/22/organic-101-what-usda-organic-label-means

TAKE A BREAK FROM FAKE: PROBLEMS WITH ULTRA-PROCESSED FOODS

1. "The True Obesity Paradox: Obese and Malnourished?," Sigismond Lasocki, *Critical Care Medicine*. https://journals.lww.com/ccmjournal/Citation/2015/01000/The_True_Obesity_Paradox__Obese_and_Malnourished__.33.aspx

2. https://d1wqtxts1xzle7.cloudfront.net/43530209/Nutritional_Deficiencies
   _in_Morbidly_Obe20160308-22374-1gblf0r.pdf?1457503103=&response
   -content-disposition=inline%3B+filename%3DNutritional_Deficiencies_in
   _Morbidly_Obe.pdf&Expires=1614366681&Signature=hAkpIznG4tsy-YBbD
   lQMcfcUasklNPr9yoUVDGikOquoXEvcY4TqA4z0pHCIPu1dGnzk-dRL8P
   mcE~AGXs67XPd9R66m6n2IkIjswn2Hfwnvjtq1vLwj1Ojy0YrMJ7V2ND9D
   3LTYrioKGQydTH4cZRiypCrjZ3PuLokykl~9jW0WuUnnHEoEf~NszGXN
   pH-1ae1RqzVJCNWBLoMWZNnmnvrogsQLRKtk9IcFM3WRu-je0xxV4Q
   Xgqn69kkEmr5nlxKCG0eTbM5Y8QdaLmXWDF7CJNEZrkZySVf7ixG0xof
   q4rMMd5DByY3B1A~C2udV2h5M~LQ9rgFvZy3unIy~C3g__&Key-Pair-Id
   =APKAJLOHF5GGSLRBV4ZA

3. "Nutritional Deficiencies in Obesity and After Bariatric Surgery," Stavra A.
   Xanthakos, *Pediatric Clinics of North America.* https://www.ncbi.nlm.nih.gov
   /pmc/articles/PMC2784422/

4. "Cell Metabolism: Ultra-Processed Diets Cause Excess Calorie Intake and
   Weight Gain: An Inpatient Randomized Controlled Trial of *Ad Libitum* Food
   Intake," *Cell Metabolism.* https://www.cell.com/action/showPdf?pii=S1550
   -4131%2819%2930248-7

5. "The share of ultra-processed foods and the overall nutritional quality of diets
   in the US: evidence from a nationally representative cross-sectional study,"
   Martinez Steele, Euridice, Barry M. Popkin, Boyd Swinburn, and Carlos
   A. Monteiro, *Population Health Metrics.* https://pubmed.ncbi.nlm.nih.gov
   /28193285/

6. "Impact of ultra-processed foods on micronutrient content in the Brazilian diet,"
   Maria Laura da Costa Louzada, et al, *Revista de Saúde Pública.* https://pubmed
   .ncbi.nlm.nih.gov/26270019/

7. "Results of the Self-Selection of Diets by Young Children," Clara M. Davis,
   Canadian Medical Association Journal. https://www.ncbi.nlm.nih.gov/pmc
   /articles/PMC537465/

8. "Hyper-Palatable Foods: Development of a Quantitative Definition and
   Application to the US Food System Database," Fazzino, Tera L., Kaitlyn Rohde,
   and Debra K. Sullivan, *Obesity Symposium.* https://onlinelibrary.wiley.com/doi
   /abs/10.1002/oby.22639

9. Mark Schatzker, *The Dorito Effect: The Surprising New Truth About Food and
   Flavor,* (New York: Simon & Schuster, 2016), 157.

10. "Food systems and diets: Facing the challenges of the 21st century," Global Panel
    on Agriculture and Food Systems for Nutrition. https://glopan.org/sites/default
    /files/ForesightReport.pdf

11. "Ultra-processed foods: what they are and how to identify them," Monteiro, Carlos
    A., et al, *Public Health Nutrition.* https://pubmed.ncbi.nlm.nih.gov/30744710/

12. "The Food System," Monteiro, Carlos A., et al, *World Nutrition.* https://archive
    .wphna.org/wp-content/uploads/2016/01/WN-2016-7-1-3-28-38-Monteiro
    -Cannon-Levy-et-al-NOVA.pdf

13. "Association between ultraprocessed food intake and cardiovascular health in US
    adults: a cross-sectional analysis of the NHANES 2011–2016," Zhang, Zefeng,

Sandra L. Jackson, Euridice Martinez, Cathleen Gillespie, and Quanhe Yang, *The American Journal of Clinical Nutrition*. https://academic.oup.com/ajcn/article/113/2/428/5918401?login=true

14. "Consumption of ultra-processed foods and cancer risk: results from NutriNet-Santé," Thibault Fiolet, et al, *The BMJ*. https://www.bmj.com/content/360/bmj.k322

15. "Dietary share of ultra-processed foods and metabolic syndrome in the US adult population," Euridice Martinez Steele, et al, *Preventative Medicine*. https://www.sciencedirect.com/science/article/abs/pii/S0091743519301720?via%3Dihub

16. "Ultra-Processed Foods and Health Outcomes: A Narrative Review," Elizabeth, Leonie, Priscila Machado, Marit Zinocker, Phillip Baker, and Mark Lawrence," *Nutrients*. https://www.ncbi.nlm.nih.gov/pmc/articles/PMC7399967/

17. "Ultra-processed food consumption and the risk of short telomeres in an elderly population of the Seguimiento Universidad de Navarra (SUN) Project," Lucia Alonso-Pedrero, et al, *The American Journal of Clinical Nutrition*. https://pubmed.ncbi.nlm.nih.gov/32330232/

18. "Telomeres, lifestyle, cancer, and aging," Masood A. Shammas, *Current Opinion in Clinical Nutrition & Metabolic Care*. https://www.ncbi.nlm.nih.gov/pmc/articles/PMC3370421/

19. Ibid.

20. "How Industrial Seed Oils Are Making Us Sick," Chris Kresser, Chris Kresser.com. https://chriskresser.com/how-industrial-seed-oils-are-making-us-sick/

21. "Health Implications of High Dietary Omega-6 Polyunsaturated Fatty Acids," E. Patterson, R. Wall, G. F. Fitzgerald, R. P. Ross, and C. Stanton, *Journal of Nutrition and Metabolism*. https://www.ncbi.nlm.nih.gov/pmc/articles/PMC3335257/

22. "Polyunsaturated Fatty Acids and Inflammation," Rachel Marion-Letellier, Guillaume Savoye, and Subrata Ghosh, International Union of Biochemistry and Molecular Biology. https://iubmb.onlinelibrary.wiley.com/doi/epdf/10.1002/iub.1428

23. "Lipid Peroxidation and Its Toxicological Implications," Tae-gyu Nam. *Toxicology Research*. https://www.ncbi.nlm.nih.gov/pmc/articles/PMC3834518/

24. "Environmental Obesogens and Their Impact on Susceptibility to Obesity: New Mechanisms and Chemicals," Riann Jenay Egusquiza and Bruce Blumberg, *Endocrinology*. https://academic.oup.com/endo/article/161/3/bqaa024/5739626?login=true

25. "Vitamins Hide the Low Quality of Our Food," Catherine Price, *The New York Times*. https://www.nytimes.com/2015/02/15/opinion/sunday/vitamins-hide-the-low-quality-of-our-food.html

26. "What Is a Whole Grain?," Oldways Whole Grains Council. https://wholegrainscouncil.org/what-whole-grain

27. "Ultra-processed foods and added sugars in the US diet: evidence from a nationally representative cross-sectional study," Euridice Martinez Steele, et al, *Nutrition and Metabolism*. https://bmjopen.bmj.com/content/6/3/e009892

28. "Obesogens: an emerging threat to public health," Amanda S. Janesick and Bruce

Blumberg, *American Journal of Obstetrics & Gynecology*. https://www.ajog.org /article/S0002-9378(16)00232-5/abstract

29. "The obesogenic effect of high fructose exposure during early development," Michael I. Goran, et al, *Nature Reviews Endocrinology*. https://pubmed.ncbi.nlm .nih.gov/23732284/

30. "Why artificial sweeteners can increase appetite," *Science Daily*. https://www .sciencedaily.com/releases/2016/07/160712130107.htm

31. "The Association Between Artificial Sweeteners and Obesity," Michelle Pearlman, Jon Obert, and Lisa Casey, *Current Gastroenterology Reports*. https://pubmed .ncbi.nlm.nih.gov/29159583/

32. "Neurophysiological symptoms and aspartame: What is the connection?," Arbind Kumar Choudhary, *Nutritional Neuroscience*. https://www.tandfonline.com/doi /full/10.1080/1028415X.2017.1288340

33. "Effects of chronic aspartame consumption on MPTP-induced Parkinsonism in male and female mice," Shaimaa Nasr Amin, Sherif Sabry Hassan, and Laila Ahmed Rashed, *Archives of Physiology and Biochemistry*. https://www .tandfonline.com/doi/abs/10.1080/13813455.2017.1396348?journalCode=iarp20

34. "Impact of Food Additives on Gut Homeostasis," Federica Laudisi, Carmine Stolfi, and Giovanni Monteleone, *Nutrients*. https://www.ncbi.nlm.nih.gov/pmc /articles/PMC6835893/

35. "Genetic diversity of CHC22 clathrin impacts its function in glucose metabolism," Matteo Fumagalli, et al, *eLife*. https://www.ncbi.nlm.nih.gov/pmc/articles /PMC6548504/

36. "Whole Food versus Supplement: Comparing the Clinical Evidence of Tomato Intake and Lycopene Supplementation on Cardiovascular Risk Factors," Britt M. Burton-Freeman and Howard D. Sesso, *Advances in Nutrition*. https://www.ncbi .nlm.nih.gov/pmc/articles/PMC4188219/

37. "Long-term Use of B-Carotene, Retinol, Lycopene, and Lutein Supplements and Lung Cancer Risk: Results from the Vitamins and Lifestyle (VITAL) Study," Jessie A. Satia, Alyson Littman, Christopher G. Slatore, Joseph A. Galanko, and Emily White, *American Journal of Epidemiology*. https://www.ncbi.nlm.nih.gov /pmc/articles/PMC2842198/

38. "Memory Supplements: Results of Testing for Selected Supplements," U.S. Government Accountability Office. https://www.gao.gov/assets/gao-19-23r.pdf

39. "What's in your supplements?," Robert H. Schmerling, *Harvard Health Publishing*. https://www.health.harvard.edu/blog/whats-in-your-supplements -2019021515946

WHAT'S A HEALTHY DIET? AND HOW DO WE KNOW?

1. Michael Pollan, *In Defense of Food* (New York: Penguin Press, 2008).
2. Tim Spector, *Spoon-Fed: Why Almost Everything We've Been Told About Food Is Wrong* (New York: Jonathan Cape, 2021).

3. "From a Reductionist to a Holistic Approach in Preventive Nutrition to Define New and More Ethical Paradigms," Anthony Fardet and Edmond Rock, *Healthcare*. https://www.ncbi.nlm.nih.gov/pmc/articles/PMC4934630/

4. "Dr. Weston A. Price Movietone," The Weston A. Price Foundation. https://www .westonaprice.org/about-us/dr-weston-a-price-movietone/

5. "The Secrets of Long Life," Dan Buettner, *National Geographic*. https://bluezones .com/wp-content/uploads/2015/01/Nat_Geo_LongevityF.pdf

6. http://www.unav.edu/departamento/preventiva/files/file/predimed/NEJM _PREDIMED_printed.pdf

7. http://www.predimed.es/publications.html

8. "Adherence to the Mediterranean Diet in Relation to All-Cause Mortality: A Systematic Review and Dose-Response Meta-Analysis of Prospective Cohort Studies," Sepideh Soltani, Ahmad Jayedi, Sakineh Shab-Bidar, Nerea Becerra-Tomas, and Jordi Salas-Salvado, *Advances in Nutrition*. https://www .ncbi.nlm.nih.gov/pmc/articles/PMC6855973/

9. "Welcome to the official website of the NutriNet-Santé Study," Étude NutriNet Santé. https://info.etude-nutrinet-sante.fr/en/node/2

10. "The Nutrinet-Santé Study: a web-based prospective study on the relationship between nutrition and health and determinants of dietary patterns and nutritional status," Serge Hercberg, et al, *BMC Public Health*. https://bmcpublichealth .biomedcentral.com/articles/10.1186/1471-2458-10-242

11. "Contribution of ultra-processed foods in the diet of adults from the French NutriNet-Santé study," Chantal Julia, et al, Cambridge University Press. https: //www.cambridge.org/core/journals/public-health-nutrition/article/contribution -of-ultraprocessed-foods-in-the-diet-of-adults-from-the-french-nutrinetsante -study/DAD2E5364AEC9B6424644403258F9A1A

12. "Association of Frequency of Organic Food Consumption With Cancer Risk," Julia Baudry, et al, *JAMA Internal Medicine*. https://jamanetwork.com/journals /jamainternalmedicine/fullarticle/2707948

13. "Association between nutritional profiles of foods underlying Nutri-Score front-of-pack labels and mortality: EPIC cohort study in 10 European countries," Melanie Deschasaux, et al, *BMJ* https://www.bmj.com/content/bmj/370/bmj.m3173.full.pdf

14. "Milestones in human microbiota research," Nature.com. https://www.nature .com/immersive/d42859-019-00041-z/index.html

15. "The importance of feeding your microbiota," Alison Farrell, Nature.com. https://www.nature.com/articles/d42859-019-00015-1

16. "The Gut Microbiota in Immune-Mediated Inflammatory Diseases," Jessica D. Forbes, Gary Van Domselaar, and Charles N. Bernstein, *Frontiers in Microbiology*. https://www.frontiersin.org/articles/10.3389/fmicb.2016.01081/full

17. "Effect of ultra-processed diet on gut microbiota and thus its role in neurodegenerative diseases," Edwin E Martinez Leo and Maira R Segura Campos, *Nutrition*. https://pubmed.ncbi.nlm.nih.gov/31837645/

18. "Predicting Personal Metabolic Responses to Food Using Multi-omics Machine Learning in over 1,000 Twins and Singletons from the UK and US: The PREDICT I Study," Sarah Berry, et al, *Current Developments in Nutrition*.

https://academic.oup.com/cdn/article/3/Supplement_1/nzz037.OR31-01-19/5517817

19. "Human postprandial responses to food and potential for precision nutrition," Zoe. https://joinzoe.com/post/nature-medicine-predict-1

20. "Microbiome Signatures of Nutrients, Foods and Dietary Patterns: Potential for Personalized Nutrition from The PREDICT I Study," Tim Spector, et al, *Current Developments in Nutrition*. https://academic.oup.com/cdn/article/4/Supplement_2/1587/5844882

21. "PREDICT study provides personalized nutrition revelations," Nikki Hancocks, NutraIngredients.com. https://www.nutraingredients.com/Article/2020/06/08/PREDICT-study-provides-personalised-nutrition-revelations

22. "Perspective: Design and Conduct of Human Nutrition Randomized Controlled Trials," Alice H. Lichteinstein, et al, *Advances in Nutrition*. https://academic.oup.com/advances/article/12/1/4/5983119

23. Ibid.

24. "Ancestors' dietary patterns and environments could drive positive selection in genes involved in micronutrient metabolism—the case of cofactor transporters," Silvia Parolo, Sebastian Lacroix, Jim Kaput, and Marie-Pier Scott-Boyer, *Genes & Nutrition*. https://www.ncbi.nlm.nih.gov/pmc/articles/PMC5628472/

25. "Evolution of lactase persistence: an example of human niche construction," Pascale Gerbault, et al, *Philosophical transactions of the Royal Society of London*. https://www.ncbi.nlm.nih.gov/pmc/articles/PMC3048992/

26. "Lactose Intolerance: Information for Health Care Providers," U.S. Department of Health and Human Services. https://www.nichd.nih.gov/sites/default/files/publications/pubs/documents/NICHD_MM_Lactose_FS_rev.pdf

27. "Diet and the evolution of human amylase gene copy number variation," George H. Perry, et al, *Nature Genetics*. https://www.ncbi.nlm.nih.gov/pmc/articles/PMC2377015/

PARALYSIS OF ANALYSIS: WHEN GETTING HEALTHY BECOMES AN OBSESSION

1. Steven Bratman, *Health Food Junkies* (New York: Broadway, 2001).

2. "Definition and diagnostic criteria for orthorexia nervosa: a narrative review of the literature," Hellas Cena, et al, *Eating and Weight Disorders: Studies on Anorexia, Bulimia and Obesity*. https://link.springer.com/article/10.1007/s40519-018-0606-y

3. "The Authorized Bratman Orthorexia Self-Test," Orthorexia.com. http://www.orthorexia.com

4. Bratman, *Health Food Junkies*, 30-31.

5. "On orthorexia nervosa: A review of the literature and proposed diagnostic

criteria," Thomas M. Dunn and Steven Bratman, *Eating Behaviors*. https://www
.sciencedirect.com/science/article/abs/pii/S1471015315300362?via%3Dihub

6. www.orthorexia.com

YOUR BODY'S SELF-CLEANING PATHWAYS

1. "Conventional Laboratory Tests to Assess Toxin Burden," Joseph Pizzorno, *Integrative Medicine*. https://www.ncbi.nlm.nih.gov/pmc/articles/PMC4712864/

2. "Detoxing Your Liver: Fact Versus Fiction," Johns Hopkins Medicine. https://www.hopkinsmedicine.org/health/wellness-and-prevention/detoxing-your-liver-fact-versus-fiction

3. "What's Your Liver Got to Do with Losing Weight? Only Everything!," Jonny Bowden, *Clean Eating Magazine*. https://www.cleaneatingmag.com/clean-diet/disease-prevention/whats-your-liver-got-to-do-with-losing-weight/

4. "Nutritional Aspects of Detoxification in Clinical Practice," John C. Cline, *Alternative Therapies*. https://nutmed.com.br/storage/resources/5/2249/Artigo_2_-_Nutritional_Aspects_of_Detoxification_in_Clinical[1].pdf

5. "Digestive (liver detox, nutrition, weight loss)," Carahealth. https://www.carahealth.com/health-articles/digestive-liver-detox-nutrition-weight-loss/phase-1-2-liver-detoxification

6. "Modulation of Metabolic Detoxification Pathways Using Foods and Food-Derived Components: A Scientific Review with Clinical Application," Romilly E. Hodges and Deanna M. Minich, *Journal of Nutrition and Metabolism*. https://www.ncbi.nlm.nih.gov/pmc/articles/PMC4488002/

7. "Alcohol in the body," Alex Paton, *BMJ*. https://www.ncbi.nlm.nih.gov/pmc/articles/PMC543875/

8. "Exploring Alcohol's Effects on Liver Function," Jacquelyn J. Maher, *Alcohol Health and Research World*. https://www.ncbi.nlm.nih.gov/pmc/articles/PMC6826796/

9. "Nonsteroidal anti-inflammatory drugs: effects on kidney function," A. Whelton and C. W. Hamilton. *The Journal of Clinical Pharmacology*. https://pubmed.ncbi.nlm.nih.gov/1894754/

10. "The Kidney Dysfunction Epidemic, Part 1: Causes," Joseph Pizzorno, *Integrative Medicine*. https://www.ncbi.nlm.nih.gov/pmc/articles/PMC4718206/

11. "Chronic kidney Disease in the United States, 2021," Centers for Disease Control and Prevention. https://www.cdc.gov/kidneydisease/publications-resources/ckd-national-facts.html

12. "The Kidney Dysfunction Epidemic, Part 2: Intervention," Joseph Pizzorno, *Integrative Medicine*. https://www.ncbi.nlm.nih.gov/pmc/articles/PMC4818073/

13. "Cerebral hypoxia," MedlinePlus. https://medlineplus.gov/ency/article/001435.htm

14. "Pathophysiology and clinical effects of chronic hypoxia," D J Pierson, *Respiratory Care*. https://pubmed.ncbi.nlm.nih.gov/10771781/

15. "How is brain hypoxia diagnosed?," Healthline. https://www.healthline.com/health/cerebral-hypoxia#diagnosis

16. "Is vaping better than smoking for cardiorespiratory and muscle function?," Mohammad Z. Darabseh, James Selfe, Christophe I. Morse, and Hans Degens, *Multidisciplinary Respiratory Medicine*. https://www.ncbi.nlm.nih.gov/pmc/articles/PMC7348661/

17. "Indoor Air Quality and Health," Alessandra Cincinelli and Tania Martellini, *International Journal of Environmental Research and Public Health*. https://www.ncbi.nlm.nih.gov/pmc/articles/PMC5707925/

18. "Your lungs and exercise," *Breathe*. https://www.ncbi.nlm.nih.gov/pmc/articles/PMC4818249/

19. "Effects of breathing exercises on lung capacity and muscle activities of elderly smokers," Hyun-Ju Jun, Ki-Kong Kim, Ki-Won Nam, and Chang-Heon Kim, *The Journal of Physical Therapy Science*. https://www.ncbi.nlm.nih.gov/pmc/articles/PMC4932035/

20. "Nutrition and Respiratory Health—Feature Review," Bronwyn S. Berthon and Lisa G. Wood, *Nutrients*. https://www.ncbi.nlm.nih.gov/pmc/articles/PMC4377870/

21. https://www.ncbi.nlm.nih.gov/pmc/articles/PMC2861991/ https://pdskin.com/blogs/skin-fun-facts/

22. "The skin function: a factor of anti-metabolic syndrome," Shi-Sheng Zhou, Da Li, Yi-Ming Zhou, and Ji-Min Cao, *Diabetology & Metabolic Syndrome*. https://www.ncbi.nlm.nih.gov/pmc/articles/PMC3567429/

23. "Skin Exposures & Effects," The National Institute for Occupational Safety and Health. https://www.cdc.gov/niosh/topics/skin/default.html

24. "Recent Developments in Sweat Analysis and Its Applications," Saima Jadoon, et al, *International Journal of Analytical Chemistry*. https://www.ncbi.nlm.nih.gov/pmc/articles/PMC4369929/

25. "Arsenic, Cadmium, Lead, and mercury in Sweat: A Systematic Review," Margaret E. Sears, Kathleen J. Kerr, and Riina I. Bray, *International Journal of Environmental Research and Public Health*. https://www.ncbi.nlm.nih.gov/pmc/articles/PMC3312275/

26. "Blood, Urine, and Sweat (BUS) Study: Monitoring and Elimination of Bioaccumulated Toxic Elements," Stephen J. Genuis, Detlef Birkholz, Ilia Rodushkin, and Sanjay Beesoon, *Archives of Environmental Contamination and Toxicology*. https://link.springer.com/article/10.1007%2Fs00244-010-9611-5

27. "The skin function."

28. "Decreased skin—mediated detoxification contributes to oxidative stress and insulin resistance," Xing-Xing Liu, et al, *Experimental Diabetes Research*. https://pubmed.ncbi.nlm.nih.gov/22899900/

29. "Lymphatic system acts as a vital link between metabolic syndrome and inflammation," Sanjukta Chakraborty, Scott Zawieja, David C. Zawieja, and Mariappan Muthuchamy, *Annals of the New York Academy of Sciences*. https://www.ncbi.nlm.nih.gov/pmc/articles/PMC2965625/

30. "Lymphedema and nutrition: a review," Attilio Cavezzi, et al, *Veins and Lymphatics*. https://www.pagepressjournals.org/index.php/vl/article/view/8220/8246

31. "Lymphatic System Flows," James E. Moore and Christopher D. Bertram, *Annual Review of Fluid Mechanics*. https://www.ncbi.nlm.nih.gov/pmc/articles/PMC5922450/

32. "The Truth About Dry Brushing and What It Does For You," Cleveland Clinic. https://health.clevelandclinic.org/the-truth-about-dry-brushing-and-what-it-does-for-you/

33. "Brain Drain," Maiken Nedergaard and Steven A. Goldman, *Scientific American*. https://www.ncbi.nlm.nih.gov/pmc/articles/PMC5347443/

34. "Understanding the Glymphatic System," Neuronline. https://neuronline.sfn.org/scientific-research/understanding-the-glymphatic-system

35. "The Glymphatic System: A Beginner's Guide," Nadia Aalling Jessen, Anne Sofie Finmann Munk, Iben Lundgaard, and Maiken Nedergaard, *Neurochemistry International*. https://pubmed.ncbi.nlm.nih.gov/25947369/

36. "Enzymatic Activities and Compostional Properties of Whole Wheat Flour," Rachana Poudel, University of Nebraska-Lincoln. https://digitalcommons.unl.edu/cgi/viewcontent.cgi?referer=https://www.google.com/&httpsredir=1&article=1099&context=foodscidiss

37. "Undigested Food and Gut Microbiota May Cooperate in the Pathogenesis of Neuroinflammatory Diseases: A Matter of Barriers and a Proposal on the Origin of Organ Specificity," Paolo Riccio and Rocco Rossano, *Nutrients*. https://www.ncbi.nlm.nih.gov/pmc/articles/PMC6893834/

38. Ibid.

39. "Modulation of Intestinal Functions by Dietary Substances: An Effective Approach to Health Promotion," Makoto Shimizu, *Journal of Traditional and Complementary Medicine*. https://www.ncbi.nlm.nih.gov/pmc/articles/PMC3942919/

40. "Undigested Food and Gut Microbiota."

41. "Impact of Dietary Fibers on Nutrient Management and Detoxification Organs: Gut, Liver, and Kidneys," Dorothy A. Kieffer, Roy J. Martin, and Sean H. Adams, *Advances in Nutrition*. https://www.ncbi.nlm.nih.gov/pmc/articles/PMC5105045/

42. "Small Intestinal Bacterial Overgrowth," Andrew C. Dukowicz, Brian E. Lacy, and Gary M. Levine, *Gastroenterology & Hepatology*. https://www.ncbi.nlm.nih.gov/pmc/articles/PMC3099351/

43. "Influence of bowel habits on gut-derived toxins in peritoneal dialysis patients," Natalia Barros Ferreira Pereira, et al, *Journal of the American Society of Nephrology*. https://pubmed.ncbi.nlm.nih.gov/32737690/

44. "The Characterization of Feces and Urine: A Review of the Literature to Inform Advanced Treatment Technology," C. Rose, A. Parker, B. Jefferson, and E. Cartmell, *Critical Reviews in Environmental Science and Technology*. https://www.ncbi.nlm.nih.gov/pmc/articles/PMC4500995/

45. "Effect of dietary fiber on constipation: A meta analysis," Jing Yang, Hai-Peng Wang, and Chun-Fang Xu, *World Journal of Gastroenterology*. https://www.ncbi .nlm.nih.gov/pmc/articles/PMC3544045/

WHAT'S FOOD GOT TO DO WITH IT?

1. "Modulation of Metabolic Detoxification Pathways Using Foods and Food-Derived Components: A Scientific Review with Clinical Application," Romilly E. Hodges and Deanna M. Minich, *Journal of Nutrition and Metabolism*. https://www.ncbi .nlm.nih.gov/pmc/articles/PMC4488002/
2. "Plants Consumption and Liver Health," Yong-Song Guan and Qing He, *Evidence-Based Complementary and Alternative Medicine*. https://www.ncbi.nlm .nih.gov/pmc/articles/PMC4499388/
3. "Nutritional Aspects of Detoxification in Clinical Practice," John C. Cline, *Alternative Therapies*. https://nutmed.com.br/storage/resources/5/2249/Artigo_2 _-_Nutritional_Aspects_of_Detoxification_in_Clinical[1].pdf
4. "The One Food To Eat To Avoid Heart Disease, According to RDs," Kiersten Hickman, Eat This, Not That!. https://www.eatthis.com/one-food-to-avoid-heart -disease/
5. "How to live longer: Blueberries may reduce age-related diseases to boost longevity," Jessica Knibbs, *Express*. https://www.express.co.uk/life-style/health /1398527/how-to-live-longer-blueberries-boost-longevity
6. "Daily Blueberry Consumption May Help Manage Diabetes, Study Finds," Lauren Manaker, Verywell Health. https://www.verywellhealth.com/blueberries -type-2-diabetes-5083083
7. "From Improving Gut-Health to Managing Diabetes, 6 Reasons Why You Must Eat Blueberries," Somdatta Saha, NDTV. https://food.ndtv.com/food-drinks /from-improving-gut-health-to-managing-diabetes-6-reasons-why-you-must -eat-blueberries-2251555
8. "Blueberry-enriched diet may help women's muscle growth, repair: Study," *Hindustan Times*. https://www.hindustantimes.com/health/blueberry -enriched-diet-may-help-women-s-muscle-growth-repair-study/story -IcnNmQLp1o2HVCSkv1EnGK.html
9. "Single dose of blueberry polyphenols boost cognitive performance in middle aged adults," Hank Schultz, Nutra Ingredients. https://www.nutraingredients -usa.com/Article/2020/08/05/Single-dose-of-blueberry-polyphenols-boosts -cognitive-performance-in-middle-aged-adults
10. "How People Came to Believe Blueberries Are the Healthiest Fruit," James Hamblin, *The Atlantic*. https://www.theatlantic.com/health/archive/2017/11 /blueberries/545840/
11. "Detox diets for toxin elimination and weight management: a critical review of the evidence," A. V. Klein and H. Kiat, *Journal of Human Nutrition and Dietetics*. https://pubmed.ncbi.nlm.nih.gov/25522674/

12. "Fill up on phytochemicals," Harvard Health Publishing. https://www.health
.harvard.edu/staying-healthy/fill-up-on-phytochemicals

13. "A Review of the Science of Colorful, Plant-Based Food and Practical Strategies
for 'Eating the Rainbow,'" Deanna M. Minich, *Journal of Nutrition and
Metabolism.* https://www.hindawi.com/journals/jnme/2019/2125070/

14. "Biological Activities of Stilbenoids," Bolanle C. Akinwumi, Kimberly-Ann M.
Bordun, and Hope D. Anderson, *International Journal of Molecular Sciences.*
https://www.ncbi.nlm.nih.gov/pmc/articles/PMC5877653/

15. "Chemistry and Biochemistry of Dietary Polyphenols," Rong Tsao, *Nutrients.*
https://www.ncbi.nlm.nih.gov/pmc/articles/PMC3257627/

16. "Phytochemicals That Influence Gut Microbiota as Prophylactics and for the
Treatment of Obesity and Inflammatory Diseases," Lucrecia Carrera-Quintanar,
et al, *Mediators of Inflammation.* https://www.hindawi.com/journals/mi/2018
/9734845/

17. "Naturally Lignan-Rich Foods: A Dietary Tool for Health Promotion?," Carmen
Rodriguez-Garcia, et al, *Molecules.* https://www.ncbi.nlm.nih.gov/pmc/articles
/PMC6429205/

18. "Phenolic acids: Natural versatile molecules with promising therapeutic
applications," Naresh Kumar and Nidhi Goel, *Biotechnology Reports.* https://www
.ncbi.nlm.nih.gov/pmc/articles/PMC6734135/

19. "Chemistry and Biological Activities of Flavonoids: An Overview," Shashank
Kumar and Abhay K. Pandey, *Scientific World Journal.* https://www.ncbi.nlm.nih
.gov/pmc/articles/PMC3891543/

20. "Neurohormetic phytochemicals: Low-dose toxins that induce adaptive neuronal
stress responses," Mark P. Mattson and Aiwu Cheng, *Trends in Neurosciences.*
https://pubmed.ncbi.nlm.nih.gov/17000014/

21. "Exercise, oxidative stress and hormesis," Zsolt Radak, Hae Y. Chung, Erika
Koltai, Albert W Taylor, and Sataro Goto, *Ageing Research Reviews.*
https://pubmed.ncbi.nlm.nih.gov/17869589/

22. "Inflammaging, hormesis and the rationale for anti-aging strategies," Aurelia
Santoro, et al, *Ageing Research Reviews.* https://pubmed.ncbi.nlm.nih.gov
/32814129/

23. "Plant polyphenols as dietary antioxidants in human health and disease," Kanti
Bhooshan Pandey and Syed Ibrahim Rizvi, *Oxidative Medicine and Cellular
Longevity.* https://www.ncbi.nlm.nih.gov/pmc/articles/PMC2835915/

24. "Chapter 2: Antioxidants in Herbs and Spices," Ingvild Paur, Monica H.
Carlsen, Bente Lisa Halvorsen, and Rune Blomhoff, *Herbal Medicine:
Biomolecular and Clinical Aspects, 2nd ed.* https://www.ncbi.nlm.nih.gov/books
/NBK92763/

25. Ibid.

26. "Enzymes: How they work and what they do," Medical News Today. https://www
.medicalnewstoday.com/articles/319704

27. "The gut virome: the 'missing link' between gut bacteria and host immunity?,"
Indrani Mukhopadhya, et al, *Therapeutic Advances in Gastroenterology.*
https://www.ncbi.nlm.nih.gov/pmc/articles/PMC6435874/

28. Tim Spector, *Spoon-Fed: Why Almost Everything We've Been Told About Food Is Wrong* (New York: Jonathan Cape, 2021).

29. "Impact of Dietary Fibers on Nutrient Management and Detoxification Organs: Gut, Liver, and Kidneys," Dorothy A. Kieffer, Roy J. Martin, and Sean H. Adams, *Advances in Nutrition.* https://academic.oup.com/advances/article/7/6/1111/4568672?login=true

30. "Nutritional aspects of detoxification in clinical practice," John C. Cline, *Alternative Therapies in Health and Medicine.* https://pubmed.ncbi.nlm.nih.gov/26026145/

INTERMITTENT FASTING: A POWERFUL
SELF-CLEANING TOOL

1. "Effect of Alternate-Day Fasting on Weight Loss, Weight Maintenance, and Cardioprotection Among Metabolically Healthy Obese Adults," John F. Trepanowski, et al, *JAMA Internal Medicine.* https://jamanetwork.com/journals/jamainternalmedicine/fullarticle/2623528

2. "The cardiovascular, metabolic and hormonal changes accompanying acute starvation in men and women," J. Webber and I. A. Macdonald, *British Journal of Nutrition.* https://pubmed.ncbi.nlm.nih.gov/8172872/

3. "A randomized pilot study comparing zero-calorie alternate-day fasting to daily caloric restriction in adults with obesity," Victoria A. Catenacci, et al, *Obesity.* https://www.acesototalhealth.com/wp-content/uploads/2020/07/alternate-day-fasting-vs-low-calorie-in-obese.pdf

4. "Hallmarks of Aging: An Autophagic Perspective," Maria Carolina Barbosa, Ruben Adrian Grosso, and Claudio Marcelo Fader, *Frontiers in Endocrinology.* https://www.frontiersin.org/articles/10.3389/fendo.2018.00790/full

5. "Autophagy as a promoter of longevity: insights from model organisms," Malene Hansen, David C. Rubinsztein, and David W. Walker, *Nature Reviews Molecular Cell Biology.* https://www.ncbi.nlm.nih.gov/pmc/articles/PMC6424591/

6. "Circadian rhythm of autophagy proteins in hippocampus is blunted by sleep fragmentation," Yi He, et al, *Chronobiology International.* https://pubmed.ncbi.nlm.nih.gov/27078501/

7. "Autophagy fights disease through cellular self-digestion," Noboru Mizushima, Beth Levine, Ana Maria Cuervo, and Daniel J. Klionsky, *Nature.* https://www.ncbi.nlm.nih.gov/pmc/articles/PMC2670399/

8. "On the Fly: Recent Progress on Autophagy and Aging in Drosophila," Tamas Maruzs, Zsofia Simon-Vecsei, Viktoria Kiss, Tamas Csizmadia, and Gabor Juhasz, *Frontiers in Cell and Developmental Biology.* https://www.frontiersin.org/articles/10.3389/fcell.2019.00140/full

9. "A Comprehensive Review of Autophagy and Its Various Roles in Infectious, Non-Infectious, and Lifestyle Diseases: Current Knowledge and Prospects for Disease Prevention, Novel Drug Design, and Therapy," Rekha Khandia, et al, *Cells.* https://www.ncbi.nlm.nih.gov/pmc/articles/PMC6678135/

10. "Autophagy and Metabolism," Joshua D. Rabinowitz and Eileen White, *Science*. https://www.ncbi.nlm.nih.gov/pmc/articles/PMC3010857/

11. "Effects of Intermittent Fasting on Health, Aging, and Disease," Rafael de Cabo and Mark P. Mattson, *The New England Journal of Medicine*. https://www.nejm.org/doi/full/10.1056/nejmra1905136

12. Ibid.

13. Ibid.

EXTRA CREDIT: MORE TOOLS FOR SELF-CLEANING

1. "Sauna as a Valuable Clinical Tool for Cardiovascular, Autoimmune, Toxicant-induced and other Chronic Health Problems," Walter J. Crinnion, *Environmental Medicine*. http://archive.foundationalmedicinereview.com/publications/16/3/215.pdf

2. "In reply: Sauna Bathing and Healthy Sweating," Jari A. Laukkanen, Tanjaniina Laukkanen, and Setor Kunutsor, Mayo Clinic Proceedings. https://www.mayoclinicproceedings.org/article/S0025-6196(18)31013-9/fulltext

3. "Sauna bathing is inversely associated with dementia and Alzheimer's disease in middle-aged Finnish men," Tanjaniina Laukkanen, Setor Kunutsor, Jussi Kauhanen, and Jari Antero Laukkanen, *Age and Ageing*. https://academic.oup.com/ageing/article/46/2/245/2654230?login=true

4. "Environmental Toxins and Neurodegenerative Diseases," Beate Ritz, *Epidemiology*. https://www.ncbi.nlm.nih.gov/pmc/articles/PMC3643974/

5. "A meta-analysis of massage therapy research," Christopher A. Moyer, James Rounds, and James W. Hannum, *Psychological Bulletin*. https://pubmed.ncbi.nlm.nih.gov/14717648/

6. "Massage therapy for cardiac surgery patients—a randomized trial," Lesley A. Braun, et al, *The Journal of Thoracic and Cardiovascular Surgery*. https://pubmed.ncbi.nlm.nih.gov/22964355/

7. "Investigating the Short-Term Effects of Manual Lymphatic Drainage and Compression Garment Therapies on Lymphatic Function Using Near-Infrared Imaging," Catalina Lopera, Peter R. Worsley, Dan L. Bader, and Deborah Fenlon, *Lymphatic Research and Biology*. https://www.liebertpub.com/doi/10.1089/lrb.2017.0001?url_ver=Z39.88-2003&rfr_id=ori:rid:crossref.org&rfr_dat=cr_pub%20%200pubmed

8. "Effectiveness of different styles of massage therapy in fibromyalgia: A systematic review and meta-analysis," Susan Lee King Yuan, Luciana Akemi Matsutani, and Amelia Pasqual Marques, *Manual Therapy*. https://www.sciencedirect.com/science/article/abs/pii/S1356689X14001829

9. "Massage Therapy Improves the Management of Alcohol Withdrawal Syndrome," Margaret Reader, Ross Young, and Jason P. Connor, *The Journal of Alternative and Complementary Medicine*. https://www.liebertpub.com/doi/10.1089/acm.2005.11.311?url_ver=Z39.88-2003&rfr_id=ori:rid:crossref.org&rfr_dat=cr_pub%20%200pubmed

10. "Chair massage for treating anxiety in patients withdrawing from psychoactive drugs," Shaun Black, et al, *Journal of Alternative and Complementary Medicine.* https://pubmed.ncbi.nlm.nih.gov/20799900/

11. "The beneficial effects of massage therapy for insomnia in postmenopausal women," H. Hachul, D.S. Oliveira, L.R.A. Bittencourt, M.L. Andersen, and S. Tufik, *Sleep Science.* https://www.ncbi.nlm.nih.gov/pmc/articles/PMC4521661/

12. "The Neuroprotective Aspects of Sleep," Andy R. Eugene and Jolanta Masiak, *MEDtube Science.* https://www.ncbi.nlm.nih.gov/pmc/articles/PMC4651462/

13. "About Sleep's Role in Memory," Bjorn Rasch and Jan Born, *Physiological Reviews.* https://www.ncbi.nlm.nih.gov/pmc/articles/PMC3768102/

14. "Blocking nocturnal blue light for insomnia: A randomized controlled trial," Ari Schechter, Elijah Wookhyun Kim, Marie-Pierre St-Onge, and Andrew J. Westwood, *Journal of Psychiatric Research.* https://www.ncbi.nlm.nih.gov/pmc /articles/PMC5703049/

15. "Blue light has a dark side," Harvard Health Publishing. https://www.health .harvard.edu/staying-healthy/blue-light-has-a-dark-side

16. "Red Light and the Sleep Quality and Endurance Performance of Chinese Female Basketball Players," Jieziu Zhao, Ye Tian, Jinlei Nie, Jincheng Xu, and Dongsen Liu, *Journal of Athletic Training.* https://www.ncbi.nlm.nih.gov/pmc/articles /PMC3499892/

17. "Blocking nocturnal blue light for insomnia."

18. "How the human body uses electricity," Amber Plante, University of Maryland Graduate Student Association. https://www.graduate.umaryland.edu/gsa/gazette /February-2016/How-the-human-body-uses-electricity/

19. "Anatomy and Function of the Heart's Electrical System," Johns Hopkins Medicine. https://www.hopkinsmedicine.org/health/conditions-and-diseases /anatomy-and-function-of-the-hearts-electrical-system

20. "Chapter 2: Electrical Signals of Nerve Cells," *Neuroscience, 2nd ed.* https://www .ncbi.nlm.nih.gov/books/NBK11053/

21. "Electricity in the body," The University of Western Australia. https://www.uwa .edu.au/science/-/media/Faculties/Science/Docs/Electricity-in-the-body.pdf

22. "Integrative and lifestyle medicine strategies should include Earthing (grounding): Review of research evidence and clinical observations," Wendy Menigoz, Tracy T. Latz, Robin A. Ely, Cimone Kamei, Gregory Melvin, and Drew Sinatra, *Explore: The Journal of Science and Healing.* https://pubmed.ncbi.nlm.nih.gov /31831261/

23. "The Importance of 'Grounding' Electrical Currents," Platinum Electricians. https://www.platinumelectricians.com.au/blog/importance-grounding-electrical -currents/

24. "Earthing: Health Implications of Reconnecting the Human Body to the Earth's Surface Electrons," Gaetan Chevalier, Stephen T. Sinatra, James L. Oschman, Karol Sokal, and Pawel Sokal, *International Journal of Environmental Research and Public Health.* https://www.ncbi.nlm.nih.gov/pmc /articles/PMC3265077/

25. "Can electrons act as antioxidants? A review and commentary," James L

Oschman, *Journal of Alternative and Complementary Medicine*. https://pubmed
.ncbi.nlm.nih.gov/18047442/

26. "Health Effects of Alkaline Diet and Water, Reduction of Digestive-tract Bacterial
Load, and Earthing," Haider Abdul-Lateef Mousa, *Alternative Therapies in Health
and Medicine*. https://pubmed.ncbi.nlm.nih.gov/27089527/

27. "Integrative and lifestyle medicine strategies."

28. "Introduction to Indoor Air Quality," United States Environmental protection
Agency. https://www.epa.gov/indoor-air-quality-iaq/introduction-indoor-air
-quality

29. "Air Cleaners and Air Filters in the Home," United States Environmental
Protection Agency. https://www.epa.gov/indoor-air-quality-iaq/air-cleaners-and
-air-filters-home

30. "Plants and indoor Air Quality," Nick Gromicko and Kate Tarasenko,
International Association of Certified Home Inspectors. https://www.nachi.org
/plants-indoor-air-quality.htm

31. "Plants Clean Air and Water for Indoor Environments," NASA Technology
Transfer Program. https://spinoff.nasa.gov/Spinoff2007/ps_3.html

32. "Using plants and soil microbes to purify indoor air: lessons from NASA and
Biosphere 2 experiments," Bill C. Wolverton and Mark Nelson, *Field Actions
Science Reports*. https://journals.openedition.org/factsreports/6092

THE PRECAUTIONARY PRINCIPLE

1. "The precautionary principle: protecting public health, the environment and the
future of our children," World Health Organization. https://www.euro.who.int/__data
/assets/pdf_file/0003/91173/E83079.pdf

2. "Benefits and Limitations of the Precautionary Principle," P.F. Ricci and J. Zhang,
Encyclopedia of Environmental Health. https://www.sciencedirect.com/topics
/earth-and-planetary-sciences/precautionary-principle

3. "Turning Science Into Junk: The Tobacco Industry and passive Smoking,"
Jonathan M. Samet and Thomas A. Burke, *American Journal of Public Health*.
https://www.ncbi.nlm.nih.gov/pmc/articles/PMC1446866/

4. "Smokescreen: The Truth Behind the Tobacco Industry Cover-up," Robert N.
Proctor, *JAMA*. https://jamanetwork.com/journals/jama/article-abstract
/408415

5. "The precautionary principle in environmental science," D. Kriebel, et al,
Environmental Health Perspectives. https://www.ncbi.nlm.nih.gov/pmc/articles
/PMC1240435/

6. "The precautionary principle," A. Wallace Hayes, *Archives of Industrial Hygiene
and Toxicology*. https://pubmed.ncbi.nlm.nih.gov/15968832/

EAT (MOSTLY) CLEAN

1. "Organic Production Enhances Milk Nutritional Quality by Shifting Fatty Acid Composition: A United States–Wide, 18-Month Study," Charles M. Benbrook, Gillian Butler, Maged A. Latif, Carlo Leifert, and Donald R. Davis, *PLOS One*. https://www.ncbi.nlm.nih.gov/pmc/articles/PMC3857247/

2. Ibid.

3. "Food Safety Facts," University of Maine. https://extension.umaine.edu /publications/4336e/

4. "Comparison of life cycle environmental impacts from meal kits and grocery store meals," Brent R. Heard, Mayur Bandekar, Benjamin Vassar, and Shelie A. Miller, *Resources, Conservation and Recycling*. https://www.sciencedirect.com /science/article/abs/pii/S0921344919301703?via%3Dihub

5. "Hyperinsulinemic syndrome: the metabolic syndrome is broader than you think," Christopher T. Kelly, et al, *Surgery*. https://pubmed.ncbi.nlm.nih.gov /24962189/

6. "Comparison of the mineral content of tap water and bottled waters," A. Azoulay, P. Garzon, and M. J. Eisenberg, *Journal of General Internal Medicine*. https://pubmed.ncbi.nlm.nih.gov/11318912/

7. "Bottled Water Everywhere: Keeping it Safe," U.S. Food & Drug Administration. https://www.fda.gov/consumers/consumer-updates/bottled-water-everywhere -keeping-it-safe

8. "Health Effects of Alkaline Diet and Water, Reduction of Digestive-tract bacterial Load, and Earthing," Haider Abdul-Lateef Mousa, *Alternative Therapies in Health and Medicine*. https://pubmed.ncbi.nlm.nih.gov/27089527/

9. "Natural mineral waters: chemical characteristics and health effects," Sara Quattrini, Barbara Pampaloni, and Maria Luisa Brandi, *Clinical Cases in Mineral and Bone Metabolism*. https://www.ncbi.nlm.nih.gov/pmc/articles /PMC5318167/

10. "Polyethylene Terephthalate May Yield Endocrine Disruptors," Leonard Sax, *Environmental Health Perspectives*. https://www.ncbi.nlm.nih.gov/pmc/articles /PMC2854718/

11. "How consumers of plastic water bottles are responding to environmental policies?," Caroline Orset, Nicolas Barret, and Aurelien Lemaire, *Journal of Alternative and Complementary Medicine*. https://pubmed.ncbi.nlm.nih.gov /28117128/

12. "Leaching of the plasticizer di(2-ethylhexyl)phthalate (DEHP) from plastic containers and the question of human exposure," Hanno C. Erythropel, Milan Maric, Jim A. Nicell, Richard L. Leask, and Viviane Yargeau, *Applied Microbiology and Biotechnology*. https://pubmed.ncbi.nlm.nih.gov/25376446/

13. "Phthalate Esters and Their Potential Risk in PET Bottled Water Stored under Common Conditions," Xiangqin Xu, Gang Zhou, Kun Lei, Gerald A LeBlanc, and Lihui An, *International Journal of Environmental Research and Public Health*. https://pubmed.ncbi.nlm.nih.gov/31878152/

LIVE (MAINLY) CLEAN

1. "PTFE-coated non-stick cookware and toxicity concerns: a perspective," Muhammad Sajid and Muhammad Ilyas, *Environmental Science and Pollution Research*. https://pubmed.ncbi.nlm.nih.gov/28913736/

2. "63 million Americans exposed to unsafe drinking water," Agnel Philip, Elizabeth Sims, Jordan Houston, and Rachel Konieczny, *USA Today*. https://www.usatoday .com/story/news/2017/08/14/63-million-americans-exposed-unsafe-drinking -water/564278001/

3. "Plastic and Wooden Cutting Boards," Dean O. Cliver, University of California, Davis, Food Safety Laboratory. https://www.terrygrimmond.com/res/uploads /2015/01/Cliver-UC-Davis-Food-Safety-Laboratory_-Cutting-Board-Research -Overview-2005.pdf

4. "Cutting Boards," U.S. Department of Agriculture. https://www.fsis.usda.gov /food-safety/safe-food-handling-and-preparation/food-safety-basics/cutting -boards

5. "Flame Retardants in Furniture," Green Science Policy Institute. https://greensciencepolicy.org/our-work/furniture/

6. "Can ornamental potted plants remove volatile organic compounds from indoor air? A review," Majbrit Dela Cruz, Jan H. Christensen, Jane Dyrhauge Thomsen, and Renate Muller, *Environmental Science and Pollution Research*. https://pubmed.ncbi.nlm.nih.gov/25056742/

7. "Phytoremediation of VOCs from indoor air by ornamental potted plants: A pilot study using *a palm species* under the controlled environment," Hakimeh Teiri, Hamidreza Pourzamani, Yaghoub Hajizadeh, *Chemosphere*. https://www.sciencedirect.com/science/article/abs/pii/S0045653518300869 ?via%3Dihub

8. "The basic roles of indoor plants in human health and comfort," Linjing Deng and Qihong Deng, *Environmental Science and Pollution Research*. https://link .springer.com/article/10.1007/s11356-018-3554-1

9. "Particle emission characteristics of filter-equipped vacuum cleaners," S. Trakumas, et al, American Industrial Hygiene Association. https://pubmed.ncbi .nlm.nih.gov/11549143/

10. "Green Label Plus: A Higher Standard for Indoor Air Quality," The Carpet and Rug Institute. https://carpet-rug.org/testing/green-label-plus/

11. "What are volatile organic compounds (VOCs)?," United States Environmental Protection Agency. https://www.epa.gov/indoor-air-quality-iaq/what-are-volatile -organic-compounds-vocs

12. "Pyrethroid Insecticides Alter Honey Bee Behavior," Entomology Today. https://entomologytoday.org/2015/05/29/pyrethroid-insecticides-alter-honey -bee-behavior/

GETTING YOUR FAMILY ON BOARD

1. "Prevalence of picky eaters among infants and toddlers and their caregivers' decisions about offering a new food," *Journal of the American Dietetic Association*. https://www.researchgate.net/publication/8937338_Prevalence_of_picky_eaters _amongInfants_and_toddlers_and_their_caregivers'_decisions_about_offering _a_new_food

2. "The science of getting your kids to eat more vegetables," Akshat Rathi and Jenny Anderson. Quartz. https://qz.com/701128/the-science-behind-getting-your-kids -to-eat-everything/

3. "Influences on the Development of Children's Eating Behaviours: From Infancy to Adolescence," Dr. Leann Birch, Jennifer S. Savage, and Alison Ventura, *Canadian Journal of Dietetic Practice and Research*. https://www.ncbi.nlm.nih.gov /pmc/articles/PMC2678872/#R35

4. "Children eat more food when they prepare it themselves," Jasmine M. DeJesus, Susan A. Gelman, Isabella Herold, and Julia C. Lumeng, *Appetite*. https://www .ncbi.nlm.nih.gov/pmc/articles/PMC6768385/

5. "Garden-Based integrated Intervention for Improving Children's Eating Behavior for Vegetables," Seon-Ok Kim and Sin-Ae Park, *International Journal of Enrivonmental Research*

INDEX